Pediatrician's Guide to Discussing Research with Patients

Christina A. Di Bartolo · Maureen K. Braun

Pediatrician's Guide to Discussing Research with Patients

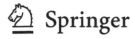 Springer

Christina A. Di Bartolo
The Child Study Center
NYU Langone Medical Center
New York, NY
USA

Maureen K. Braun
Department of Pediatrics
Icahn School of Medicine at Mount
    Sinai Hospital
New York, NY
USA

ISBN 978-3-319-49546-0   ISBN 978-3-319-49547-7   (eBook)
DOI 10.1007/978-3-319-49547-7

Library of Congress Control Number: 2016959518

Printed on acid-free paper

This Springer imprint is published by Springer Nature
The registered company is Springer International Publishing AG
The registered company address is: Gewerbestrasse 11, 6330 Cham, Switzerland

Preface

The past few decades have witnessed a remarkable shift in the doctor–patient relationship. Beginning in the late twentieth century, patients began assuming increasingly active roles in their medical care. While shared decision-making and patient-centered care convey benefits, they are not without challenges. The Internet, with a plethora of easily accessible information, contributes to the wave of patients visiting their physicians with preconceived notions of their diagnosis and preferred treatment course. When patients read accurate information from reputable sources, their increased knowledge and understanding expedites the consultation by reducing the time needed for patient education. However, the poor quality of information available to the lay public causes many patients to become misinformed, confused, and fearful. Physicians, compelled to respond accordingly, are then tasked with correcting misconceptions.

Results of research studies, complicated and nuanced by nature, are regularly presented over-broadly or incorrectly on the Internet. Viral Internet content is taken as fact. Basic science research results are commonly presented in the media as if they directly apply to patients. Clinical outcomes studies commonly test differences between large groups of research subjects, limiting the applicability of their conclusions for the individual patient. Without comprehending this context, patients ask their doctors how these recent results will affect their treatment.

In this landscape, clear communication between physicians and their patients is imperative. This book is designed to facilitate conversations about research studies between pediatricians and patients by two means. Part I of the book assists physicians in promoting research literacy among their patients. When patients do not have the research literacy skills needed to discern fact from fiction, confusion and disagreement easily occur. Informed consumers of online content understand basic facts about research and the factors that influence the relevance of a study's findings. These first five chapters explain how patients can easily determine the validity and applicability of the information they encounter online and elsewhere. Because complex concepts are described, these chapters include sample language that pediatricians can use as models for their own explanations to patients. These sections are demarcated with headers, "To Explain to a Patient."

While not suggesting that pediatricians use this language verbatim, the samples provide accurate distillations of the concepts for pediatricians to explain in their own words.

Part II of the book is comprised of research reviews in special topic areas. The authors used their clinical observations of parents' common questions in pediatric health and mental health outpatient settings to select the topics. The nine resulting chapters distill the relevant information to address common parental concerns and misconceptions. Each chapter opens with an overview of the topic. The chapter then discusses common parental concerns, misconceptions, and findings from current research. Because of the constantly unfolding nature of the scientific process, this part of the book is meant to serve solely as a base for pediatricians to hold these conversations. The skills taught in the Part I of the book should be applied to any emerging research findings in these areas.

Ms. Di Bartolo and Dr. Braun would like to thank those who supported them in preparing this book. We are grateful to Springer for coordinating the project. Michael Wilt provided essential editing and compilation assistance. Colleague Jess P. Shatkin, M.D., M.P.H. prompted the pursuit of the goal, while F. Xavier Castellanos, M.D. judiciously grounded the aspiration in practical realities. Advice from mentors, Howard Abikoff, Ph.D., Richard Gallagher, Ph.D., and Timothy Verduin, Ph.D., was constantly referenced throughout the project. Opening-shift employees at a particular coffee shop played a direct role in turning this book from idea into reality. Argelinda Baroni, M.D., colleague, sounding board, and friend, knew when to check in and when to leave well enough alone. Thank you to family and friends for their interest, especially James P. Di Bartolo, for his unflagging enthusiasm.

Finally, this book could not exist without the countless researchers who devoted lifetimes to the pursuit of scientific inquiry and the research participants who gave their time without expectation of direct return. Thank you.

New York, NY, USA   Christina A. Di Bartolo
                                                                                   Maureen K. Braun

Contents

Chapter 1
Introduction: Evidence-Based Practice in Patient-Centered Care

Paternalistic Medicine

The concept of medicine, the practice of helping another individual prevent and cure ailments, has existed for thousands of years. While original practitioners focused on religion, philosophy, and art within their practice, the alleviation of suffering was the ultimate goal. Today's medical practices place a heavier emphasis on knowledge and science to achieve that same end. While healing methods have changed throughout the millennia, the dynamic between doctors and patients remained fixed for nearly 2400 years [1]. From this historical standpoint, an abrupt paradigm shift occurred within the past century, forever changing how doctors and patients relate to one another [1].

Hippocrates is credited with establishing the dominant doctor-patient relationship model that persisted for those millennia [1]. His model is based on the value of beneficence, or actions to maximize the patients' good [1]. In Hippocrates' time, because doctors were granted special knowledge, the thinking followed that they should use their knowledge to make all care decisions for their patients [1]. Ultimate physician discretion is called **paternalism** [1]. Given that doctors made every choice, Hippocrates absented from his guide any precepts for physicians to communicate their knowledge or reasons for their decisions to their patients. On the contrary, Hippocrates considered deception and lying appropriate if the doctors felt these strategies were necessary to achieve their ultimate healing aims [1]. Along with the other aspects of the Hippocratic tradition, modern medicine continued to sanction the practice of doctors lying to their patients.

Doctors suffered a public relations setback as medical practice moved gradually from predominantly religious and philosophical healing to the somewhat more rational and scientific methods produced by the Enlightenment [1]. While doctors could identify for themselves who were true practitioners of this new kind of medicine, they did so based on their specialized training and knowledge.

© Springer International Publishing AG 2017
C.A. Di Bartolo and M.K. Braun, *Pediatrician's Guide to Discussing Research with Patients*, DOI 10.1007/978-3-319-49547-7_1

Prospective patients had no such method to distinguish between doctors and charlatans. Without knowing more about the mode of medicine, there was very little apparent difference between doctors and snake oil salesmen who capitalized on the confusion [1]. Eventually there would be a standardization of the medical education and profession, but in the meantime, doctors needed to act. They responded to this skepticism by establishing a set of professional guidelines for everything from their appearance to their manner in delivering treatments [1]. Doctors intended these new guidelines to reassure patients that they were seeking treatment from a legitimate source of knowledge. To mollify a confused and decidedly uncertain public, doctors emphasized their confidence and assurance. For doctors to provide any less than their unequivocal diagnoses and recommendations would have fed into the already rampant skepticism of their profession. They utilized Thomas Percival's codified endorsement of the Hippocratic tradition of paternalism, *Medical Ethics*, published at the start of the nineteenth century [2, 3].

At this stage in medicine, paternalism included more than doctors making active decisions as to treatment course. As Hippocrates established and Percival reiterated for a modern audience, doctors sometimes withheld information from patients [1]. In addition to excusing patients from making decisions, doctors sometimes left patients unaware that a decision was even being made [1]. For example, upon finding that a newborn had a significant birth defect (such as spina bifida), doctors might report to the parents that the child was stillborn [1]. It was also common practice for doctors to withhold diagnostic findings if they thought sharing the news would upset a patient [4]. Doctors withheld treatments that might prolong patients' lives if the doctors felt the medications would adversely affect patient quality of life [1]. The common thread among these decisions to withhold or deceive is that doctors followed beneficence as their predominant value. They believed the best medical practice would maximize patients' wellbeing. Sometimes curative medicine maximized patient wellbeing, but when it was not expected to, doctors attempted to absorb the responsibility of making challenging ethical and moral decisions on their patients' behalf.

Such paternalistic practices sound jarring to many practitioners' ears today, particularly when not situated within the overall context of how medicine was typically practiced. Before the high cost of health care and numerous physician options, patients typically saw one doctor for the entirety of their lives [5]. This longitudinal time frame allowed doctors to develop consistent, ongoing, and close relationships with their patients [5]. Before the advent of hospitals and doctor's offices, doctors generally treated patients in the patients' own houses. Traveling to where patients lived and venturing into their homes provided doctors a great amount of insight into their lives [5]. Doctors developed a broad understanding of the social, economic, and familial factors affecting their patients. Also, by treating multiple generations within the same family, physicians cultivated a vast amount of knowledge that clinicians now term "family history" [5]. Rather than ask a patient to check off on a checklist which relatives had various ailments at the start of a consultation, doctors at that time had a working knowledge of the patients' family risk factors.

Even within this context, certainly doctors did not always make decisions for their patients that the patients would have made for themselves if granted the opportunity. But doctors were making decisions based on a more intimate view of their patients' lives than they typically have today. In this way, the practice of doctors making decisions for their patients was not so different from parents making medical decision on behalf of their minor children, or powers of attorney designated by patients to make medical decisions should the patients become incapacitated. These two examples show that in the twenty-first century, we maintain the view that decisions can be made on another's behalf [6]. We simply do not hold as strongly the degree to which doctors should make decisions for their patients when their patients have the capacity to do so. The difference between these paternalistic practices in historical medicine and our current state is a matter of degree, not one of kind.

Compliance Under Paternalism

Under the paternalistic view of medicine, a clear power differential sets the doctor apart from the patient. The doctor is presumed to have knowledge and the ability to make decisions. Therefore the clinicians decide and prescribe while the patients comply or not. The 1970s brought about discussions about patient compliance, defined as, "the extent to which the patient's behavior (in terms of taking medication, following diets, or executing other lifestyle changes) coincides with medical or health advice" [7, 8].

As such, physicians and researchers began studying health outcomes as a function of patient compliance. The thinking ran that if the doctor prescribed a course of treatment, it would, by definition, be the "correct" one [9]. Subsequently, patients who did not comply could reasonably be assumed to have poorer outcomes, whereas compliant patients would reap the benefits of following doctors' orders [9]. In some cases, nothing could be more accurate. Not taking certain medications through to their final dosage, or conversely, taking a medication past its needed state can result in terrible health outcomes [10]. Overall, studies reported that medication regimens followed as prescribed led to better health outcomes, increased patient safety, and improved quality of life [8]. Particularly with carefully tested and calibrated medication regimens, patients who follow those guidelines are more likely to see the desired health outcome [10].

Within the paternalistic framework, noncompliance is necessarily viewed as a flaw in the patient. Either the patient never agreed with the course of action and chose to override the physician through passive noncompliance, or the patient agreed but then failed to follow through [11]. Neither explanation portrays the patient in a particularly positive light. While these two interpretations are possible, they are not the only ones. The compliance view assumes the optimal medical health outcome, irrespective of other patient values, is the top priority. What then, to make of a patient who chooses not to take medication that causes significant weight gain as a side effect? Or the patient who does not follow medical advice to avoid travel due to an important out of town family event? Or, as is unfortunately the case for many, the patient who cannot afford treatment in addition to other financial obligations, and instead chooses to pay rent? Rather than placing the outcome of the treatment at the fore, patients in these situations might reasonably conclude that other priorities (in these examples, other health and well-being, social, and financial) will take precedence over their doctors' instructions.

Despite these logical interpretations behind a patient's noncompliance, entire journals were established to publish findings as to patients' compliance levels and outcomes as a function of compliance. This area of research inquiry exploded from 1975 through the mid-nineties [6]. These descriptive accounts present a dire image: roughly half of patients with chronic illness are noncompliant with their medical regimens [6]. It would take the rise and promulgation of the autonomy movement to finally put compliance aside in favor of a different construct.

Patient-Centered Care

The paternalistic view of medicine never aligned particularly well with the American culture of independence and freedom [1]. Even though Americans largely placed their trust and faith in their doctors during the mid-nineteenth century, paternalism was never completely accepted [1]. The field of applied ethics grappled with the thorny issues that arise as a result paternalism [12]. Americans warily accepted paternalism, but the end of World War II elicited growing distrust of medicine and medical research. Nazi doctors committed atrocities in the name of science [5]. Researchers on American soil violated human rights in travesties that appalled the public, such as withholding proven treatments from individuals during the Tuskegee Syphilis Study [5].

These injustices ushered in a new era of participant consent for research studies. First addressed at Nuremberg and then later through the Belmont report, the doctrine of informed consent became law in the field of medical research [5]. No longer could researchers lawfully involve an individual in untested practices without their consent. After informed consent became a staple of medical research proceedings, the public increasingly asserted their right to consent to medical care in clinical settings as well [5]. Now that a new paradigm existed, patients wanted it implemented in the clinical realm.

A number of factors and movements bolstered the public's demand for informed consent. First, as has been stated, paternalism and American culture were never an ideal fit. It is perhaps not surprising that once the idea of informed consent was presented to the American public as part of research practices, they advocated for such a freedom in their clinical care. Informed consent reflects well the value of autonomy, a value much more aligned with overall founding principle of the United States [5]. Ethicists had been tackling the paternalism-autonomy dichotomy in the theoretical realm for years. Once a famous case of challenging ethical decision-making (Baby Doe) reached the public's eyes, Americans became aware that doctors were regularly making decisions without their knowledge or consent [5]. The burgeoning bioethics movement influenced the American Medical Association to dispense with the main tenets of paternalism in 1980.

Second, it is unlikely a coincidence that the drive for patient rights occurred at the same time as the civil rights movement. Rights of the individual, the ability to stand up to established authority systems, and increased advocating were in the air [5]. The bioethics movement likely benefitted from the kinds of conversations that occurred as a direct result of the Freedom Riders and their crusade to promote equality in America.

A third driving factor is that while doctors often assumed to know their patients' values and preferences, they were quite commonly incorrect [13]. With the "doctor knows best" model proven not to be true with regard to patients' actual preferences, the public clamored for change. The consumerist movement in the United States aided that change by encouraging individuals to seek out control over their life choices, particularly with regard to purchasing from different businesses. Health care was seen as a business predicated on information transferal, so patients began to view themselves as consumers of health care [14].

Fourth, part and parcel with the consumer movement came new advertising models and the flow of information to potential purchasers. The rise of 24-hour television news programming, advertising targeted directly to the consumer, and high-speed Internet connections that allow easy access to sophisticated search engines created a burst of information [14]. With patients now feeling more informed about their consumer choices than ever, doctors lost their position as the main source of health information. Of course, whether or not the information presented is accurate or complete is another matter entirely. Patients' ability to parse out fact from fiction or find the relevant information for their decision is a meta decision-making process that requires a great deal of education, effort, and time. However, the public *felt* as thought they had information at their fingertips. This heightened feeling of empowerment supplanted their previous tendency to accept doctors' recommendations at face value.

Fifth, in addition to expanding knowledge, viable treatment options expanded. One cannot be said to make a decision when only one option exists (other than the decision to accept that option or not) [5]. As research and medical advances surged forwards, patients found they had more than one treatment available to them. Consumers could now choose from a number of medical treatments as they had become accustomed to choose from a number of household cleaning products.

Finally, the legal system oversaw a surge in medical malpractice lawsuits. Once malpractice litigation became common, the trust patients placed in doctors during the "golden age of medicine" effectively ended [5]. Many cited the rise of malpractice suits as a direct cause in contributing to the increased practice among doctors of obtaining signed informed consent from their patients as part of their new defensive practice [5].

Due to these factors and likely others, informed consent was now a standard aspect of clinical care. So what, exactly, was this right to informed consent that patients fought for? Informed consent consists of an individual understanding the risks and benefits of their involvement in a particular medical procedure [15]. Therefore, a transfer of information is a required staple of informed consent. If informed consent in research required the transfer of information from researcher to participant, informed consent within the clinical world requires even more so the flow of information from doctor to patient. The natural outgrowth of a policy of informed consent is one of choice. If doctors now need patients' informed consent, the clear implication is that patients have a choice. The concepts of autonomy and informed consent are intertwined [16]. If one does not have information, one is not considered able to make a choice at all.

Embedded within the principle of autonomy is the freedom to act unrestrained by coercion or manipulation. For an individual to make a completely autonomous choice, the patient would have to understand the information and feel completely free to make any decision without influence or coercion [15]. If doctors do not provide information for patients to decide whether or not to consent, they are essentially coercing patients. Physicians providing only certain pieces of relevant information are also considered to be manipulating patients. As coercion strikes at the heart of autonomy within medicine, clinicians are urged to provide all the information a reasonable person would need to make their healthcare decision. After processing the information provided, patients can now refuse care at all levels of their encounter with their doctors or medical establishments. Caveats to informed consent exist in emergency circumstances or in limited situations wherein patients are found not to be of sound mind, or are in danger of harming themselves or others. In those cases, the value of beneficence regains precedence once again over the value of autonomy. But physicians are now, under most circumstances, required to obtain their patients' affirmative informed consent before initiating a test, beginning a treatment regimen, or implementing a medical procedure. As a result, the shift from paternalism to patient-centered care was all but cemented as the new way of practicing medicine [17].

Coercion still occurs within the patient-centered model, particularly when a physician feels strongly that a specific course of action is the best but a patient refuses to consent. While some practitioners ask patients to sign a form stating that they are declining a recommended treatment "Against Medical Advice," this is not legally required and in fact goes against the principles of informed consent and shared decision-making [18]. The practice of using such forms represents a number of ethical breaches: it demonstrates a rupture in the patient-doctor relationship, a communication breakdown, and—given findings that show patients are less likely to return for care after signing such a form—this practice undermines the physicians' oath to "do no harm." These forms also include legalese that can intimidate and therefore coerce patients.

The preferred model under the autonomy movement is for physicians to provide information to patients and assist them as they weigh their options. This process, diametrically opposed to paternalism, is called **shared decision-making** [8]. In 2011 the National Heart Foundation of Australia supplied this description of shared decision-making when well-performed: a decision made jointly between doctor and patient, taking the patient's opinion into account only once the patient has been adequately informed [11]. The informed approach falls somewhere in the middle of these two, describing situations in which doctors inform their patients of their conditions and the upcoming treatment but do not leave room for the patient to decide [18].

While autonomy is a crucial aspect of this new medical framework, it is not all-encompassing. As we shall soon see, many patients do not want to be "autonomous" in the strictest sense. However, they would like some amount of information and level of control, which falls under the umbrella term "patient-centered care." We will use this term throughout to describe the new model of medicine we find ourselves in today.

Adherence Under Patient-Centered Care

Above we discussed compliance under the patriarchal model, as well as the dismal outcomes. The emergence of patient-centered care necessitated a new construct to define patients' usage of prescribed medical care. By definition, one cannot be noncompliant with a self-made decision. Once patients contributed to the decision-making process, the more apt term became **adherence**. Rather than using a term that implies the doctor is more "powerful" than the patient, as compliance does, adherence is meant to reflect the supposedly equal relationship between patient and doctor, particularly with regard to decision-making. The ensuing literature uses the term as defined by the World Health Organization: "the extent to which a person's behavior—taking medication, following a diet, and/or executing lifestyle changes, corresponds with agreed recommendations from a health care provider" [19]. In the body of adherence literature, there is room to acknowledge a patient could intentionally not take or use prescribed medical care as originally prescribed. The argument follows that if patients make a decision to enter into a treatment regimen, they are equally able to decide to discontinue it or use it not as planned.

If patients can make their own medical decisions, and if using prescribed care not as designed is now a choice, why would this concept need a term at all? Firstly, to observe and note it when such situations occur. The next logical question becomes, why would one want to observe it and mark when it occurs? Patients deciding to use medical treatments not as designed have implications for their clinical outcomes. From a medicolegal standpoint, this decision also has ramifications on the doctors' practice. If a patient were to sue a doctor for a poor health outcome, the legal defense would include information as to how the patient followed through on the decided treatment plan. Particularly as doctors have been sensitized to practice defensive medicine, tracking adherence represents a small "insurance policy" for the doctor should the patient experience poor outcomes as a result of their nonadherence.

Secondly, adherence is relevant for medical interventions in which specific usage, dosage, frequency, and length of treatment are known entities in the presence of robust medical research literature. If enough patients were not adherent with a specific medication guideline, outcomes would imply the medications did not work as designed without rates of adherence to explain the discrepancy between medication and outcome.

Finally, adherence rates remain crucial for treatments or prevention decisions that affect society as a whole [9]. While patient-centered care focuses on individual choices and outcomes, medicine as a whole remains committed to promoting a healthy society and reducing waste in the healthcare system. If enough individuals do not adhere to clinical recommendations intended to benefit a group, this could only be addressed if measured in the first place.

Researchers and healthcare providers are also interested in the underlying reasons for nonadherence. Above we proposed a few scenarios in which patients may choose not to adhere. But nonadherence can occur for many reasons, including patients' lack of comprehension of the severity of their illness, whether they truly believe the treatment will be effective, and whether the patient is able to access the treatment in their current setting. For example, a patient might initially agree to a course of medication for a blood-diagnosed thyroid problem, but if the patient had not experienced any side effects prior to medication treatment, the patient may eventually stop treatment from a lack perceived benefit. Some patients understand that the treatment is needed, but do not have overall faith that it will work, such as chemotherapy in cases of cancer. Finally, some patients want to adhere but have trouble doing so due to environmental or financial constraints, such as finding a dialysis center within a reasonable travel distance from their home. Naturally these need not be separate patients, but some amount of these issues is present in any individual attempting to adhere to care. Presumably if a treatment is known to be effective, the medical profession has an interest in promoting adherence for better health outcomes. Tackling reasons for nonadherence to help more patients achieve these desired outcomes can only occur if the reasons are collected and analyzed.

Patient Response to Consumer Choice

Given the work required to shift the medical profession and associated legislation from paternalism to patient-centered care, one might assume that patients are relieved and pleased with the new state of the situation. As with most assumptions, this one is not uniformly accurate. Until now, we have described patient-centered care as a model in which patients make their decisions after hearing information from their doctors without influence. This clear delineation between sharing information up until the decision point is not the preferred state for most patients. They do not want to shoulder the decision-making process alone. Multiple studies indicate that patients appreciate obtaining more medical information from their doctors and that some might even prefer more [20]. Research shows that in some cases, the addition of patient choice changes patterns of care, and others indicate that patient control over choice may lead to better psychological outcomes [20]. With so many patients accessing health information regardless, one can easily imagine a feeling of reassurance to discuss the wide and often confusing information with a trusted source.

However, not all patients embrace ultimate responsibility for their healthcare decisions. In one large cross-sectional survey conducted among the American public, results uncovered diverse responses regarding shared decision-making approach. Specifically, 62% of respondents preferred shared decision-making, 28% preferred the autonomous or consumerist approach, and 9% preferred paternalism [21]. Other studies back up these findings, with one small study finding that less than 2% of their respondents preferred a truly autonomous role [17]. Again, the preferred choice was shared decision-making [17]. Differences among patients emerged, including socioeconomic status and acuteness of illness as factors. Among those of low socioeconomic status, this study's patients tended to prefer either of the two extreme forms—autonomy or paternalism. As to acuity, patients with chronic illnesses are, on average, more interested in taking a consumerist approach to their care [17, 20]. After coming to understand their illness over a course of time and gradually learning and incorporating the knowledge into their working understanding, it is hypothesized that these patients are more likely to assume an active role in the management of their illness. Acutely ill patients however, can find themselves overwhelmed, in medical crisis, in pain, and in an unfamiliar setting (hospital as compared to a consulting office). Given that decision-making is mentally and physically taxing, it follows that patients already burdened by acute illness or pain do not feel inclined to take on this additional task [16].

Other factors influence patients to reject responsibility for making decisions regarding their care. One psychological factor lies in that people often do not want the knowledge that they made the choice when they experience negative outcomes (e.g., treatment does not go as planned, challenging side effects) associated with that choice. Another factor includes patients' varying levels of resistance to "look behind the curtain" at just how tentative the evidence is for a multitude of medical treatments. Decision-making in informed consent requires full awareness of the choices and possible outcomes, including the probabilities of success and possible risks associated with the choices. Some patients understandably want to simply accept what is available without confronting the uncertainties.

Patients are concerned with their ability to understand the full decision in front of them. As many medical conditions and treatments are complex, it is unfair to assume that all patients are always capable or willing to consider what is essentially advanced graduate-level knowledge before receiving care for a myriad of ailments they will undoubtedly encounter in their lives. Efforts to gauge the public's understanding of scientific information have met with limited success [20]. In the same large study described above assessing patients' preferences for decision-making, the researchers asked patients how often they feel they have adequate access to health care information, a seeming prerequisite to feeling comfortable with being placed in a decision-making role [21]. While approximately 60% reported feeling that they had information at least "most of the time," 40% reported they had the needed information either "some of the time" or "never" [21]. Both low educational attainment and minority race (in this study, Blacks and Hispanics) were more likely to report not having the needed information to make a decision [21]. Another study found similar results among their less-educated patients, who were also more likely to choose a paternalistic approach [17]. Overall, patients who gave high ratings to their doctors' care also indicated that they felt as though they had the needed information [17].

Literacy skills in the average patient present a logistical and theoretical hurdle to informed consent. Critics of the autonomous version of decision-making point to the inadequacy of literacy skills among a typical patient [22]. The issue becomes further compounded when the introduction of medical concepts into literacy is introduced. One researcher conducted a small survey in which patients were asked to interpret what a reduction in 25% was equivalent to [23]. His findings were discouraging: 39% of patients did not know 25% was equivalent to one in four [23].

Finally, patients' response to decision-making is often affected by their relationship with their doctor, as well as the doctor's actions (or lack thereof) during the decision-making process. Perhaps not surprisingly, patients who rated their doctors as delivering better care and patients with regular doctors were more likely to say they preferred shared decision-making [21]. Those patients who trust their physicians tend to prefer shared decision-making to paternalism is nevertheless an interesting finding when one considers trust is crucial for an effective paternalistic approach as well. Additionally, doctors who present information but then assist the patient in deciding leave the patients feeling more supported. As one medical sociologist noted, "When a doctor says 'Here are your options,' without offering expert help and judgment, that is a form of abandonment" [24]. Patients experience this interaction as such. Research on the use of decisional aids found similar results—these tools were not well received by patients without an additional consultation from a medical professional [14].

The autonomy movement was built upon the concept that individuals should have freedom over their bodies and what is done to them. This freedom necessitates some choice, which then necessitates understanding. For most, understanding comes from the imparting of knowledge from their doctors, but patients find this is not sufficient to make them comfortable in their decision-making process. The movement for more patient autonomy has therefore resulted in patients and doctors now requiring more from each other in terms of their relationship and interactions. This need for enhanced relationships and interactions occurs within the context of shorter office visits, less knowledge on the doctors' part of their patients' overall lives, and a burgeoning body of literature and misinformation regarding medicine which could easily overwhelm patient and doctor alike [20].

Patient Understanding Key to Decision-Making

Despite most patients' preference for shared decision-making, United States law stipulates the information doctors need to tell patients based on the autonomous model. Prior to patient-centered care, doctors were tasked with making clinical decisions using the standard of considering what a reasonable and prudent physician would do when given the same information about a case. When deciding what information to disclose within the patient-centered movement, the new standard compels doctors to ask themselves whether or not that information would be material (that is, relevant) to the decision-making process among reasonable patients. This distinction has actionable ramifications, based on the noted difference between a "reasonable physician" and a "reasonable patient" [15]. The information doctors want before deciding a course of treatment includes what percentage of the population benefits from the treatment, the relative risk versus benefit ratio, and importantly, how other clinical and demographic patient features will interact with the treatment to either enhance or undermine its effects [25]. Patients, on the other hand, display a greater interest in knowing their risk profile for developing a particular condition, hearing how that condition would specifically affect them and their lives, and the risks and costs of a particular treatment [25]. The difference between the information needs of a reasonable doctor and a reasonable patient matters if doctors are not aware of the discrepancy. Clinicians may tell patients what they themselves would want to know, as opposed to what the patient needs to make a decision.

Perhaps most interestingly, patients voice a greater preference for more information than they do for then deciding based on that information [18]. As a result, physicians tend to underestimate how much information their patients want and overestimate how much control patients want in deciding. It has been noted that shared decision-making is a technical misnomer, while informed decision-making is more accurate [22]. While a doctor recommends, the patient experiences the ramifications of the decision [22]. As far as distribution of risk goes, shared decision-making (or informed decision-making) still best addresses the imbalance. Physicians also report affinity for shared decision-making as well; with 75% preferring shared decision-making, 14% a paternalistic approach, and 11% a consumerist approach [26].

Physician Response to Patient-Centered Care

Understandably, physicians can be in a difficult situation when their patients arrive into their examination room with preconceived notions of their illness and the best treatment course. In one small review of practices from 1992, nearly one quarter of incidents in which doctors reported feeling uncomfortable with their prescription choice, antibiotics were implicated [27]. Out of a total of 307 incidents outlined in the study, doctors identified antibiotics as a cause for concern in 138 [27]. While this is simply one example, most physicians can think of a time when patients insisted on a medical interpretation they knew to be false or premature.

Indeed, doctors' discomfort is well founded if their patients are mistaking preference in treatment options during decision-making for situations in which preference is irrelevant (termed by some as "problem-solving," as these situations reflect a clear problem that has one solution) [17]. To provide an extreme example, a patient with a broken arm cannot make a decision to heal the bone by taking oral calcium supplements in lieu of wearing a cast. Regardless how strong the patient's preference, the cast is the correct solution to the problem. Patient preference becomes extraneous information to the clinical prescription [22].

Other moral instances in which patient preference is not given as full weight is when the choice would confer net loss for society as a whole [20]. The sufficient population vaccination rate needed to achieve herd immunity is one such obvious example. Other individual patient preferences within the broader context of society's health exist regarding communicable diseases.

While doctors report preferring patient-centered care over the previous paternalistic model, they reasonably understand the additional hurdles in providing this kind of care. Transfer of information is one such challenge. One of the first challenges doctors encounter is describing the rationale behind the different treatment options when studies show that only a small amount of medical recommendations are backed by scientifically rigorous evidence [28]. Rigorous scientific studies have simply not addressed all conditions and patient populations [20, 22]. Even when well-executed studies exist, outcomes that patients care about other than clear indicators of disease remission (e.g., mortality, physical and biometric indicators) are often not included. In particular, patients are interested in quality of life, functional status, and perception of health as a result of the treatment. Researchers study these outcomes, as well as long-term outcomes and adverse event information with far less frequency [20]. The information from these studies that doctors can present to patients often implicitly assumes that disease remission is the patients' only metric used in making a decision. Doctors cannot provide their patients with other outcomes they truly want to know.

Even when treatments have a rigorous evidence base, the obligation lies with doctors to find out the information. The scientific literature constantly changes and shifts. Peer-reviewed journals publish new findings on a daily basis. In the course of a day, doctors generate at least one clinical question per patient [29]. Obtaining the needed information from databases compiling this overwhelming body of literature is a logistical nightmare. In the course of a busy day, clinicians do not find themselves logging onto PubMed or a similar database to find answers to their questions. Preferring readily available information, physicians most frequently reach out to colleagues [30]. Referring to printed materials such as textbooks or reference books is the next most commonly used option [30]. These formats may not necessarily hold the most scientifically rigorous, recent, or relevant information, but their accessibility trumps other considerations. Consulting with colleagues also confers the psychological benefit of support [30]. Without accessible and applicable information, doctors commonly proceed with patient care without obtaining answers to their clinical questions [30]. Physicians are most likely to pursue clinical questions when there is urgency for their patients' conditions or when they feel confident the information they need is available [30]. Patients' request for more information is not a leading influence in doctors seeking out information [30].

Doctors with up-to-date information on treatment options then confront how to best communicate information to their patients. Risk ratios present a special conundrum. Unlike other clinical questions, risk ratio information is widely available, leading doctors to feel responsible for communicating it to their patients [31]. Many patients concur, considering the communication of this information part of their doctors' role [14]. With both doctors and patients agreeing on the importance of discussing risk, these conversations remain difficult to conduct. Risk probabilities focus on statistical likelihood, and the human brain is poorly equipped to handle statistical thinking [32]. Scientists derive risk probabilities from samples of people, meant to represent the entire clinical population. Doctors are then tasked with interpreting those findings for one specific person—the patient in front of them. From person to person, individuals interpret risks differently and are not necessarily aware of their implicit biases when listening to the statistics [31]. A doctor and patient with different risk profiles can therefore think they are speaking about the same amount of risk, but are in fact viewing the same situation from two different perspectives. Some go so far as to argue that patients' inability to properly apply population risk study results to their individual case flies in the face of the theoretical underpinnings of informed consent [22]. One cannot know with certainty the true risk versus benefit on an individual level. The application of statistical information to an individual defies the precepts of statistics, which are predicated upon a sample of individuals rather than one [22]. Therefore patients can only be fully informed as to the population's probabilistic outcome; they cannot be fully informed as to their individual response without a crystal ball [22].

Risk studies presented in the media in oversimplified form without this desperately needed context present a particular conundrum. Following such releases, doctors then strive to explain the intricacies conveniently left out of the nightly news report to their patients during their time-limited office visits [31]. The media's frequently overstated claims thus serve to undermine the relationship of trust doctors have worked to build with their patients [31].

Electronic Propagation of (Mis)Information

At least as far back as the late 1950s, doctors became increasingly concerned about the source of patients' medical information. We have now established that patients consistently display an interest in obtaining a fair amount of information about medicine. When this information is not made formally available, patients transmit and receive information through informal networks (giving rise to old wives' tales and other forms of technically untested information). In the mid-twentieth century, widespread dissemination of information propagated through increasingly popular publications such as *Reader's Digest* as well as electronic sources in radio and television [33]. Patients had more access than ever to the medical information they craved. Inevitable hand wringing occurred in the medical profession over patients' inability to develop "any real understanding about his illness" [33]. Given this rise in information occurred prior to the autonomy movement, doctors concluded that "[g]reater profit therefore, will be earned if the doctor affords time to talk to each patient" [33]. The paternalistic view of medicine still predominating, one can only assume these conversations with patients about what they read or heard elsewhere regarding their condition were intended to increase compliance for whatever treatment the doctor would then inevitably prescribe. This stands in contrast to the kinds of conversations that would occur after the autonomy movement took shape, in which doctors informed their patients in order to help them understand what they had read and then decide.

Research Literacy Education

The shift from paternalism to patient-centered care in medical decision-making places additional requirements on patients and doctors alike. Patient responsibilities include providing informed consent and endeavoring to understand the decisions they sign their names to. The responsibility lies with the doctors to communicate the information their patients would deem relevant to their decision-making. As malpractice lawsuits continue to affect doctors' practice, physicians benefit from support to uphold their responsibilities in the partnership. This section has outlined the constraints on doctors' implementation of their side of informed consent. Logistical constraints (time, money, availability of research) reveal systems-wide inefficiencies requiring legal and policy initiatives, and are therefore outside the scope of this work. However, the struggle to impart knowledge of research studies and the conversations needed to increase patient literacy can be handled in a written format.

The following four chapters will broadly outline the research considerations physicians may choose to become familiar with before entering into informed consent conversations with their patients about such findings. The latter half of this book reviews, summarizes, and outlines updated relevant research literature to address the practicing clinician's struggle to stay abreast of ever-evolving studies. Naturally this information will become incomplete by the time the book is put on the shelf. However, this jumping off point allows physicians to start conversations with patients and then reference additional work in these areas as information is updated.

References

1. Will JF. A brief historical and theoretical perspective on patient autonomy and medical decision making: part I: the beneficence model. Chest J. 2011;139(3):669–73.
2. Percival T. Medical ethics, or, a code of institutes and precepts, adapted to the professional conduct of physicians and surgeons. The Classics of Medicine Library; 1985.
3. Faden RR, Beauchamp TL, King NM. A history and theory of informed consent.
4. Sokol DK. How the doctor's nose has shortened over time; a historical overview of the truth-telling debate in the doctor-patient relationship. J R Soc Med. 2006;99(12):632–6.
5. Will JF. A brief historical and theoretical perspective on patient autonomy and medical decision making: Part II: the autonomy model. CHEST Journal. 2011;139(6):1491–7.
6. Trostle JA. The history and meaning of patient compliance as an ideology. In Handbook of Health Behavior Research II 1997. Springer US. pp. 109–24.
7. Sackett DL, Haynes RB. Compliance with therapeutic regimens.
8. Ahmed R, Aslani P. What is patient adherence? A terminology overview. Int J Clin Pharm. 2014;36(1):4–7.
9. Sandman L, Granger BB, Ekman I, Munthe C. Adherence, shared decision-making and patient autonomy. Med Health Care Philos. 2012;15(2):115–27.
10. Lehane E, McCarthy G. Medication non-adherence—exploring the conceptual mire. Int J Nurs Pract. 2009;15(1):25–31.
11. Aslani P, Krass I, Bajorek B, Thistlethwaite J, Tofler G. Improving adherence in cardiovascular care. A toolkit for health professionals. National Heart Foundation of Australia. 2011:19–36.
12. Dworkin G. The Stanford Encyclopedia of Philosophy.
13. Tuckett AG. On paternalism, autonomy and best interests: Telling the (competent) aged-care resident what they want to know. International journal of nursing practice. 2006;12(3):166–73.
14. Woolf SH, Chan EC, Harris R, Sheridan SL, Braddock CH, Kaplan RM, Krist A, O'Connor AM, Tunis S. Promoting informed choice: transforming health care to dispense knowledge for decision making. Ann Intern Med. 2005;143(4):293–300.
15. Kapp MB. Patient autonomy in the age of consumer-driven health care: informed consent and informed choice. J legal Med. 2007;28(1):91–117.
16. Rodriguez-Osorio CA, Dominguez-Cherit G. Medical decision making: paternalism versus patient-centered (autonomous) care. Curr Opin Crit Care. 2008;14(6):708–13.
17. Deber RB, Kraetschmer N, Urowitz S, Sharpe N. Do people want to be autonomous patients? Preferred roles in treatment decision-making in several patient populations. Health Expect. 2007;10(3):248–58.
18. Elwyn G, Edwards A, Kinnersley P. Shared decision-making in primary care: the neglected second half of the consultation. Br J Gen Pract. 1999;49(443):477–82.
19. Sabaté E. Adherence to long-term therapies: evidence for action. World Health Organization; 2003.
20. Entwistle VA, Sheldon TA, Sowden A, Watt IS. Evidence-informed patient choice: practical issues of involving patients in decisions about health care technologies. Int J Technol Assess Health Care. 1998;14(02):212–25.
21. Murray E, Pollack L, White M, Lo B. Clinical decision-making: Patients' preferences and experiences. Patient Educ Couns. 2007;65(2):189–96.
22. McNutt RA. Shared medical decision making: problems, process, progress. JAMA. 2004;292(20):2516–8.
23. Ellis SJ, Matthews C, Weather SJ. Informed consent is flawed. Lancet. 2001;357(9250):149–50.
24. Hoffman, J. (2005). Awash in information, patients face a lonely, uncertain road. New York Times, 14.

25. Chatterton HT. Efficacy, risk, and the determination of value: shared medical decision making in the age of information. J Fam Pract. 1999;48(7):505.
26. Murray E, Pollack L, White M, Lo B. Clinical decision-making: physicians' preferences and experiences. BMC Fam Pract. 2007;8(1):1.
27. Bradley CP. Uncomfortable prescribing decisions: a critical incident study. BMJ. 1992;304(6822):294–6.
28. Naylor CD. Grey zones of clinical practice: some limits to evidence-based medicine. Lancet. 1995;345(8953):840–2.
29. Smith R. What clinical information do doctors need? BMJ. 1996;313(7064):1062–8.
30. Gorman PN, Helfand M. Information seeking in primary care how physicians choose which clinical questions to pursue and which to leave unanswered. Med Decis Making. 1995;15(2):113–9.
31. Edwards A, Matthews E, Pill R, Bloor M. Communication about risk: diversity among primary care professionals. Fam Pract. 1998;15(4):296–300.
32. Patel N. Why your brain struggles with probability. Inverse. 2016. https://www.inverse.com/article/6339-why-people-suck-at-understanding-probability. Accessed 21 March 2016.
33. Evans W. Faults in the diagnosis and management of cardiac pain. Br Med J. 1959;1(5117):249.
34. Alfandre D, Schumann JH. What is wrong with discharges against medical advice (and how to fix them). JAMA. 2013;310(22):2393–4.

Part I
Overview of Research Concepts and Literacy

Chapter 2
Funding and Bias

Information Dissemination

The patient-centered movement in the medical profession reinforces patient autonomy while patients make their health care decisions. Truly autonomous decision-making relies crucially on informed consent, and in turn, informed consent requires information [1]. All this begs the question: where does this information come from? Put another way, how do the results of researchers' studies reach patients? The information chain from researcher to patient is comprised of multiple players, including: the researcher, the funder of the research, the medical journal editor, the journalist whose interpretation of the study appears in popular media, the doctor reading the study, and the patient reading the journalist's article. Together, these players serve to fund, research, disseminate, and implement new medical advances. How effective is this process in transporting a clear message from start (researcher) to finish (patient)? Consider the playground game of "Telephone," in which children sit in a row and whisper a message from one end of the line to the other. As in the game, even when no one intentionally distorts the message, the end result the patient hears is often radically different than the one the researcher meant to deliver. Distortion can occur without necessarily malicious intent because each player in the process brings his or her own biases into the process.

Bias

Now is the time to define the word bias, for both physician and patient. Bias carries a negative connotation in the popular lexicon. In everyday language, only judgmental, close-minded people are biased. This chapter will heavily review how

© Springer International Publishing AG 2017
C.A. Di Bartolo and M.K. Braun, *Pediatrician's Guide to Discussing
Research with Patients*, DOI 10.1007/978-3-319-49547-7_2

explicit kinds of biases affect research studies. However, from a psychological standpoint, the construct of a bias can also refer to a neutral process. **Biases** are our brains' automatic and unconscious processes that occur without our intent [2]. In the field of psychology, everyone is biased. Biases operate to affect our thinking and subsequent behavior without conscious awareness. This category of biases is said to be "implicit" [2]. Cognitive psychologists refer to a bias when they describe any particular systematic "lean" of our brains. Psychologists consider these biases systematic because they function in a relatively predictable fashion; that is, they are not random.

To Explain to a Patient

Biases can be thought of as sunglasses for our brains. Sunglasses are not inherently bad. They might even serve some goals well: to look attractive, to filter out harmful UV rays, or to reduce the discomfort of bright light. Sunglasses accomplish all these goals by way of distortion. Biases in our brains are the same. They create slight distortions to serve a goal (e.g., to react quickly, to reduce cognitive burden, to simplify disparate details into a cohesive story). When people wear sunglasses for a long time, they eventually "forget" they are wearing them. Their brains stop consciously noting that the environment looks darker, and they begin to operate as if this is the way the world always looks. Anyone who has ever forgotten to remove their sunglasses even once they have entered a building has experienced how easy it is to lose track of a distortion. This is what biases do. They provide distortions for such a prolonged time that your brain does not notice them. Biases are systematic, in that they are not random; they work in one way. Similarly, one pair of sunglasses can also only make things look darker. They do not sometimes make things darker, other times lighter, and other times tinted green or yellow. However your sunglasses distort, they distort this way every time. Each bias is like that, too. Even though we often do not notice them, they behave in a predictable fashion.

Biases exist in everyone's brains and affect our behavior. Because the chain of information from researcher to patient involves a myriad of people, all of those biases gradually distort the message as it winds its way through the chain. We will examine different biases that occur among the parties to affect their behaviors within the research process.

A bias affecting people who are involved in research projects spanning years is called the **sunk cost fallacy**. This bias exists because people do not make each decision in their lives independently of others they have already made. Instead, people perform something called "mental accounting," in which they take their previous decisions into account when making a new one. This bias is designed to keep people on track with their goals. For example, when someone is deciding whether or not to eat a piece of cake, that individual will factor into their decision that they already indulged in ice cream and cookies earlier in the day. The true decision is not whether to eat cake or not eat cake, the decision is whether to eat cake in addition to the other sweets consumed that day. In this fashion, mental accounting can be helpful.

However helpful mental accounting may be, the sunk cost fallacy bias that distorts thinking and prompts people to put more energy into an endeavor if they have already put some energy into it previously [2]. It takes a great deal of effort for people to realize their project is not reaping benefits, and that subsequently, stopping is the most cost-effective choice. In deciding whether or not to stop, people utilize mental accounting and factor in everything they have already poured into the project. They want the work to pay off to justify all of their previous efforts. As much as this makes sense on the surface, the logic is only a result of our faulty mental accounting. In truth, once something is done, it becomes a "sunk cost." It cannot be recouped at any point regardless of the next move. Take, as an example of a sunk cost, startup costs for a company. The money spent to start the company is spent before the company can generate a return. It is gone, regardless of whether the company makes money or does not.

> **To Explain to a Patient**
>
> Ask your patient if they have ever spent more time on something than they originally intended to because by the time they realized it was not going well, it felt too late to stop. If they found themselves putting in more time and energy into something that was not going well than they normally would, ask them if it was because they had already spent time on it. This is the sunk cost fallacy.

Researchers are not immune to the sunk cost fallacy. Initial interest prompts researchers into their fields of study. This interest represents an emotional investment in their work. They complete many years of advanced schooling to enter positions for conducting their research. These years—of at least forgoing income while studying, if not also paying outright for tuition—represent time and financial costs. Once finally able to begin conducting their own studies, researchers have already invested considerable cost into their work. The sunk cost fallacy is ripe to unconsciously distort their behaviors at this stage. No matter how objective researchers consciously strive to remain, the sunk cost fallacy urges them to unconsciously hope for one outcome over another.

Funders with a vested interest (i.e., financial incentive) in one outcome over another are also prone to sunk cost fallacy. Pharmaceutical companies consider the money they stand to make should a study go well, and the money they will lose if study results are delayed or disappointing. In some cases, the desire for a return on investment is more than simply an implicit bias—it is a conscious anxiety that affects pharmaceutical companies' choices, which we will see later in detail.

Another bias in research affecting people who have an idea that one outcome is more likely than another is the **confirmation bias** [2]. All people with ideas experience confirmation bias. Whenever people have a preconceived opinion about something, the confirmation bias leads them to selectively look for evidence in favor of their opinion and discount information that does not fit their opinion. Just as with other implicit biases, confirmation bias is not intentional.

To Explain to a Patient

Ask your patient how they perform searches on the Internet. For example, imagine they have been worried about how much juice is safe to give their child. Do they enter, "Recommended daily juice intake for children" or do they enter, "How much juice is too much for children?" Many patients will enter the latter. That is because we search for information based on what we already expect to find. But confirmation bias is not finished yet. After performing the search, most people would skim over results that indicate any possible health benefits of some juice intake and click on the links that highlight overconsumption and the effects thereof. This selective searching and acquisition of new information is confirmation bias.

Researchers, certain funders, academic journal editors, pediatricians, and patients alike experience confirmation bias. Researchers want to find a positive outcome, whether that outcome is a cure for a disease or a new neuronal explanation for a disorder. The modern scientific process depends on researchers first theorizing and choosing a hypothesis before starting their study. Requiring researchers to first form a hypothesis is a direct path to confirmation bias. Pharmaceutical companies have a somewhat more explicit confirmation bias at play, and we will review the behavioral outcomes of the bias in this group. Academic journal editors decide what papers to accept based on how the study will be received by the medical community. Making this determination can only be done if those editors have their own ideas about hypotheses and trends in science. They then accept papers that reinforce their ideas. When physicians and patients read about new studies (whether in the medical literature or in the media), confirmation bias prompts them to spend more time reading studies that reinforce what they already believe or hope to be true. When individuals read studies refuting their hypotheses, skepticism increases. Skepticism prompts them to initiate searches for flaws in the design or other information that will help them discount the study findings.

The last bias affecting essentially everyone in the research chain is the **novelty preference**. This bias operates in humans because we are primed to attend to stimuli that are new and different for the purposes of learning [3]. (Of course at other times people evince a familiarity bias; the two seem to serve different purposes.) New events or knowledge represent a possible source of benefit or harm beyond people's typical experiences. The novelty preference helps individuals pay attention to learn whether this new stimulus is helpful or harmful. Psychologists describe things that command an outsize place of precedence in our minds as being **salient**. Newness is highly salient.

To Explain to a Patient

Ask your patients to imagine their houses in their minds. Most pieces of furniture and decorations are in the same place every day. Has the patient ever, one day, moved something? What happened when they came back home later that day or woke up the next day? Did they suddenly "notice" that piece of furniture or decoration in a way they hadn't before they moved it? That is novelty preference. There is no reason for their notice of this item beyond the novelty of the location. The novelty preference means we pay more attention to something just because it is novel and not because that novelty is necessarily good or bad.

The field of research seeks to uncover new information. Even historians, who research past events, search for new developments in their field. Other than replication studies—a necessary part of the scientific process—all studies conducted are rooted in the idea that the results will uncover some new, as of yet unknown information. The novelty preference leads researchers to believe their findings are inherently important and worthy of attention because they are new. Pharmaceutical companies use patients' novelty preference to sell "me too" drugs: medications essentially the same as the preexisting medications. Marketers easily sell these kinds of medications to consumers based solely on their newness [4]. Medical journal editors are tasked with publishing innovative findings. The general public reads newspapers or online media to find out what has recently happened. Readers are not interested in yesterday's news. Journalists prefer writing about new treatments, aware that these articles will garner more reader interest than if they were to write about established treatments.

The implicit biases discussed here are, with a few exceptions, largely blameless. Implicit cognitive biases influence how all people operate their lives. These barely perceptible distortions naturally influence the chain of communication from researcher to patient. Because implicit biases operate below our consciousness, patients are likely unaware how such biases influence what they seek out and read about research. Discussing these implicit biases can help patients remove their metaphorical sunglasses, if only temporarily.

In addition to implicit biases, explicit biases influence the research process and are not morally neutral. Explicit biases function in conscious awareness and can result in everything from neglect and carelessness to outright fraud. The remainder of this chapter focuses on one of the greatest sources of conscious bias in research:

funding bias. While the medical profession is designed to help people, the pharmaceutical industry is designed to earn a profit for shareholders and CEOs. This divergence of goals has not escaped many patients' notice. Yet self-interest is not the all-powerful motivator some believe it to be [5]. Patients can benefit from an increased understanding as to how funding is more or less likely to affect study outcomes. Armed with this knowledge, they can more accurately calibrate their opinions on the research results they encounter.

Before discussing how funding can influence outcomes, we will preview how outcomes are typically reached in research studies. The next chapter provides a complete review of how studies are run and conclusions drawn. Many studies seek to determine if a new treatment provides better health outcomes than the preexisting treatment (if one exists). As such, researchers directing these studies look for evidence of a difference between the treatments. Differences are observed through the use of inferential statistics. These statistics are based on a concept of disputing the null hypothesis, which is a concept that presupposes there will be no difference between the groups. Studies showing evidence in favor of a difference between the groups are said to be "significant." Notably, statistical significance and clinical significance are separate issues, which we will discuss in depth later in this book. Much as how the American legal system is based on a presumption of innocence (placing the burden on the plaintiff or prosecution to supply enough evidence of wrongdoing), research studies presume no difference between two groups, and the results of the research study shoulder the responsibility of rejecting the null hypothesis. The null hypothesis is rejected on the basis that it is statistically extremely unlikely that the difference observed between the two groups is by chance. The null hypothesis itself can never be proven, because in this case, it is not possible to prove a negative (this is relevant when discussing the limitations of research studies with parents).

Funding Sources

Funding in medical research can be divided into two large categories: publicly funded and privately funded. Public funds come from sources such as the government or charities, where money (typically from taxes or donations) is disbursed with the aim of funding the activities that constitute a civil society. Public funds are designed to promote the public good and are not intended to have a specific agenda. People who give their dollars to charities do not do so with the aim of getting more money in return (although some may hope their charitable donations curry favor or win them influence).

Private funds come from privately held companies, in which individuals invest their money with the stated aim of seeing a return on their investment. The goal for dollars from private funding is to earn more dollars. For example, a company that invests its own money in research and development is anticipating eventually selling the resulting product at a profit.

The main source of public funding in medical research is the National Institute of Health (NIH) [6]. The United States founded the NIH the late nineteenth century. It now disburses approximately 30.1 billion dollars annually [6]. Funded with taxpayer dollars, the NIH is government-run and nonprofit. The NIH does not take in money based on its research efforts, although a small percentage of its research dollars fund grants and contracts through Small Business Innovation Research and Small Business Technology Transfer initiatives [7]. Therefore, NIH-funded research trials are fairly unlikely to be influenced by financial motives. The dedicated cynic will point out that it is impossible to be truly disinterested in money. Nevertheless, influence due to money is observed to occur less in publicly funded trials than in privately funded ones, as discussed below.

Private funding for medical research overwhelmingly comes from pharmaceutical companies [8]. While the NIH continues to be the primary funder for basic research science, in the mid-1980s pharmaceutical companies surpassed the NIH as the primary funder of biomedical research [8, 9]. In 2013, the top pharmaceutical company spent over 8 billion dollars in research and development [10]. Even as far back as a decade ago, estimates found that for-profit entities sponsored 75% of clinical research [8].

As corporate entities, the goal of a pharmaceutical manufacturer is to make money, ideally as quickly as possible. If shares of the company are traded on the stock market, their earnings are reported quarterly. This produces a near-constant pressure to perform well (i.e., make money). This pressure causes myopia of goals, prioritizing short-term monetary outcomes over long-term health gains.

Conducting research is a costly and time-consuming effort. Given their profit motives, it seems paradoxical that pharmaceutical companies would fund research at all. Yet they do not have a choice. By law, prior to selling a new medicine or treatment, companies must prove to the Food and Drug Administration (FDA) that the product passed efficacy and safety standards [11]. This proof is available only through research. Hence, pharmaceutical companies find themselves involved simultaneously in two activities—marketing and research—with divergent goals. The goal of marketing is to make money, and making money requires that the information be in the product's favor. The goal of research is to expand knowledge in the field (whatever that knowledge may show), and in doing so, it expends vast sums of money. These goals are not quite diametrically opposed, but there is significant tension between them. This tension creates an inherent conflict of interest that serves as a common thread running through all pharmaceutical research.

For a multitude of practical reasons, pharmaceutical companies typically do not conduct research in-house [11]. Instead, these companies previously relied heavily on academic researchers to assist in conducting their trials [11]. Including academic researchers was thought to mitigate the pharmaceutical company's desire for money by offsetting it with the researcher's desire to be perceived well in the field by striving to conduct objective, bias-free, pure research. Academic researchers viewing their careers through a long-term lens are incentivized to keep their priorities from shifting to the short-term focus of the pharmaceutical companies. By assigning each entity in the process its own goal, this arrangement was established as a kind of checks and balances system. High-profile academic names tied to pharmaceutical studies benefitted the companies because of the implicit assumption that academic researchers' quest for knowledge placed them above the desire for money, however unrealistic this perception may be [11, 12]. Of course researchers are not immune to the influence of money. Pharmaceutical companies provide equity ownership of their companies, consultancy positions, and funding to researchers. All of these activities cost money to pharmaceutical companies. As they are not charities, companies continually spending money in this fashion can be assumed to lead to a direct benefit for the companies [12].

While there is great prestige for companies when they involve academic researchers, this partnership comes at a cost. As stated, academic research is costly and takes notoriously long to conduct. Various approvals processes in academic centers, such as the Institutional Review Board (established to protect the rights of human participants) and Sponsored Programs Administrations (which oversee the distribution and use of funds awarded for research purposes), are required before study activities can begin. In some cases, companies found that it took too long to recruit enough patients to reach the numbers needed for the study [11]. These delays directly impact the pharmaceutical companies' bottom line. Delays in research mean delays in obtaining FDA approval. Each day a drug cannot be sold costs the company approximately 1.3 million dollars [11].

These costly delays prompted pharmaceutical companies to partner elsewhere for their research needs [11]. Contract-research organizations (CROs) and site-management organizations (SMOs) cropped up to meet this need of the pharmaceutical companies [11]. CROs are centers specifically designed to conduct research studies [11]. When a commercial advertises a product as "clinically proven," they are likely referring to a clinic such as can be found in a CRO. The purpose of a CRO is to make money, and they do so by obtaining contracts from pharmaceutical companies who need their products tested. SMOs are similar in that they are involved in testing, but they are often contracted with CROs, so that they become subcontracted with pharmaceutical companies. As the pharmaceutical company pays the CRO, it becomes the customer in the arrangement. The phrase "the customer is always right," is often bandied about in modern customer service. The sentiment in this phrase is remarkably apt when the customer (the pharmaceutical company) has orders of magnitude more money and influence than the entity they are choosing to send their business to. CROs competing with one another for pharmaceutical companies' business have every financial incentive to keep the pharmaceutical companies satisfied with their tests' findings.

One can see how this arrangement between the large pharmaceutical companies and the relatively weaker CROs could lead to subpar research quality. From the start, the pharmaceutical company typically creates a study design and gives it to the CRO to follow, like a chef handing a recipe off to a line cook. There is no independent oversight of these study designs to ensure that they are properly powered, ethical, and valid [11].

Just as in academic research studies, pharmaceutical companies typically establish protocols whereby two groups of people are compared—those who get the new treatment, and those get something else (either nothing, a placebo, or a pre-existing treatment for the same ailment). Despite this key similarity, many meaningful differences have been consistently observed between privately funded and publicly funded studies. Privately funded studies often use surrogate outcome measures rather than actual clinical outcomes [4]. For example, a study of executive functioning in children might examine whether children become better at a study measure such as playing computer games (theorized by the treatment developer to represent underlying executive functioning abilities) rather than whether or not the child is actually turning in more of their homework on time (the functional outcome most parents and teachers care about). Such a study would conclude that the client's program helps children's executive functioning, when in reality is only helps them get better at playing a game.

Many privately funded studies exist for the purposes of FDA approval, a one-time goal. Therefore, they do not spend the copious amounts needed to fund long-term trials, examining what happens to the people in their trials after years have passed. By not conducting such longitudinal studies, long-term health effects of the treatment or medication, including adverse events, are not included in test results [4]. Subsequently, some extreme adverse events, such as toxicity, have occurred in the general population taking a drug because it had never been tested for long-term safety before the drug came to market [4]. For this reason alone, statistically speaking, an old drug that is still used by the medical profession is more likely to be safe than a newer one [13]. If a drug has been used clinically for a generation, the range of likely adverse events is already known.

Privately funded studies are also more likely to compare new drugs to a placebo than are NIH-funded trials, which are more likely to compare to another active treatment [14]. It is obviously easier to find a difference between two treatments when one of the treatments is a sugar pill. By using placebos more often than other active treatments, privately funded studies are designed to more easily find the difference they need for FDA approval. Even when privately funded studies use an active treatment as a comparator, investigations have found they often underdose the comparator when compared to the new treatment [15]. Similar to the placebo issue, it is easier to conclude a drug is successful when comparing it to a drug that is less effective due to underdosing [15].

Privately funded studies are also more likely to use participants who are not true users of the drug [4]. For example, a blood pressure medicine, which would give the most relief to the elderly, was tested in healthy young participants [4]. A study using people who are already healthy can skew results of the drug, making it appear the healthy outcomes are more due to the drug than they really are. Another effect of recruiting young people for studies is that they are known to experience fewer adverse side effects to drugs in general [11]. The researchers can then honestly state they found few adverse events among participants in their study. When actually ill patients take the drug after approval, they will experience more adverse events than were reported in a set of healthy participants [11].

In addition to these design flaws that are clearly employed to yield more favorable outcomes, privately funded studies also occasionally violate the principles of ethical research involving human participants. Specifically, it has been shown that privately funded studies have stopped prematurely due solely to cost concerns [8]. This violates the risk/benefit ratio agreements made with participants when they consented to participate [8]. Publicly funded studies can be stopped prematurely as well, but the reasons must be limited to emerging data that changes the risk/benefit ratio for participants. For example, if another researcher acting independently concludes that the treatment being studied is not as effective as current treatment, or is harmful, this represents a change in the risk/benefit ratio originally presented to possible participants when they were deciding whether or not to participate. The new ratio might change their willingness to continue to participate, so they must be informed. In some cases, the study is halted altogether in light of the new information. In these cases, a clinical population of participants would naturally want to know that so they could discontinue the study and resume the current treatment. Notice that the early termination of the study is done to benefit the participants, not the researcher. Stopping a study due to cost concerns benefits solely the researcher and could be at the expense of the participants.

Once a privately funded study is complete and the data have been collected, pharmaceutical companies often invite academic researchers to put their name on the study, despite the fact that the researcher was not involved in the study design or execution [11]. These requests for academic researcher names are motivated by the same reasons that pharmaceutical companies used to work with academic centers in the first place. Private studies aim for prestige and an appearance of being more scholarly and objective than commercially minded. When academic researchers choose to lend their names to studies like this, they are required to follow the International Committee of Medical Journal Editors' (ICMJE) standards for making sure they met authorship criteria [11, 16]. Academic researchers do not always follow these standards [11]. One study revealed that of the manuscripts reviewed, 19% had authors who did not meet the criteria [17]. The practice of ghostwriting, in which the pharmaceutical company contracts someone to write the article, provides another violation of the ICMJE guidelines [11]. The same study found that 11% of articles employed a ghostwriter [17]. These misrepresentations of authorship further complicate the task of determining the validity of the study.

In some cases, pharmaceutical companies engaged in suppression of study results when they were either neutral (i.e., they were inconclusive and therefore could not be used to support the new drug) or actively detrimental (i.e., they showed the new drug was either ineffective or detrimental) [11]. In one instance, a drug company began arbitration in response to one of their academic collaborators who published undesirable findings from a research trial of their product [18]. Pharmaceutical companies have published other findings from the same contested study while the original draft is being held up in arbitration [11]. Most tragically, important safety information has been withheld for years [11].

Pharmaceutical-funded studies have produced more results favoring new therapies than publicly funded trials have [19]. Some argue that **publication bias**, wherein journals are more likely to publish significant results rather than nonsignificant ones, drives this phenomenon. Because publication bias affects publicly funded trials as well as pharmaceutically funded ones, this bias cannot explain the difference between funding styles. A better explanation is that in most cases, pharmaceutical companies save money by only conducting research on drugs that have already shown some promise in-house [4].

While this practice makes sense in practical terms, it is not justified under the scientific method. A strict interpretation of the scientific method holds that two interventions can only be compared using statistics if the null hypothesis maintains there is no difference between the two interventions. The presumption of no difference must be made prior to testing, with the study then required to show if there is one. This uncertainty that a difference exists is what necessitates a research study in the first place, at least academically speaking. For pharmaceutical companies to study interventions they already have evidence in favor of against an older intervention violates this uncertainty principle [14]. While, it makes sense on a cost basis to only test what is likely to be effective, this is the scientific equivalent to "stacking the deck." It reveals that the companies are only using research for the purposes of gaining FDA approval, not for truly understanding more about the drug.

Pharmaceutical companies do produce advances in technology [12]. They have provided products, treatments, and drugs that have improved, lengthened, and saved the lives of countless people. The products they develop are often helpful, despite the fact that their studies are most certainly biased. An extensive meta-review of the literature shows that the issue is largely resolved when it comes to the question of bias in funding [20]. Rather than spend more time and money researching whether the bias exists, the time has come to begin to prevent it where possible and respond to it. Recommendations to improve the situation should be directed toward stakeholders and decision makers. Patients are certainly stakeholders, but unless they are interested in policy and advocacy work, they are not decision makers. Instead, physicians can help patients understand the biases that influence research into medical advances so that they can respond with appropriate skepticism.

Conflicts of Interest

By now, it should be clear that conflicts of interest exist in the running of research studies, particularly when great sums of money are on the line. Regulatory bodies have attempted to reduce the effects of these influences by requiring disclosures of interest [21]. The function of the disclosure is to satisfy "caveat emptor," or, "let the buyer beware." In order for people to avoid being deceived, they must have information about conflicts. Then, it is presumed they can decide if the conflict is one they will tolerate. The rationale is that once the discloser has revealed the extent of their conflict, consumers are then educated enough in the facts to make an educated decision for themselves. Responsibility shifts from seller to buyer [21].

Disclosure is required in a number of settings, including in published papers and presentations [21]. However, disclosures can have a paradoxical effect on the people making them [21, 22]. Once a disclosure has been made, the discloser feels a reduced burden for any future possible negative outcomes [21]. Having warned the consumer, they feel relieved of further responsibility. The consumer is supposedly making an "informed" choice due to the disclosure. Disclosures can also have a paradoxical effect on the people reading them. Research shows that after hearing a disclosure, people trust the discloser even more [21].

This paradoxical effect does not operate to the same extent among educated consumers of the information. When people educated in a specific area read disclosures, doing so does not reassure them about the validity of the work, but rather increases their skepticism [21]. In one study, doctors reading disclosures of financial interest downgraded their assessment of the rigor of trials based on the disclosure of conflict alone [22]. These doctors were technically inaccurate in downgrading the rigor based on this information alone. A disclosure is not inherently tied to methodology, and rigor pertains to methodology alone. However, this bias among educated consumers of disclosures might, practically speaking, counteract the influence that conflicts have clearly been seen to have over research outcomes. In this case, the old adage about two wrongs not making a right might be incorrect. Experts unfairly downgrading the rigor of studies unfairly propped up due to financial interest may be an instance of the checks and balances system working.

Skepticism

Responding to the mounting skepticism of privately funded trial results, academic journal editors began setting more rigorous publication criteria for pharmaceutical companies' studies [23]. Some patients are aware of the specific biases pertaining to funding in the pharmaceutical industry. In general, people maintain skepticism of corporations and seek to determine motivations for corporate actions [24]. Consumers know that the primary goal of corporations is to make a profit. These consumers feel more comfortable when they can readily identify a profit motive for companies' activities, because these motives fit easily within their notions about companies. When corporations act in ways not directly tied to making a profit (or in actions that would seem to undercut their profit, as in the case of a cigarette company launching an anti-smoking campaign for teens), people's skepticism increases. They begin searching harder for a profit motive to explain the action, putting the company's actions under further scrutiny.

We have been speaking of skepticism in a general sense. In the medical literature, skepticism is defined as the level of one's doubts that medical intervention can appreciably change one's health status [25]. Highly skeptical patients tend to have certain characteristics compared to those with lower skepticism: they are younger, identify their race as white, earn lower incomes, attain less years of education, and perceive their own health status as better than their less skeptical peers, despite lower healthcare utilization and less healthy lifestyle [25]. While we cannot infer causation, skeptical patients are observed to lead less healthy lifestyles, experience poorer mental health, engage in fewer preventative medical activities, and utilize less medical care overall [25]. Additionally, skeptical patients were found to engage in other risky or health-reducing behaviors, such as smoking. The study authors surmised that these behaviors might have contributed to the skeptics' subsequent higher five-year mortality rates compared to non-skeptics [26], although again, a directly causal link was not tested. These authors propose a potential model to explain their findings: high levels of skepticism lead to less engagement with medical care and poorer health choices, which in turn, affected their mortality rates.

Clearly people's skepticism affects how they view the health care industry and their medical choices stemming from it. Pediatricians encounter parents who object to giving their children medications on the basis that the medications only exist to serve the pharmaceutical industry's profit motive. While, we have explored how this can be true in some cases (particularly with "me too" drugs), this blanket skepticism as to motives is not entirely fair. Health care providers have more effective and safe treatment options at their disposal, and they have them more rapidly than they would have without the pharmaceutical industry and privately funded trials.

Addressing skepticism is a matter of public health. If those who are skeptical of medical interventions engage in fewer health-promoting behaviors and have higher mortality rates, doctors will want to address those concerns. This daunting task must occur within a complicated context, given evidence that some medical interventions are, in fact, not necessary or less safe than established alternatives.

However, well-placed skepticism of medical research findings is in some cases, the skepticism often manifests in behaviors that can only be described as illogical. For example, it is established that privately funded trials do not test new drugs or methods over long periods of time to assess their longitudinal safety and efficacy, making them inherently riskier than preexisting models. Yet skeptical patients often evince wariness of well-established methods rather than new ones. For example, lately a vocal minority of patients became concerned that the amount of vaccines recommended for their child is influenced more by the pharmaceutical companies' profit motives than safety for their children. These patients subsequently decided to withhold vaccines (most commonly via spreading out doses over longer periods of time or outright refusal) from their children based on this presumption. Becoming concerned about profit motives but responding to that concern by avoiding well-established practices is an erroneous conflation of ideas. While it is true that pharmaceutical companies want to make a profit, vaccines delivered according to the well-researched guidelines for timing and dosage are inherently safer than individually experimenting with their own children's vaccination schedule. Exposing a child to risks by conducting individual "experiments" negligibly affects the pharmaceutical companies' bottom lines and ignores the fact that the riskiest medicines are marketed as new and innovative. A patients' skepticism would be more logically applied if a parent were to refuse a newer version of a treatment for their child when an older one is available. This behavior corresponds to an actual, proven source of skepticism rather than a misplaced one.

Direct to Consumer Advertising

Other patients are not nearly as skeptical as they could be. Pharmaceutical companies frequently message individuals to acclimate them to new products with direct-to-consumer advertising (DTCA). DTCA began in 1708, when Nicholas Boone purchased an advertisement in a newspaper for a patent medicine [13]. The newspaper provided the information about the product directly to the people who might use it, rather to the doctors who would prescribe it. Since that early time, pharmaceutical companies have now come to spend twice as much on advertising as they do on research [10]. The top pharmaceutical company spent upwards of 17 billion dollars on marketing in 2013 [10]. Even though companies still spend comparatively more of their marketing budgets selling to physicians, the movement from paternalism to consumerism helped companies increasingly benefit from DTCA strategies [10, 13]. If these profit-driven companies spend so much of their operating budget on DTCA, it presumably works.

Disappointingly, surveys show that many people think that messages in DTCA have been pre-reviewed and approved by the FDA [13]. The same study revealed that this false assumption led them to believe that the promoted drugs were safer due to this supposed governmental intervention, that medications with serious side effects were banned from being marketed in this manner, and that only drugs that are "extremely effective" could be marketed in this fashion. None of these facts are true [13].

This perception of regulation where there is none is troubling. DTCA works: patients come to their doctors' offices requesting specific drugs. When doctors explain that the drug is not as well-established as older versions, they are confronted with first undoing patients' misconceptions [13]. It is inherently harder to undo a misconception than to educate someone from a neutral starting point. Clearing up these misconceptions also has an opportunity cost: it takes time away from discussing the patient's specific symptoms and other treatment options that might be more suitable for this individual [13]. Despite the challenges stemming from DTCA, patients still rate physicians as their most trusted interpersonal source of health information [27]. This trust should be carefully guarded, and doctors have an obligation to correct misconceptions their patients raise resulting from advertising.

Media

Advertising is not the only point of contact patients have with new treatment options. Patients read about research in the media they consume. Journalists working for publications with editorial oversight are expected to follow a journalistic code of ethics set forth by the Society of Professional Journalists. By agreeing to this code, journalists voluntarily assume some responsibility for their role in the accurate dissemination of information. Medical journalists reporting the results of research studies are no different in this regard, and their reporting has wide-ranging effects. When journalists present dramatic research findings, the public responds. As an illustration, news articles reporting long-term results of hormone replacement therapy sufficiently alarmed the public, promoting widespread abandonment of the treatment [28]. Regrettably, research shows that many articles presenting study results do not include adequate information to situate the findings within a meaningful context [29].

Part of the responsibility can be placed with the researchers who interact with journalists about their published studies. Many researchers utilize press releases to spread the word about their work. Researchers use press releases because they work-statistics show journalists are more likely to cover a study if has a press release [30]. While journalists are tasked with reporting more than the content of the press release, as many as one-third of all medical articles published report no more than the information contained in the original press release [30]. Of course this lack of additional reporting is technically the responsibility of the journalist. But now that this neglect is common knowledge, researchers should assume the responsibility of providing more context themselves in the release.

Researchers can certainly improve in this area. One study examined press releases written by the original study author and found an overarching tendency to overstate the importance of a particular research finding and understate (or outright ignore) the limitations of the study's design and conclusions [30]. The bias of researchers distributing press releases overstating their work can be tied to the sunk cost fallacy and their emotional ties to their work. Researchers have often invested years of their careers into particular studies. They are also emotionally invested, influencing them to overstate their work's importance [31].

Like others in the chain of research, journalists are subject to funding bias. The media is comprised of companies with bottom lines, just like pharmaceutical companies. Media outlets make most of their profits from advertising [13]. Advertisers trying to get their message to as many people as possible pay more for outlets providing a large audience. Knowing this, the media is financially motivated to secure as many readers as possible to review their publications. While individuals within the media machine may be ethical, they experience a wide array of pressures to get the most "clicks," "likes," "shares," and "retweets." Knowing as we do that people prefer novelty, journalists write articles about research that they think readers will find new and exciting [32]. These funding biases would affect the chain of communication about research even if no specific individual in this chain were acting reproachfully. It would be as fruitless to blame journalists for trying to make their work interesting as it would be to blame an individual person for choosing to read an article based on its "click-bait" headline.

While the responsibility rests with researchers and journalists to monitor the information they disseminate, neither a pediatrician nor a parent can compel them to do so. They can only be aware that practices of misrepresentation exist and respond by applying critical thinking skills when reading about studies. Pediatricians can review the study itself, if they have access to the medical journal in which it was originally published. Most pediatricians are unlikely to have investigated a specific study prior to their patient coming into inquire about it. As discussed in the introduction, doctors would ideally keep informed of new research advances, but time constraints make this extremely challenging. To supplement investigating studies themselves whenever possible, pediatricians can encourage their patients to examine the validity of the reporting themselves.

Almost any individual reading a news report of a study can conduct a cursory assessment to determine if it is worthwhile to look into it further. Woloshin and Schwartz recommend some basic rules of thumb for patients to gauge if studies have any applicability to their lives:

- **Animal studies**: Animal studies are, by their very nature, preliminary. They tend to be closer to "basic science" rather than having any clinical applicability.
- **Small studies**: Thirty or fewer participants represent a very small sample size, so any study with fewer than 30 should be judged to have limited inferential ability.
- **Studies that were controlled but not randomized**: If people were not assigned at random to one treatment/condition over another, the inferences from these studies are also limited due to confounding factors.
- **Studies that are described as "preliminary" or not published in a scientific journal**: Again, preliminary studies represent a step in the research process towards learning new information. This new information is not likely to have any direct bearing on a patient's life at this stage.
- **Studies that do not include mention of adverse events**: Without knowing the adverse outcomes, patients could not make an informed decision.

Provided a study passes these rules of thumb, patients (with the help of their doctors) can examine how well the reporting of the study has been placed in the overall context of medical research. Australian researchers developed a set of ten considerations to guide a critical reading of a popular media outlet's take on a research study [28]. Ask patients to print out a copy of the article or pull it up on their phone during an office visit to review the article with them using this checklist. The considerations are as follows, and each will be discussed specifically below:

1. genuine novelty of the treatment
2. availability of treatment
3. discussion (or at least mention) of alternative treatments

4. no evidence of "disease mongering"
5. objective evidence in favor of treatment
6. benefits framed in absolute terms rather than relative
7. mention of harms
8. mention of costs
9. mention of conflicts of interest
10. article includes reporting beyond the press release.

1. *Genuine novelty of the treatment*
   Help patient determines if this treatment is truly novel, or simply a re-hashing of a preexisting treatment. Some studies are replication studies, specifically tasked with investigating if they can find the same positive results as a previous study. Reporters, not realizing this, can publish replication studies as if they are new treatments. Other times, a treatment has been studied in one format, but researchers adapt it slightly for a new population or diagnostic subcategory. Although the study may be testing a new focus, the treatment itself is not actually novel.

2. *Availability of treatment*
   Some articles excitedly report findings of a groundbreaking new treatment, proclaiming its promise for saving lives. But if the treatment is so new as to be offered in only one location, the research results are, for intents and purposes, irrelevant.

3. *Discussion (or at least mention) of alternative treatments*
   Medical journalists should include a mention of what treatments are already available to treat the condition the new treatment addresses. If they have not, they leave this task to doctors.

4. *No evidence of "disease mongering"*
   Moynihan defines the methods of disease mongering: re-characterizing common ailments into medical problems, overstating mild symptoms as serious ones, interpreting personal problems as medical illnesses, conflating risk with disease, and stating the higher end of prevalence estimates to maximize potential markets. No matter which method is employed in disease mongering, the overall goal is to sell more products to people who otherwise would not have purchased them. Disease mongering essentially frightens people into purchasing treatments. Suggest that patients look for signs that the creators of the treatment or the journalists are using fear to prompt them to action.

5. *Objective evidence in favor of treatment*
   Help patients find studies reporting objective evidence, which are more convincing than those use subjective outcomes. Look for studies using objective outcomes whenever possible (e.g., a measure of blood pressure is more objective than asking how stressed someone is feeling). Also look for studies where the conclusions presented result from statistical analysis, rather than a qualitative review of the data. Objectivity of outcomes is not always possible (e.g., social science research, like psychology, often must employ subjective

measures—indeed, subjective experience is what people care about). But studies that use subjective measures where objective ones are available deserve careful scrutiny.

6. *Benefits framed in absolute terms rather than relative*

   The human brain is not well suited for probabilities. Articles reporting outcomes in relative terms require the reader to employ probabilistic thinking. Using relative terms makes differences sound larger or more meaningful than they really are. Describing the influence of a drug as helping to reduce symptoms by 50% sounds good. It becomes less interesting when realizing that if the overall prevalence of symptoms of the disease is extremely low, a 50% symptom reduction can, in some cases, be quite negligible. This is just an example, of course, but it shows how journalists describing benefits in relative terms make the story sound more interesting without giving the reader a clear picture of what's happening for the patient. Stating the benefits in absolute terms is much more clear for patients so they can decide if the benefit is worthwhile, e.g.: "participants taking the new drug had two outbreaks per month, whereas the control group had four."

7. *Mention of harms*

   Patients considering a new treatment should want to know what the potential harms are. If the article omits this information, patients cannot possibly make an informed decision about the treatment.

8. *Mention of costs*

   Similar to availability, patients should know what the costs of the treatment are—ongoing costs as well as initial. Prohibitively expensive treatments, or treatments so new that they cannot be covered by insurance, are once again, irrelevant to individual patients.

9. *Mention of conflicts of interest*

   While disclosures of financial interest are problematic, the scientific community is obligated to report them. Reporters familiar with writing medical research articles are aware of this obligation. Articles that omit disclosures indicate some oversight. Where disclosures of financial interest are reported, help patients decide if this conflict would bias anyone in the research chain (implicitly or explicitly) to present the findings as more important or relevant than they are to an individual patient.

10. *Article includes reporting beyond the press release*

    We saw that as many as one-third of articles include no additional reporting beyond the press release contents. When physicians have access to the press release, they can help patients compare the release to the article. Ask patients what they think it means if the two documents are identical. See if they can identify the problems discussed above that arise when journalists act as a medium for the researchers to spread their message at no cost, with no examination from the press. If the original press release is not available, examine the length of the article with patients. The shorter the article, the less information it includes. The more likely it is to be almost completely derived from the press release.

Investigate Source of Information

Pediatricians can encourage patients to apply various litmus tests to infer funding sources when they are unclear. Many people now get their information from the Internet. Website extensions provide a quick and easy way to begin to examine funding. Websites ending with ".com" are automatically disclosing their primary interest: commerce [33]. Any .com site faithfully represents itself as for-profit. Websites beginning with .gov are run by the government and are inherently designed to be free from as many conflicts as possible [33]. Of course conflicts can still exist, but at the very least, the government is nonprofit. Websites ending with .edu are primarily focused on education [33]. As with the government, education is not always free from conflict, by any means. Recent lawsuits against for-profit higher educational companies reveal institutions that placed profit motives above educational goals. Reputable educational organizations proceed at least somewhat cautiously with the information they present to the public. This caution protects their reputation and—in the cases of nonprofit institutions—their tax-exempt status. Websites with .org extensions are less clear at the outset as to their goals, given "org" stands simply for "organization" [33]. If patients find themselves on .org websites, they should proceed to the next litmus test.

Most websites of repute have some kind of "About Us" page outlining the entity's goals and missions. These pages list leaders among the organization, sometimes with short biographical details. A quick search on a search engine of these names will reveal important facts about the leaders that patients can consider. Is the leader of the organization a business leader or an academic leader? If the leader heads a charitable organization, how did they come to be dedicated to this cause? What experiences do they highlight as important or transformational moments in their lives? These experiences sometimes reveal an emotional investment that is subject to bias.

If patients cannot find an About Us section, they should look for any kind of oversight of the website at all. They might be on a personal blog, a questionably moderated forum, or a site created with the specific intention of spreading misinformation. Sites like these of course can create legitimate looking About Us sections, but the information therein would not hold up to further scrutiny with a subsequent online search.

To Explain to a Patient

Have you ever received an unanticipated phone call or email from your bank or credit card company, during which the message asks you to call them at a certain number? If you were to call that number, it would likely ask you for personal information, as these are commonly phishing attacks to obtain your personal data for identity theft. After getting a call or email like this, if you searched the phone number they wanted you to call or called your institution directly using the number posted on their official website, you would quickly learn that the original call or email was a scam. Websites operate the same way. They can present themselves initially as legitimate, but they do not typically hold up when you try to confirm their authenticity from simply one or two other verifiable sources.

Finally, if patients want basic information about the study that was not included within the article, direct them to search for the study on ClinicalTrials.gov. This database was created in 1997. Over the years, it has increased the amount of information required of all researchers to post about their studies. As a result of International Committee of Medical Journal Editors policies, researchers must now report key elements of the data, basic results, and adverse events on ClinicalTrials.gov prior to publication. If patients cannot find the study on ClinicalTrials.gov, they should maintain skepticism until they obtain sufficient information as to its authenticity from a trusted source.

References

1. Kapp MB. Patient autonomy in the age of consumer-driven health care: informed consent and informed choice. J Legal Med. 2007;28(1):91–117.
2. Kahneman D. Thinking, fast and slow. Macmillan; 2011.
3. Snyder KA, Blank MP, Marsolek CJ. What form of memory underlies novelty preferences? Psychon Bull Rev. 2008;15(2):315–21.
4. Montaner JS, O'Shaughnessy MV, Schechter MT. Industry-sponsored clinical research: a double-edged sword. Lancet. 2001;358(9296):1893–5.
5. Miller DT, Ratner RK. The power of the myth of self-interest. In current societal concerns about justice. US: Springer; 1996. p. 25–48.
6. Grants & Funding. National Institutes of Health (NIH). 2016. http://www.nih.gov/grants-funding Accessed 24 Mar 2016.
7. FAQs | NIH Small Business Innovation Research (SBIR) and Small Business Technology Transfer (STTR) Programs. Sbir.nih.gov. 2016. https://sbir.nih.gov/faqs#intellectual-property-req1 Accessed 24 Mar 2016.
8. Chopra SS. Industry funding of clinical trials: benefit or bias? Jama. 2003;290(1):113–4.
9. Schwarz RP. Maintaining integrity and credibility in industry-sponsored clinical research. Control Clin Trials. 1991;12(6):753–60.
10. Swanson A. Big pharmaceutical companies are spending far more on marketing than research. Washington Post. 2016. https://www.washingtonpost.com/news/wonk/wp/2015/02/11/big-pharmaceutical-companies-are-spending-far-more-on-marketing-than-research/ Accessed 23 Mar 2016.
11. Bodenheimer T. Uneasy alliance. N Engl J Med. 2000;342(20):1539–44.
12. Angell M. Is academic medicine for sale? Quaderns de la Fundació Dr. Antoni Esteve. 2012(24):59–62.
13. Glascoff DW. Direct-to-consumer prescription drug advertising: trends, impact and implications. Mark Health Serv. 2000;20(1):38.
14. Djulbegovic B, Lacevic M, Cantor A, Fields KK, Bennett CL, Adams JR, Kuderer NM, Lyman GH. The uncertainty principle and industry-sponsored research. Lancet. 2000;356(9230):635–8.

15. Rochon PA, Gurwitz JH, Simms RW, Fortin PR, Felson DT, Minaker KL, Chalmers TC. A study of manufacturer-supported trials of nonsteroidal anti-inflammatory drugs in the treatment of arthritis. Arch Intern Med. 1994;154(2):157–63.

16. ICMJE | Recommendations| Defining the Role of Authors and Contributors. Icmje.org. 2016. http://www.icmje.org/recommendations/browse/roles-and-responsibilities/defining-the-role-of-authors-and-contributors.html Accessed 23 Mar 2016.

17. Flanagin A, Carey LA, Fontanarosa PB, Phillips SG, Pace BP, Lundberg GD, Rennie D. Prevalence of articles with honorary authors and ghost authors in peer-reviewed medical journals. Jama. 1998;280(3):222–4.

18. Niiler E. Company, academics argue over data. Nat Biotechnol. 2000;18(12):1235.

19. Davidson RA. Source of funding and outcome of clinical trials. J Gen Intern Med. 1986;1(3):155–8.

20. Sismondo S. Pharmaceutical company funding and its consequences: a qualitative systematic review. Contemp Clin Trials. 2008;29(2):109–13.

21. Cain DM, Loewenstein G, Moore DA. The dirt on coming clean: perverse effects of disclosing conflicts of interest. J Legal Stud. 2005;34(1):1–25.

22. Kesselheim AS, Robertson CT, Myers JA, Rose SL, Gillet V, Ross KM, Glynn RJ, Joffe S, Avorn J. A randomized study of how physicians interpret research funding disclosures. N Engl J Med. 2012;367(12):1119–27.

23. Lexchin J, Bero LA, Djulbegovic B, Clark O. Pharmaceutical industry sponsorship and research outcome and quality: systematic review. Br Med J. 2003;326(7400):1167–70.

24. Szykman LR. Who are you and why are you being nice?: Investigating the industry effect on consumer reaction to corporate societal marketing efforts. Adv CONSUM RES. 2004;31:306–13.

25. Fiscella K, Franks P, Clancy CM. Skepticism toward medical care and health care utilization. Med Care. 1998;36(2):180–9.

26. Fiscella K, Franks P, Clancy CM, Doescher MP, Banthin JS. Does skepticism towards medical care predict mortality? Med Care. 1999;37(4):409–14.

27. DeLorme DE, Huh J, Reid LN. Direct-to-consumer advertising skepticism and the use and perceived usefulness of prescription drug information sources. Health Mark Q. 2009;26(4):293–314.

28. Smith DE, Wilson AJ, Henry DA. Monitoring the quality of medical news reporting: early experience with media doctor. Med J Aust. 2005;183(4):190.

29. Schwitzer G. How do US journalists cover treatments, tests, products, and procedures? An evaluation of 500 stories. PLoS Med. 2008;5(5):e95.

30. Woloshin S, Schwartz LM, Casella SL, Kennedy AT, Larson RJ. Press releases by academic medical centers: not so academic? Ann Intern Med. 2009;150(9):613–8.

31. Woloshin S, Schwartz LM, Kramer BS. Promoting healthy skepticism in the news: helping journalists get it right. J Natl Cancer Inst. 2009;101(23):1596–9.

32. Wilkes MS, Kravitz RL. Medical researchers and the media: attitudes toward public dissemination of research. Jama. 1992;268(8):999–1003.

33. Wald HS, Dube CE, Anthony DC. Untangling the web—the impact of internet use on health care and the physician–patient relationship. Patient Educ Couns. 2007;68(3):218–24.

Chapter 3
Study Design

Study Rigor

By this point, it should be clear which kinds of studies warrant an in-depth look from pediatricians and patients. First, an obvious and meaningful conflict of interest (whether disclosed outright or inferred based on funding streams) should be absent. Second, patients have performed their own due diligence: applying guiding principles, ascertaining the legitimacy of the Web site presenting the study, or reviewing the overview of the study on ClinicalTrials.gov. Physicians and patients must next determine if the study's design is rigorous enough to incorporate its conclusions into the shared decision-making process.

Broadly, rigor is an assessment of the methodologies used in a particular study. We touched on rigor when discussing the experiment examining how conflict of interest disclosures affect doctors' perceptions of the quality of the study [1]. The quality of a study can be defined in many ways, but rigor is a key determinant. Not all studies can or even should follow the same design.

To Explain to a Patient

Think of research studies like custom-made suits, and methodologies like the information the tailor uses to craft the suit. Each suit needs certain measurements, like sleeve length and shoulder width. They can also be customized according to the wearer's needs or preferences (extra pockets, double-breasted, single vent or two, etc.). While each one is a suit, they will not all look the same. In fact, one of the defining characteristics of a custom-made suit is that it is expected to vary from wearer to wearer. However, a suit should still fit the wearer. A poorly designed research study is like a

---

© Springer International Publishing AG 2017
C.A. Di Bartolo and M.K. Braun, *Pediatrician's Guide to Discussing Research with Patients*, DOI 10.1007/978-3-319-49547-7_3

custom-made suit that fits poorly. It is still a suit, but would you want to buy it? Examining the rigor of a study is like checking to see if the custom-made suit fits.

More precisely, rigor represents how easy or challenging it is for a study to report significant and meaningful results. The researchers choose methodologies that directly influence the study's rigor.

To Explain to a Patient

Think of methodological rigor as hurdles of various heights, and a significant result as a jumper who makes it over a hurdle. We award more points to a jumper who clears a high hurdle. We should place more consideration in significant results when they come from a study with a highly rigorous design. A hurdler who clears a high hurdle can obviously clear a lower one as well. While a jumper who clears a low hurdle is still technically successful, we award fewer points to that jumper. We have limited information about the overall skill of that hurdler. We don't know if he would have cleared a higher one. We have less confidence in that jumper. On the other hand, a jumper who knocks a hurdle of any height over represents a non-significant result. It doesn't matter how high the hurdle was; not clearing it earns the jumper no points anyway.

Study rigor ranges from none at all to the highest level the scientific process currently has available. The lowest level of rigor would be equivalent to no study. Patients, for example, often present to their pediatricians anecdotal statements such as the following: "My friend started giving her son linseed oil for teething; do you think I should do that?" This is an example of the lowest level of rigor. Anecdotal evidence does not constitute a study, it therefore has no rigor.

At this stage in science, the highest level of rigor at researchers' disposal is the randomized controlled trial (RCT). If researchers have RCTs—the highest hurdle that will award their jumper the maximum number of points should it be cleared—at their disposal, patients often implicitly wonder why they do not employ it every time. It appears neglectful to choose a less rigorous methodology when RCTs exist. This is essentially the question patients ask when they assert that until an RCT is conducted disproving their personal viewpoints; they will continue to believe in an unproven treatment or scientific hypothesis.

The answer lies in that RCTs are *not* always available: they can be impractical, impossible, unlikely to be implemented with proper fidelity, or unethical. Again, research methodologies are not a one-size-fits-all scenario. Later in this chapter, we will review in detail how RCTs can be unavailable to researchers who would otherwise want to perform their study with the highest rigor level.

Given that RCTs are not always possible, patients are left to determine the level of rigor of studies they encounter. We will outline the various signposts patients can use to approximate the level of rigor. The signposts stem from the mathematical tools underlying the scientific method. Patients who would like to understand the specific details can access resources written for a general audience, such as *Naked Statistics* [2]. Here, we will discuss the signposts and rationale for their importance.

Inferential Statistics

In statistics, a **population** refers to the set of individuals implicated in a phenomenon. For example, the typical population in cancer studies is patients with cancer. Some phenomena affect a large number of individuals, while others implicate far fewer people. Consider how many more people have cancer than, for example, the number of people with a rare genetic disorder. Many researchers are interested in wide-scale phenomena, such as children with ear infections, mothers who breast-fed, or fathers who were over forty when their first child was born. Because researchers cannot observe everyone in those populations, they use **inferential statistics** to learn more about the phenomena. In inferential statistics, researchers must first select individuals that represent the entire population. This selection is called the **sample.** One foundation of inferential statistics is that a properly drawn sample will represent its population well. After selecting participants to comprise their sample, researchers observe them. Once sufficient observations have been collected, the researchers use statistical methods to infer conclusions about the population based on the sample's data.

Inferential statistics derive from the assumption that two samples (or two groups) will not differ from each other if they come from the same population. Statistics provides the likelihood that any observed difference between the two groups is due to chance. A difference attributed to chance is the null hypothesis, which we discussed in Chap. 2. The alternative option is the likelihood that the difference is a result of the two groups coming from different populations. This is called the experimental hypothesis. The careful reader will notice that statistics cannot definitively state whether or not a difference is due to chance or a difference in population.

Individuals within a sample will not be identical. There will be some amount of variability which can be measured and factored into analyses. Because individuals within a sample differ, statistics provides simplifying metrics to describe the sample as a whole. This simplifier permits researchers to compare one group to another, despite the individuals' variability within each group. These simplifying metrics are called "measures of central tendency," and they serve to reduce data from multiple individuals from a sample into one number. The measure of central tendency patients are most familiar with is the mean, or average.

Statistics assumes that truly different populations will have means that differ from one another. The further apart the means of two groups, the less likely the difference is due to chance. Put another way, the farther apart the means of two samples are, the less likely the null hypothesis is to be true. Therefore, large differences between the means represent an increased likelihood that the difference is due to an underlying difference in the populations that the samples are representing.

Combining these two foundations together, researchers can infer that two samples come from different populations without being able to infer one step further: to infer from one individual's information to which population they belong. Statistics can only tell us the likelihood that an observed difference is due to chance. While this is a crucial limitation, statistics is still the most powerful and valuable tool available in the field of research. Yet because inferential statistics have serious limitations, physicians need to be clear about these limits with their patients.

To Explain to a Patient

Statistics is powerful, but limited. Statistics can tell us that on average, adult males are taller than adult females. This means the average height of a group of males is very likely to be taller than the average height of a group of females. But that doesn't mean that all groups of men will be taller than all groups of women. Sometimes men are short and women are tall. If you sample enough groups of men and women, over and over again, eventually, by chance alone, you'll find one group of men who is, on average, shorter than your group of women. This is because height varies among individual women and individual men. If we know the height of a person is 5 ft, 7 in., statistics cannot definitively tell whether that person is a man or woman.

Acceptable Uncertainty

When determining whether or not an observed difference between two samples is likely due to an underlying difference of populations, statisticians must decide what the word *likely* stands for. Perceptions of likelihood change depending on the circumstances. An individual packing for a trip to Kansas or Seattle might consider the likelihood of rain when choosing whether or not to bring an umbrella. There may reasonably be a lower threshold for likeliness when packing for the Seattle trip, given how notoriously wet the Pacific Northwest is. The traveler might accept only 0% chance of rain in the forecast as the umbrella threshold for Seattle, whereas at least 50% chance of rain in the Kansas forecast would be warranted to pack the umbrella.

It would be terribly confusing if each researcher used his or her own threshold for likelihood. Accordingly, statisticians commonly use one agreed-upon threshold as their definition of likelihood. This threshold is that if an observed difference could be due to chance (and not an actual difference in the populations) 5 times out of 100 or less, researchers typically report they found a "significant" result. The probability of 5 times out of 100 is commonly reduced to decimal format: .05. Any observed difference that could be due to chance only .05 or less is called a "significant" result. Because the scientific community has agreed upon this threshold, a result below .05 allows researchers to reject the null hypothesis and proclaim a difference between the two groups as likely to be due to a difference in underlying populations.

The word *significant* in this case is defined very precisely. Its meaning is limited to the likelihood that the observed difference is due to chance less than .05. In research parlance, significance is not synonymous with importance, or even clinical relevance. We devote the next chapter to this foundational distinction.

The statistical measure of significance is called the *p*-value. The *p*-value is akin to the weather forecast. Saying the researchers "used a *p*-value of 0.05" mirrors the traveler deciding "I will only pack my umbrella if the forecast says at least 50% chance of rain." The traveler's significance threshold, 0.5, is relatively low. The commonly used statistical threshold, a *p*-value of 0.05, is sufficiently difficult to overcome. As far as hurdles go, it's fairly high. A *p*-value of, for example, 0.01, is even harder to overcome. A *p*-value of 0.01 represents a likelihood of 1 in a 100 that the observed difference is due to chance. The researcher would have decreased even further the likelihood that the observed difference was due to chance, placing more confidence in a result that surpassed the threshold. The significance threshold could of course be set even more strictly for more assurance that an observed difference is truly part of an underlying difference of populations.

Yet researchers do not regularly set the threshold at 0.01. This was a decision born of a desire to avoid the occurrence of false negatives. In statistics terminology, a false negative is called a **Type II error**. What most researchers aim for—finding a true difference between groups to reject the null hypothesis—is the target. The threshold for the *p*-value is the size of the bull's eye. The smaller the threshold *p*-value, the smaller and smaller the area of the bull's eye shrinks. Accordingly, it becomes harder and harder for the data to show a difference between two groups that meets this strict criteria. With strict criteria (such a *p*-value of 0.01), the torturously small bull's eye could show a "miss," even when the data truly do represent a true underlying population difference. The drawbacks, or even dangers, of setting the *p*-value threshold too low are all associated with situations when missing phenomena that *could* be there would be detrimental.

In some circumstances, misses are the least-preferred outcome. If a child remains nonverbal at age 3, there is a chance that the child will still develop speech in future without any additional intervention. There is also a chance the child has some specific problem that lies outside the population norms of typical development. If there is a problem, finding it via evaluation represents a "hit." Failing to observe a problem where there is one would be a "miss." Physicians must decide whether to set the threshold high and require that a child age further before intervening with evaluations and services, or set a low threshold and evaluate right away.

Most parents would agree to a lower testing threshold. They do not tolerate much chance their child might have a true difficulty that they miss. This miss would be more likely to occur when the threshold for significance is too strict. Setting the threshold is more than a statistical exercise. It represents the tradeoff between the confidence someone can place in a "hit" result, versus their concerns that they not "miss" something that may be there and require attention.

A "miss" is an error reporting nothing is there when something is. But errors can report the opposite: that something is there when nothing is. Statisticians call these kinds false positives **Type I errors**. A Type I error occurs when the bull's eye is too large. A large p-value (say, accepting that an observed difference is due to chance 50 in 100 times, or 0.5) is the equivalent of a large bull's eye. The data can score a point for "significance" due to the large bull's eye even when there is no true difference in the two groups. We have seen that setting the p-value threshold too low is problematic when the risk of missing is intolerable. There are also situations when the risk of false positives takes precedence.

False positive results lead to over-intervention for the many in service of catching a problem for the few. Situations where the burden of over-intervention of the many is unacceptable require setting the p-value threshold sufficiently low. As with misses, what burden is too large is not a challenge for statisticians; rather, it is a challenge for the people who use statistics to inform their decision-making.

An example of well-intentioned people deciding what amount of false positives to accept is the recent revision of the American Cancer Society's recommendations for women's breast cancer screenings. The previous rationale held that more screenings were better, following a "better safe than sorry" approach. The many false positives (Type I errors) seemed preferable than a few misses (Type II errors). Oncologists deliberated over the harm of few more painful mammogram procedures, a few more weeks of worry while more precise results come back. What they failed to adequately grasp was that this "few more" was multiplied by the millions of women across the country. Over the years, the answer to this perplexing question took shape. Women with benign tumors were undergoing painful, health-damaging, and costly procedures for tumors that otherwise would not have an impact on their lives. The stress of women being asked back for more scans, the lost productivity as they took time off of work and other duties for these visits, and the anxious waiting for results are all now recognized as an unfair burden to place on otherwise healthy women in the interest of a very few who might benefit from such aggressive screening. Once the data painted a clearer picture of the tradeoff between testing and not testing, the American Cancer Society revised its recommendations for screening to reduce these Type I errors [3].

Sample Size

While specific numbers vary depending on what statistics are applied to the samples, a general rule of thumb is that even the most basic inferential statistical test requires at least 30 participants per group to provide adequate confidence in the results. Inferential statistics are generally not required when studying extremely rare phenomena. In those cases, the researcher would simply observe those entities and describe the phenomenon based on the observations.

On an intuitive level, it follows that the larger the sample studied of a given population, the more faith we can place in the conclusions drawn from that sample. As the sample size gets larger, it gradually approaches the total number of individuals in the population. Some populations are bigger than others, so studies of smaller populations may employ smaller sample sizes and still be considered adequately rigorous. Technically, the aspect of the sample size patients should care most about is how close it is to the population total, so as to not discount studies with small populations. But the shorthand becomes: the larger the sample size, the better. Many studies reported in the popular media, if one digs deeper, studied only a handful of people. For example, in addition to the outright fraud involved in Andrew Wakefield's autism research, a basic design flaw is that he studied only 12 children [4].

While large sample sizes are generally preferable, they do not automatically convey more confidence in a study's results. Large sample sizes increase the likelihood that researchers reject the null hypothesis. Increasing the sample size is another way of making the "bull's eye" larger, and the result is a higher chance of Type I errors, or false positives. The next chapter will cover this in close detail.

Variables and Level of Control

The next methodological choice in a study is the level of control. **Control** refers to the researcher's ability to either direct or account for variability among their sample. In theory, the scientific method is designed to test the impact of one variable on another variable. The first variable, the one that researchers are interested in examining the effects of, is called the **independent variable**. The second variable, the one that researchers then observe the first variable's effects on, is called the **dependent variable**.

To Explain to a Patient

Think back to your fourth grade science class—maybe you conducted an experiment on bean plants with sunlight. Your teacher asked you to put one plant in the window under direct sunlight, another plant elsewhere in the classroom to receive diffuse light, and the third in the supply closet, which was dark. Even small children can exert control in this study. Children assigned the plants to various levels of light, the independent variable. After 1 week, your fourth grade teacher asked you and your classmates to measure the height of the bean plants. The height is the dependent variable, because children cannot directly influence the height of a plant the way they can directly influence the sunlight it receives. The variable is dependent on other actions for its outcome.

The plant experiment is effective for teaching learners of all ages about the basics of research because it has clear independent and dependent variables. The teacher chooses those variables to manipulate (the independent variable) and observes (the dependent variable). There are of course, others. Instead of light, she could have directed the class to manipulate the amount of water the plants received. In this version of the experiment, all the plants would be placed on the windowsill, but one plant receives 1/2 cup of water, the second 1/3 cup, and the third none at all. In this example, our fourth grade researchers must place all the plants in the same amount of sunlight to examine the effects of water. If they exposed the three different plants to varying levels of water *and* light, then any resulting differences in height would be just as much a mystery as before the experiment began. The class would not know if the shortest plant was stunted because it did not receive enough light, because it got too much water, etc.

Choosing to alter only one variable and keep all others consistent is a level of control. Control aims to reduce, as much as possible, any variability other than the independent variable. Even the plant experiment, which at first glance appears tightly controlled, is subject to variability that was not taken into account. A particularly savvy fourth grader might comment, as her teacher is concluding for the class that more light is better for plants because the tallest plant was the one on the windowsill, that the windowsill plant also received the most heat. The conclusion that more light leads to taller plants could very well be erroneous—maybe the real driving force in the plants' height differences was the amount of heat they received. The variable of "heat" in this experiment is neither the independent variable nor the dependent one. Such a variable, which undermines the amount of control in a study, is referred to as a **confounding variable**.

Some researchers can control practically every variable other than their independent variable. These researchers tend to work in basic science, which involves a tight level of control made possible due to the nature of the phenomena they study. Clinical research trials have inherently less control. Clinical researchers study human beings who introduce their own unique qualities to the experiment that researchers cannot possibly control. Many confounding variables influence clinical trials. Even with confounding variables, researchers attempt to exert as much control over their sample as they can. They do this knowing that our fourth grade know-it-all, now grown up, is ready to read and critique their study as a peer reviewer. The peer reviewer will surely bring up the influence confounding variables. Expert researchers do their best to pre-empt these challenges to their work and conclusions.

Researchers in clinical trials are confronted with the challenge of limiting the influence of confounding variables at the outset of their study. These researchers must choose the best level of control available to them. For studies that involve assigning people to different treatments or interventions, researchers can at least make sure the variability of these confounding influences is evenly distributed among their groups via randomization. Randomization, which we will cover shortly, is a powerful technique for mitigating the influence of confounding variables.

Some studies, for various reasons, cannot use randomization to mitigate the effects of confounding variables. In those cases, before beginning the experiment, researchers should make educated predictions as to what variables might confound their study. To hold these variables to account, the researchers then measure those confounding variables as well as their dependent variable. After the study is complete, they input into the statistical analysis the information about the confounding variables they measured in their sample. When they report their findings, they comment that their outcomes hold after "controlling for" the confounding variables. Take Dubner and Levitt's review of the Early Childhood Longitudinal Study's data, presented in their popular book *Freakonomics* [5]. The ECLS data collected by the National Center for Education Statistics shows a correlation between the number of books in a child's home and their test scores even when "controlling for" other relevant variables, like parental education and income levels (which also correlated with child test scores). The ECLS researchers could not randomly assign children to parents of varying education and income levels. Instead, they measured the parental variables and factored them into their analyses. This is an example of researchers exerting control over the variables in a study after the fact. Once the statistical analysis incorporates these confounding variables, the peer reviewer will have a significantly harder task of attributing the results observed in the dependent variable to the confounding variables. The analyses already factored in the confounding variables and quantified just how much influence they had or didn't have over the outcomes. The amount of influence confounding variables exert over the dependent variable is not reported as a binary yes or no. Researchers report how much of the differences observed in the dependent variable could be explained by the confounding variable. If the influence is sufficiently small, researchers conclude that while the confounding variable may have contributed to the observed results, it could not be the sole cause of the difference between the two groups. Researchers can acknowledge the effects of confounding variables while still concluding that the independent variable is the main driver of the observed results.

Researchers cannot always predict what the confounding variables will be at the outset of a study. After reviewing their baseline data, they may find a difference between the groups that randomization did not sufficiently distribute or that they did not account for. We will review proper sampling further down, but for the purposes of this section, we will assume the researchers properly sampled and *still* observed a difference between their two groups once the study was already underway.

To Explain to a Patient

Let's return to the plant experiment. By the end of the experiment, one student has noticed that a white film is growing over the soil around one of the plants. This student realizes that the soil quality could be a confounding variable, and he alerts the teacher. The class returns to the original data and investigates the origin of the plants. The poor quality soil plant is from a discount plant warehouse, while the other two came from a boutique plant shop. Their experiment now has two more possible variables—source of plant (a binary variable: warehouse or boutique) and soil quality. If our fourth grade class had a statistical software package, they would input these new variables into the dataset to include them in their analysis. The source of plant variable becomes a moderator, because it was present at the outset of the study and presumably influenced how the independent variable acted on the dependent variable. The soil quality becomes a mediating variable, because it intervened to mediate the effects of the independent variable.

The more control researchers exert over their studies, the more confidently we can conclude that the independent variable is the explanation for observed differences in the dependent variable. The more control, the better. Patients should look for control at various points in the study—before the study begins or after it concludes.

To Explain to a Patient

Let's say you are concerned that statewide testing is not an accurate assessment of a child's learning. Why do you think that the dependent variable (state test scores) is not a very good reflection of a child's learning? There are many possible reasons—some kids have better teachers than others, some kids have higher IQs to begin with, some kids have learning disabilities, some kids get test anxiety—these are all examples of confounding variables. People instinctually understand control is important before taking conclusions seriously. Look for confounding variables in research to determine if researchers have considered the confounders that matter to you.

Participant Representativeness

Generally speaking, the larger the number of participants in a study, the more rigorous the design. However, sample size is not the only participant factor contributing to the rigor of a study. Another factor is how **representative** the sample is of the population under consideration. In short, the sample should well represent the larger whole. If the sample is not representative of the population, then regardless of the conclusions of the sample, those conclusions cannot be used to infer knowledge about the population as a whole. Even a study with a sample size of 1,000 children with adequate muscle tone is not a rigorous study if the population of interest is children with low muscle tone. In our discussion of pharmaceutical companies in

Chap. 2, we reviewed how drugs intended for the infirm (the population) are often tested on young and healthy individuals (the sample). Nonrepresentative samples indicate poor study methodology, which results in diminished rigor.

Consequently, researchers strive to ensure that the participants they enroll are representative of the population as a whole. Steps taken to meet this goal include setting, at the very outset of a study, what their **inclusion and exclusion criteria** will be. The inclusion criteria outline those who would be appropriate participants for the study because they represent the overall population. Exclusion criteria outline those who would not be appropriate for the study because they deviate from the population of interest in some significant way (some exclusion criteria are also established, not for statistical reasons, but for the protection of participants). The more explicit and precise the inclusion and exclusion criteria are, the more clearly researchers can define their sample. These criteria also help subsequent researchers in the same area if they are interested in replicating the study and want to be sure they are also studying the same underlying population with their new sample.

Unlike criteria for say, entering college, where the criteria are set at a certain level and everyone must meet or exceed this level, inclusion and exclusion criteria define the participant pool more neutrally. For example, studies of children with Attention-Deficit/Hyperactivity Disorder will likely include in the inclusion criteria that the child must have a current DSM-5 diagnosis. When researchers are not studying a diagnostic category, their population and subsequent sample is termed "nonclinical." In nonclinical studies, specific diagnoses might become be part of exclusion criteria instead, to ensure the participants do not have any clinical diagnoses.

To Explain to a Patient

Inclusion and exclusion criteria are like ingredients in a recipe—there are no right or wrong ingredients, only ingredients appropriate or inappropriate for that recipe. Study researchers try to get the recipe as best as they can, knowing that these criteria help to establish representativeness of their sample, and by extension, the rigor of their study.

Researchers set inclusion and exclusion criteria to exert some level of assurance that the sample studied represents the population as a whole. An absolutely representative sample would allow researchers and the public to infer that whatever the study found for the sample is true for the overall population. Yet even with extremely well-defined inclusion and exclusion criteria, the sample will always deviate from the overall population in one important way—they are participating in the research study. The term for this bizarre challenge with which all researchers grapple is **self-selection bias**. Study volunteers differ from those who are not in the study in two main fashions.

First, people who sign up for studies have characteristics that are present at the outset [6, 7]. These characteristics are varied, but they demonstrate differences between those who participate in studies in general and those who do not. Compared to nonparticipants, for example, study volunteers might be interested in trying new things, interested in research, live closer to research sites, be more aware of studies in their areas, want some extra pocket money a research stipend would provide, and so on.

The second set of differences between participants and nonparticipants emerge as the study unfolds. Even in an area as seemingly objective as physics research, scientists are aware that their observation of a phenomenon could change it. Clinically, anyone with "white coat syndrome"—an increase in blood pressure as an anxious response directly elicited by having one's blood pressure taken—has direct experience with this **observer effect**. In research studies, people often subtly change their behavior in response to the knowledge that they are under observation. Any systematic changes prompted by this effect make participants less representative of the population. For example, participants wearing accelerometer wrist devices (called actigraphs) to measure their sleep are reminded about their sleep by virtue of wearing the device [8]. With just this subtle cue, participants may be primed to attempt to go to sleep earlier. The participants no longer as well represent the population of sleepers quite as well, since most sleepers do not wear an actigraph. Of course the effects are likely to be small in this case, but other studies may unintentionally produce more robust changes in their participants.

One such important example of a participation effect on a sample is food logging within nutrition research. To collect their data, nutrition researchers often ask participants to log their food. However, studies have now uncovered that the very act of logging one's food intake is a contributing factor in weight loss [9]. Logging food, in and of itself, seems to change individuals' perceptions and behaviors about food in a meaningful way. When researchers ask participants to eat certain foods and log them as confirmation of consumption, they might be studying the effects of logging food rather than the effects of the food itself.

Whenever possible, researchers should employ control groups to minimize the study participation effects. The control group could be asked to log their food, and make no other changes in their diet. Now that we expect the control group to lose weight as well, the researchers can subtract any changes that occurred in the control group (the influence of logging food) from any changes that occurred in the experimental group (who were influenced by logging food and possibly eating the food of interest). The resulting data tracks the influence due to the experimental food alone.

Randomization

Even utilizing the most rigorous levels of methodology discussed so far, there will still be differences among people in study samples. The final method we will discuss that the researchers use to minimize the impact of these differences is called

randomization. Randomization entails enrolling participants in the study and then assigning them, at random, to one arm of the study or another. Prior to advances in technology, randomization was as simple as a coin toss. Now researchers have computers with sophisticated algorithms to assign participants at random. These algorithms can randomize participants to more than two conditions. Researchers can also program their algorithms to evenly distribute key characteristics among the groups, such as sex or age. Prior to these algorithms, randomization could still result in significantly meaningful differences in the groups that occurred by chance. These differences become "group characteristics," that must then be factored into the analysis. If there is a decent chance that characteristics such as sex will lead to different responses to treatment, the sex effect should be randomly, yet evenly, distributed. With an even distribution, the results seen are more likely to be caused by the intervention and not to the characteristic differences between the two groups.

For an example of how key characteristics can affect outcomes, consider sleep medications and sex. Doctors now prescribe women dosing amounts of sleep medicine about half of what they prescribe for men. This guideline emerged after it was discovered that the female body metabolizes popular sleep medications at a meaningfully slower rate than males [10]. Researchers comparing a new sleep medicine to a placebo will want to make sure they do not have more females in the medicine group than the placebo group. If the sex characteristic meaningfully differed in this way, we could expect that their results would erroneously show the medications are much more potent than it is for the whole population (i.e., once more men are included).

We have been discussing randomization to groups without specifying what those groups could be. When researchers do not test their intervention against anything, this is called a **single-arm study**. Patients will want to discover if the effects reported in an article comment on that intervention's results or its results compared to some other group. Without comparing a treatment to something else, there is a fair likelihood that the effects would have been observed even without the intervention. For example, a developmental psychologist could study the effects of reading *Goodnight Moon* to 3-year-olds and examine how well they are able to develop their reading skills by age 5. Without comparing my treatment to anything else, this experiment would be roundly dismissed due to a lack of rigor. Many children make some kind of progress in reading between ages 3 and 5. Without some comparison group, it would be impossible to tell how much of the progress could be attributed to the intervention. The study's rigor would be so poor as to have been no better than no study at all.

At times, it is appropriate for researchers to use a single-arm design. Primarily, if researchers are truly unaware if their intervention will have any effect at all, it can be beneficial to first try the intervention with a few participants and look for any change from pre- to post-intervention. If the participants experience no change, the researchers saved time and money by not testing their useless intervention against other groups. If the participants show some change, researchers can then leverage those findings into obtaining enough funding for a study with a comparison group.

One of the simpler comparison groups researchers utilize in clinical trials is called "Treatment as usual," or TAU. In a TAU study, participants are informed that if they sign up for the study, they will be randomly assigned to either start the new treatment or continue with their current care. Participants assigned to TAU are told that they were not randomized to receive the intervention, and instead will continue their behaviors as they typically would. These studies give a good "real-world" impression of whether the new intervention yields improved outcomes over what interventions the status quo has to offer.

In some studies, researchers employ placebos. Placebo treatments are not expected to have any impact on outcomes. Placebos can only be used when the placebo is indistinguishable from the "real thing." Medication trials commonly enlist sugar pills as their placebo. At least a dozen studies have tested whether sugar makes children hyperactive by randomly assigning children to ingest small amounts of either a sugared syrup (the experimental treatment) or a nonsugared yet sweet syrup (the placebo) [11]. Parents were then told that their children received sugar, whether it was true or not. In fact, not only were parents blind as to whether or not their children received sugar, but the staff collecting the data did not know either. The studies used a **double-blind design**. Parents then rated their perceptions of their children's activity levels. Upending popular lore, children's hyperactivity was more closely tied to their parents' impressions of sugar consumption than whether they actually ingested any. The placebo was similar enough in appearances to the "active" agent to allow researchers to isolate and pinpoint the true driver of the children's hyperactivity—their parents' perceptions.

A word of caution—the odd truth is that, despite the ideas that placebos are used because they create a control condition, placebos can actually "work" in that they sometimes produce objective, clinically meaningful, outcomes. Some studies have shown that up to 30–40% of people who receive placebos experience objectively different physiological responses to the otherwise sham treatment [12].

While a placebo trial has more rigor than TAU or none at all, it is not always an option. If, for example, researchers want to study the effects of recess on children's afternoon focus, they would not be able to create a placebo that looks like recess to children but is not actually recess. Rather than dismissing any study without a placebo control, patients should try to determine what comparison group (placebo, TAU, or none at all) was possible for the study at hand. As long as the researchers used the most rigorous comparison group possible, their methodology with regard to comparison groups would not be called flawed.

Outcomes

We discussed the difference between the independent, or experimental, variable and the dependent, or outcome, variable. These scientific terms do not capture the wide-ranging clinical questions that prompt these studies. The outcomes studied range from vastly removed to directly relevant to patients' lives. Basic science researchers might study outcome variables as precise and distal as the speed of cell mutation. After completing enough of these studies, researchers can eventually use basic science findings to inform proximal clinical applications, such as oncology studies. Medical researchers investigate largely because they want to find improved health outcomes for patients. Instead of referring to "dependent variables," most studies in medicine report "outcomes."

For example, a study of children with Autism Spectrum Disorder (ASD), a disorder with marked social deficits including a lack of eye contact, may measure facial recognition and corresponding brain activity. Imaging studies such as the kinds that utilize fMRI serve to inform the field overall. But when a parent of a child with ASD reads a study reporting that children with ASD are significantly more likely to show decreased activity in the fusiform gyrus when identifying faces than typically developing children, he or she cannot do anything with this information [13]. The outcomes studied and reported may be important to the field and other researchers, but they are too removed from everyday life for patients to apply. When patients read titles of articles saying things like "Health Benefits Found for Acai Berry," some investigation will reveal that the "health benefits" reported have little to no bearing on daily life. This is because researchers often examine **proximal** outcomes, such as leptin levels in blood, while patients are more concerned with **distal** outcomes, such as health and longevity.

To Explain to a Patient

Research study results reported in the media often "leap to conclusions." Researchers tend to study outcomes that are very specific and usually have nothing to do with things people think about on a day-to-day basis. Meanwhile, people who read these articles are interested in their overall life and health. Journalists who report on research studies try to make the case why a new research finding is relevant to their readers. So you may see headlines that claim big health benefits, when really, the study may have examined something much less meaningful to you.

Outcomes can also be measured objectively or subjectively. Once again, one method is not necessarily better than another. The choice should reflect the field overall to attain maximum rigor. For example, an insomnia diagnosis includes subjective perception of sleep quality, as this perception is more important to the sleeper than the number of hours slept [14]. Contrast this with studies about, for example, diabetes. The outcomes that matter in that field include objective measures, such as blood sugar levels.

Study Length

The length of a study is also an important determinant of its rigor. The shorter the study, the easier and less expensive it is to conduct. However, most health outcomes affect patients over the course of a notable amount of time, if not their entire life span. Studies monitoring their participants' outcomes for extended periods of time can be better translated to practical medical conclusions.

Longitudinal studies, in which the same participants are monitored over a great length of time—years, primarily—are extremely expensive. Study budgets must factor in the time and effort of staff in re-contacting participants as they age, move, and change contact information. Some participants will eventually ask not to continue to be followed; others may fail to provide new contact information and be lost to the study, and still others will die. As the pool of original participants dwindles, each remaining participant becomes increasingly precious. While costly, longitudinal studies are the only way to accurately track outcomes over time.

A **cross-sectional study** design works around cost constraints but still attempts to quantify people's responses over time. For example, a study may examine educational outcomes of children placed in full-time daycare at three months compared to children placed at 1 year of age. These researchers could choose a longitudinal design, selecting a pool of participants (some of whom were placed at three months and others of whom were placed at 1 year) and tracking their outcomes at 1.5 years, 3 years, and 5 years old. This design requires a few years to collect outcomes, as the researchers would need to wait as the children age. The researchers might instead employ a cross-sectional design, recruiting three cohorts of children: one group of 1.5-year-olds, another of 3-year-olds, and the last 5-year-olds, making sure that each cohort has some children who have been in daycare since three months and others since one year. The researchers could simultaneously collect data from all 3 age groups and then test for significant differences between the groups in each cohort.

Despite the speed, ease, and cost-effectiveness of cross-sectional studies, they are not preferable to the longitudinal design. Cross-sectional analyses require an assumption that all three cohorts do not significantly differ on any variables that may affect the outcome, other than the grouping variable. This assumption clearly cannot always hold. The labeling of different generations (Great Generation, Silent Generation, Baby Boomers, Gen X, Gen Y, Millennials, etc.) reveals the implicit understanding that cohorts vary. People from different times are differentially shaped by the times they lived in. This is called the **cohort effect**. With the rapid advances in technology experienced today, one could conceive of a cohort effect even when comparing a 1.5-year-old child and a 3-year-old child. The 3-year-old may have been raised without any access to smart phones, while the 1.5-year-old may have been swiping a screen practically since birth. Educational abilities and social interaction might be reasonable outcomes in such a study. Access to smartphones within developmental timelines could reasonably be assumed to differentially impact the cohorts of children.

If a cohort effect among the children is a stretch, consider differences among the groups due to the parents who enrolled them. Parents comfortable with enrolling their 1.5-year-old in a study might differ from parents who would only do so once their child was verbal (3 years old) or markedly self-sufficient (5 years old). In a study of children placed in day care, parental comfort level with involving their children with relative strangers, day care personnel, or study researchers, might reflect some underlying qualities (e.g., openness to new experience, trust) that would affect the children among the different groups differentially.

If the groups in a cross-sectional design significantly and meaningfully differ, then some of the outcomes could be attributed to these cohort or group effects rather than the independent variable. Only a longitudinal study could ensure that those factors are not systematically distributed differently among cohorts or groups.

The Gold Standard: Randomized Controlled Trial

In a **Randomized Controlled Trial (RCT)**, researchers randomly assign participants to one of two arms: (1) the investigational (also called experimental) intervention; or (2) the comparison intervention (i.e., anything other than the experimental intervention). Some RCTs employ three (or more) arms, in which the experimental intervention goes head to head with an active comparator as well as a placebo. While the RCT design is the most rigorous, it is not always available.

RCTs can be impractical. Some research questions cannot be answered practically within the RCT framework. Researchers have studied whether children who had pets as toddlers are more or less likely to develop asthma [15]. It is unlikely researchers would find a sufficient number of families willing to consent to a research study that will direct them whether or not to get a dog for their toddler. Basing certain decisions on chance, the "randomized" part of randomized controlled trial, is not always practical.

Even if these researchers had found a number of families, all willing to leave their pet choices up to fate, researchers with other questions would not be so lucky. They may want to study phenomena that are not at all within their or their participants' control and, therefore, cannot be subject to randomization. Keeping ensuing asthma rates as the outcome, consider instead the independent variable of maternal birthplace. A researcher may study if participants whose mothers were born in warm climates have lower rates of asthma. This researcher could not randomly assign their participants to have mothers born in warm or cool climates. Whenever the independent variable cannot be distributed among the participant pool at random, an RCT design is impossible.

In other studies, an RCT design may not be impossible, but is so impractical as to be essentially impossible. For example, interventions that are unlikely to be implemented as intended present a logistical challenge to the RCT design. One example is nutrition studies, which are notoriously difficult to perform rigorously. People eat every day, multiple times a day. They eat at home, in restaurants, at friend's houses, or airports. They eat based on what they want to eat, but also what they can afford, and what is available when hunger strikes.

To illustrate the point, consider a hypothetical scenario. A possible research hypothesis is whether children who eat only GMO-free dairy products have less asthma as teenagers. GMO stands for Genetically Modified Organisms, concern for which abounds despite the current lack of conclusive research indicating detrimental outcomes for the average consumer [16]. In this case, it is plausible that parents could volunteer to be assigned to one condition or another. Randomization is possible. The researchers would then be obligated to monitor intake of GMO dairy products among the two groups of children to measure adherence to the intervention. Even with the best of intentions to follow one diet or another, the other kind of food studied will interfere. The children assigned to consume GMO-free products will inevitably encounter the ubiquitous product. Children in the control group may regularly consume GMO-free products, simply by interacting with the world around them. Researchers call instances when one group interacts with the other group's plan **contamination**. A child assigned to the GMO condition drinking GMO-free milk with his slice of cake at a friend's birthday party, from a research standpoint, constitutes contamination. While researcher attempt to account for contamination in their analyses, they can only do so if made aware the contamination occurred. Unfortunately, people (let alone young children) do not accurately report of the substances in their food. In some cases, researchers do not employ the RCT design because they know in advance the two (or more) conditions will not be followed to the fidelity needed to draw meaningful conclusions.

Finally, RCTs cannot be conducted when to do so would be unethical. There are ample opportunities for lapses in ethics, regardless of methodological rigor. RCTs' ethical concerns, as separate from other methodological concerns, lie in the randomization process. Even if possible, practical, and performed with fidelity, in some situations it would be unethical to randomize some participants to one condition and not the other. For example, researchers have studied how much the surgical experience level of a surgeon affects patient outcome [17]. Using an RCT to test a hypothesis that surgeons with 20 years of experience have lower complications rates and fewer post-operative infections than surgeons with 2 years of experience would present an untenable ethical problem. This hypothetical researcher would have to enroll participants who agreed to have their surgeons' experience level assigned to them at random. Even if participants agreed to have their children's care determined by a coin flip, it is unethical to ask participants to accept the implicit risks associated with an inexperienced surgeon when a vastly more experienced one is available. In the real world, people see doctors with limited experience all the time—doctors must gain experience as their careers develop just as do individuals in any profession. However, this is done with great oversight and on the understanding that the patient could seek care elsewhere if years of experience mattered to them. Patient access to experienced doctors is often limited due to constraints such as availability of experienced doctors in their area. Withholding of care done in the name of research presents an ethical catastrophe.

Examining a study for methodological rigor is a key piece of research literacy. Patients must be aware if the study was well designed and conducted before "buying into" the results. In the next chapter, we'll explore whether the results have any meaningful impact on the participants, and by extension, patients.

References

1. Kesselheim AS, Robertson CT, Myers JA, Rose SL, Gillet V, Ross KM, Glynn RJ, Joffe S, Avorn J. A randomized study of how physicians interpret research funding disclosures. N Engl J Med. 2012;367(12):1119–27.
2. Wheelan C. Naked statistics: stripping the dread from the data. WW Norton & Company; 2013 Jan 7.
3. Oeffinger KC, Fontham ET, Etzioni R, Herzig A, Michaelson JS, Shih YC, Walter LC, Church TR, Flowers CR, LaMonte SJ, Wolf AM. Breast cancer screening for women at average risk: 2015 guideline update from the American Cancer Society. JAMA. 2015;314(15):1599–614.
4. Rao TS, Andrade C. The MMR vaccine and autism: Sensation, refutation, retraction, and fraud. Indian J Psychiatry. 2011;53(2):95.
5. Levitt SD, Dubner SJ. Freakonomics. Sperling & Kupfer editori; 2010.
6. Karney BR, Davila J, Cohan CL, Sullivan KT, Johnson MD, Bradbury TN. An empirical investigation of sampling strategies in marital research. J Marriage Family. 1995;1:909–20.
7. Costigan CL, Cox MJ. Fathers' participation in family research: is there a self-selection bias? J Fam Psychol. 2001;15(4):706.
8. Lam JC, Mahone EM, Mason TB, Scharf SM. Defining the roles of actigraphy and parent logs for assessing sleep variables in preschool children. Behav Sleep Med. 2011;9(3):184–93.
9. Hollis JF, Gullion CM, Stevens VJ, Brantley PJ, Appel LJ, Ard JD, Champagne CM, Dalcin A, Erlinger TP, Funk K, Laferriere D. Weight loss during the intensive intervention phase of the weight-loss maintenance trial. Am J Prev Med. 2008;35(2):118–26.
10. Tavernise, S. Drug agency recommends lower doses of sleep aids for women. The New York Times. p. A14. http://nyti.ms/1ANmh7q. Accessed 11 Jan 2013.
11. Vreeman RC, Carroll AE. Festive medical myths. BMJ. 2008;18(337):a2769.
12. Hróbjartsson A, Gøtzsche PC. Is the placebo powerless? An analysis of clinical trials comparing placebo with no treatment. N Engl J Med. 2001;344(21):1594–602.
13. Harms MB, Martin A, Wallace GL. Facial emotion recognition in autism spectrum disorders: a review of behavioral and neuroimaging studies. Neuropsychol Rev. 2010;20(3):290–322.
14. American Psychiatric Association. Diagnostic and Statistical Manual of Mental Disorders: DSM-5. Man Mag; 2003 May 27.
15. Takkouche B, González-Barcala FJ, Etminan M, Fitzgerald M. Exposure to furry pets and the risk of asthma and allergic rhinitis: a meta-analysis. Allergy. 2008;63(7):857–64.
16. Saletan, W. Unhealthy Fixation. Slate Magazine. http://www.slate.com/articles/health_and_science/science/2015/07/are_gmos_safe_yes_the_case_against_them_is_full_of_fraud_lies_and_errors.html. Accessed 15 Jul 2015.
17. Sosa JA, Bowman HM, Tielsch JM, Powe NR, Gordon TA, Udelsman R. The importance of surgeon experience for clinical and economic outcomes from thyroidectomy. Ann Surg. 1998;228(3):320.

Chapter 4
Significance: Statistical Versus Clinical

Overview

A core aspect of informed consent in medical decision-making is full comprehension of research findings. We have been reviewing the criteria a study must meet before it merits consideration in medical decision-making. The implicit and explicit biases affecting research at various stages and levels are taken seriously, thus weeding out questionable results. Indicators of methodological rigor then provide insight into the overall quality of the study. Once these criteria are met, physicians and patients must still determine if the study results have any plausible clinical applicability. Some studies, despite passing these criteria, yield results that remain academic in nature only. Put bluntly, not every statistically significant research result is ecologically valid. To explain to patients which results apply clinically and which do not, physicians can make clear the difference between statistical significance and clinical significance. Only once this distinction is apparent to patients are they adequately informed to consent.

The Original Plan for Statistical Significance

Not only should statistical significance not conclude the decision-making process, it was never intended to. We caution in Chap. 3 that statistical significance has a narrow and precise definition. Statistical significance provides a guideline as to the likelihood that an observation in a study is due to chance [1]. Originally devised in 1920, statistician Ronald Fisher proposed that his p-value (the statistical metric of significance) provide an indication as to whether or not study results warrant a second examination [1]. Studies with p-values less than 0.05 might yield valuable

© Springer International Publishing AG 2017
C.A. Di Bartolo and M.K. Braun, *Pediatrician's Guide to Discussing Research with Patients*, DOI 10.1007/978-3-319-49547-7_4

information if investigated further. *P*-values higher than 0.05 were not as likely to produce additional results of importance.

> **To Explain to a Patient**
>
> A statistically significant result acts like a traffic "stop" sign. A *p*-value less than 0.05 does not signal the end of the trip. Instead, it tells the researchers to pause long enough to consider where they came from, what they have observed so far, and where they might like to go next based on what they observed.

Fisher carefully defined the limitations of the *p*-value out of a nuanced understanding of the role statistics should play in the scientific method. Fisher placed his statistic as one discrete part of the scientific process as a whole. If the process was to unfold in the ideal, researchers would review the preexisting work in the field, incorporate those previous findings into their ideas, set hypotheses, examine their resulting data, share their findings, collaborate with others in the field, and adjust their hypotheses accordingly.

This collaborative, evolving, and messy approach to science sounds foreign to many. The scientific process is often presented as completely methodical, objective, and rational. Consider instead, the scientific process as an art. If the scientific process were compared to the creation of an oil painting, statistics would represent the brushes. While crucial to the endeavor, the brushes alone do not create the resulting image. Other factors must be considered for the process to unfold as originally conceptualized. Describing a particular vein of scientific inquiry by stating that "the study has statistically significant findings" is akin to describing a painting solely by stating that brushes were used.

Popularity of Statistical Significance

In the years since Fisher first proposed that his statistical procedures be used in a limited fashion within a broader context, scientists, publishers, and journalists have removed his *p*-value from its recommended position of precision [2]. The media use his commonly misunderstood statistic as a catchall for the importance of a study's findings [2]. The scientific field has taken his statistical tool and raised it to the position of prominence in most published findings. High-impact journals display a preference for publishing papers with statistically significant results [2]. In turn, career academics value publication in high-impact journals [2]. These mutually beneficial incentives conspire to promote an overreliance on statistically significant findings [2]. We propose two reasons for the overinflated popularity of Fisher's *p*-value: One is practical and the other psychological.

One factor contributing to the popularity of the p-value within the scientific community was the practical benefit. At the time of Fisher's writing, computers with statistical capabilities were expensive, making them scarce commodities [2]. Most researchers computed their statistical analyses by hand, a painstaking process. They then compared their results to a table Fisher developed that provided data at various interval levels (e.g., $p = 0.05$, $p = 0.01$). At the time, a table with clearly delineated intervals assisted researchers in understanding whether or not their results had any merit. They simply needed to find the lowest possible interval on the table corresponding to their result.

The overreliance on tables with arbitrary guidelines, forgivable one hundred years ago, has overstayed its welcome. Computers, now ubiquitous, calculate statistical results *and* precise p-values at very little time and cost. Researchers do not need to settle for the closest interval that best describes their findings. While Fisher's p-value of 0.05 had an outsized effect on the field of statistics when he created it, the practical utility is no longer applicable.

With the practical aspect of Fisher's p-value clearly technologically outdated, the psychological need for simplicity marches on. It is as an inborn human trait. Cognitive psychologists Tversky and Kahneman studied processes the human brain utilizes to efficiently and rapidly perceive, judge, and make choices about the world [3]. These processes are called **heuristics** [3]. Compared to other organs, the brain requires a great deal of energy to operate even its most basic functions. The body therefore prefers to run the brain as efficiently as possible. Additionally, humans evolved when speed was crucial to physical survival. If the brain took too long to determine if a stimulus was dangerous, it often resulted in death. Brains, then, also prefer speed. Heuristics provide the advantages of efficiency and speed.

To assist the brain with rapid and efficient processing, heuristics simplify where complexity is encountered. Rather than examine every square inch of an object before determining its type, the human brain will identify key markers (legs, seat, back, wood, right angles, parallel lines) and identify the object as a chair. Fisher's p-value supplied the statistical equivalent of a heuristic. He provided one key marker (a p-value) by which researchers now identify their work as a whole (significant or not).

Oversimplification and Confusion

Utilizing procedures that simplify come with a cost. The limitations of the human brain mean that giving speed preference over accuracy will lead to an increased error rate. Most humans can be quick or accurate, but it is very challenging to be both. In cognitive terms, the errors that emerge due to heuristics are our biases. One bias that emerges from heuristics' tendency to simplify is oversimplification. In the case of Fisher's p-value, the temptation to oversimplify research results is strong.

Not only does relying solely on the *p*-value oversimplify findings within statistics, it also causes a similar error in the clinical interpretation of the findings. The simplicity error has wide-ranging effects due to the use of the word "significance." Even though statistics uses the word "significance," common parlance utilizes it also [4]. Unfortunately, the definitions are not the same in both settings. We will explain the confusion by first providing another example of a term with a different meaning depending on the context in which it is used: *negative*. In the medical setting, a negative finding often represents good news, such as when screening results for a disease are negative. In quotidian use, negative has the opposite meaning.

Significance suffers from this dual-definition conundrum. In the case of significance, however, the difference between the two definitions is nuanced. Authors often fail to bother at all with the distinction, or neglect to clarify when they see the word used erroneously. An indication of the strong propensity to oversimplify is the frequency with which popular media shortens "statistical significance" to "significance." For example, one news article reporting an epidemiological study result states, "postmenopausal women with gum disease and history of smoking have a significantly higher risk for breast cancer" [5]. Missing is the key word "statistically"—the researchers calculated a *statistically* significant association. Omitting this word could reflect a minor editorial decision. In fact, its absence results in the complete dismissal of Fisher's original intended use for his measure. The common definition of significance is commonly erroneously applied when the much narrower statistical definition is actually needed [6].

Overreliance on Statistical Significance in Publishing

Lay media aside, evidence of publication bias in the scientific literature depicts the field's overreliance on statistical significance. As discussed in Chap. 2, publication bias results when papers with significant findings are published at higher rates than papers with non-significant ones. The bias is so prevalent that results with statistically significant findings are colloquially referred to as "positive" and those without statistical significance as "negative" [7]. (This shorthand assessment of value is not applicable for types of studies that do not employ hypothesis testing as a matter of form, such as case studies.)

Before addressing the myriad ways publication bias detrimentally affects the field of scientific inquiry, we must first establish how its presence is observed. A number of researchers have studied the mathematical markers that serve as evidence of publication bias and have repeatedly found a great deal of evidence that the bias has infiltrated the literature [7]. Recall that biases affect outcomes in a systematic fashion. When researchers find systematic outcomes instead of the randomness they would expect, they infer the presence of a bias. There is no justifiable reason for a collection of *p*-values to cluster in any particular formation. Without publication bias, the *p*-values drawn from a sample of published papers should be randomly distributed. If a pattern of *p*-values, particularly *p*-values clustered at just below 0.05 were observed, this marker would imply that investigators mainly submit and journals mostly publish findings using Fisher's p-value as the driving criterion. Various researchers have repeatedly found this exact clustering of p-values just under 0.05. For example, one team of researchers examined articles reported in three psychology journals. They found that a disproportionately high number of papers report p-values just under 0.05 [8]. We can also observe the bias increasing over time: in 1990, 30% of papers published had negative findings; by 2013 it had dropped to 14% [9].

Costs of Publication Bias

Publication bias obstructs the actions involved in the true directive of the scientific process: knowledge acquisition. First of all, uncovering what is false is just as much a goal of science as discovering what is true, a fact publication bias blithely ignores [7]. Second, publication bias stymies scientific process via redundancy and false leads. In terms of redundancy, the lack of published negative findings presents unnecessary challenges to other researchers who would seek to examine the same phenomena. Without access to accounts of prior work that did not lead to significant results, other researchers (whether future or contemporary) repeatedly test hypotheses that their predecessors and colleagues have already examined and discarded. The time and money spent investigating paths that have already been tested and jettisoned could have been more effectively utilized if the negative findings were readily available [10].

While publication bias has always been a matter of concern, the more studies published, the more the bias affects the field overall with the introduction and permeation of false positives. In 1950, a few hundred thousand researchers worked and published [9]. Even in 1959, researchers were writing about their concerns that publication bias resulted in an abundance of false conclusions [11]. In 2013, the field grew to approximately 6–7 million researchers working and publishing [9]. Recall that a p-value of 0.05 represents a one-in-twenty probability that a finding is due to chance. The result is that even among a few dozen studies, one could reasonably anticipate that at least one of those statistically significant results is, in fact, a false positive. Therefore, as more studies are published, the number of false positive results will increase, even as the rate of false positive findings remains the same.

The larger the number of studies, the more false positives will emerge. Additionally, the larger the amount of data collected within a study, the more false positives it will produce. While a sufficiently large sample size is needed for appropriate methodological rigor, the rise of big data has also contributed to an overabundance of false positive results that pervade the literature. While it would seem that the larger the sample size, the more confidence one can place in results, this is not true [11]. What is more precisely accurate is that the more participants in a study, the more easily the data will be able to provide an outcome that reaches statistical significance. Large sample sizes' ability to detect differences between samples is called **statistical power**. However, increasing the power also increases the rate of false positives as well. Large sample sizes magnify both true and false differences. A property inherent in large datasets is great variability [12].

To Explain to a Patient

Having a large sample size in a study is like turning up the volume on your phone. You can hear the person you are speaking with more loudly, but you can hear background noise more loudly as well. Large sample sizes allow researchers to hear the voice, but they also make it more likely they will hear the background noise as well. The scientists might interpret that background noise as the voice.

With sophisticated computers, electronic medical record-keeping systems, and unprecedented documentation, the data sets at researchers' disposal have never been larger. This abundance of figures supplies an additional temptation for statisticians to draw inferences and make claims based on these mammoth datasets [12]. Researchers in some fields, such as epidemiologists or geneticists, have data sets in the hundreds or even thousands [9]. If researchers do not properly account for multiple comparisons in their analyses, a p-value of 0.05 is a woefully lax threshold. Simply examining a high number of possible outcome measures increases the likelihood that the researcher will find a result that is statistically significant [6].

Significant but spurious findings that easily flow from large datasets typically gain widespread attention, particularly in research areas of high interest to the public [12]. Common complaints that research is inconclusive and contradictory stem from this phenomenon. Investigations into hormone replacement therapy, vitamin β carotene, vitamin C, vitamin E, and countless other possible treatments have yielded findings that can only be described as "conflicted and often meaningless" [13]. Not only do these findings erode public confidence in research in general, the money spent to generate these useless conclusions could have been spent on more legitimate forms of research [13].

Editor Motivations and Actions

Given the costs of publication bias to the field of scientific inquiry, it is worth examining why and how it has persisted for decades. We will first address motivations and actions contributing to the bias from journal editors before we address these points from researchers themselves.

Journals that publish statistically significant findings benefit from an increased perception of selectivity and competitiveness via their **impact factor** [9]. Journals indexed in the *Journal Citation Reports* are assigned an impact factor. Impact factors are commonly interpreted as a proxy for a journal's reputation, with higher factors representing higher influence [14]. Impact factor calculations rest on the ratio of the number of citations a journal's articles receive in a 2-year span compared to the number of citable articles they publish [14]. Because articles reporting nonsignificant results are rarely cited, journals that publish a wealth of articles with nonsignificant findings risk tilting the ratio away from a favorable impact factor. Subsequently, publication bias leads to a meaningful imbalance between "positive" and "negative" findings.

How journal editors act to bias their publications is fairly straightforward. As the arbiters of what appears in their journals, editors can choose to publish papers with significant findings over those with nonsignificant results. As covered in Chap. 2, these decisions may not occur at the level of consciousness. It would be unfair to assume concerted, malicious intent for every instance in which a study with statistically significant results were accepted over one with nonsignificant results.

Author Motivations and Actions

Thus far we have described how editorial decisions contribute to publication bias. Study authors' decisions also play a role in the bias. Due to journals' editorial decisions preferencing the publication of statistically significant findings over nonsignificant ones, today's researchers find themselves in the situation Fisher explicitly cautioned against—acceptance for publication based primarily on low p-values. Careerism seems to be a potential motive for authors to contribute to the publication bias in the field. Publication in a prestigious peer-reviewed journal is the bare minimum researchers must achieve to obtain highly desirable incentives such as scientific rewards and coveted tenure-track positions [15]. As the number of researchers increases, more will fall prey to chasing the more interesting (i.e., significant) findings in their studies in order to publish [9]. Others suggest that some of the activities researchers engage in that promote publication bias stem from subconscious desires [15]. Psychologist Uri Simonsohn considers these biases key to understanding how even honest researchers can unintentionally engage in questionable practices to obtain a statistically significant result [15].

If we take seriously the incentives that motivate researchers to contribute to publication bias, the next question becomes how they do so. Publication bias occurs on the researcher level via two actions: selection and selective reporting [4]. Selection occurs when researchers decide not to submit negative findings for publication [4]. Selective reporting occurs when researchers decide not to accept their negative findings. Instead, they continue to manipulate and analyze their data until they find a statistically significant finding to report.

The overreliance on statistical significance has rendered the metric susceptible to researcher exploitation, whether intentionally or unintentionally. The calculations involved in reaching statistical significance are open knowledge. The capability to calculate a p-value provides the same knowledge needed to manipulate the data to produce a significant p-value. The process of exploiting data to produce statistically significant results has several names. It has been called data dredging, data snooping, data mining, and fishing [16]. This work will use the term coined by Joseph Simmons and his colleagues (including Simonsohn, mentioned above) at University of Pennsylvania: **p-hacking** [17].

P-hacking encompasses a number of unscrupulous activities performed to ensure that statistical significance is reached [4]. These activities include: reopening the study to gather data from more participants; analyzing only a subset of the data; removing outlier data; adjusting or transforming the variables; including additional variables in the data set; choosing a different variable to serve as the outcome; changing the control group; and using a different statistical test [4]. The distinction between activities that fall within the bounds of permissible statistical modeling versus p-hacking rests in the timing. Statistical decisions made before collecting data or running any analyses constitute the study's methodology. For example, deciding to enroll enough participants to gather data that could show a significant difference, if one exists, is a valid methodological choice. Conducting a study is pointless if researchers do not plan to collect enough data to properly power their studies. However, statistical actions taken after running the initial analyses indicate that researchers are dissatisfied with their results and are attempting to affect the outcome with new data.

Changing course statistically after examining the data is highly suspect. For example, in a larger study of 13 meta-reviews in the psychological literature, authors found that researchers engaged in the practice of running multiple small sample-size studies repeatedly until they found results from one that reached the $p < 0.05$ level [18]. Running a series of small studies and stopping only once statistical significance has been found, rather than running one large study, is a clear example of p-hacking.

The Replication Correction

Replication is a crucial tenet of the scientific process because it assists researchers in discovering false positive results that litter the field due to publication bias and p-hacking practices. When studies are replicated, scientists must confront the false positives head on. A biotech firm, Amgen, could reproduce only 6 of 53 "landmark" cancer studies; Bayer could reproduce only one quarter of 67 papers they published and were deemed "important" to the field; and social scientists replicated 100 psychological studies and found that more than half did not produce statistically significant results upon replication [19–21].

Despite its importance, replication is a costly endeavor and is less interesting to funders and researchers alike [9]. Many in research agree that a sufficient number of replication studies are not performed, but this conviction does not automatically lead to change. In 2015, the director of the National Institute of Mental Health, Thomas Insel, penned an editorial on the importance of reproducibility in research studies [22]. He specified that in the face of biological variability, poor methodology, questionable analytical practices, and outright fraud, reproducibility is the only way science can correct its own false positive findings. He specifically cites p-hacking as a contributing factor in the current challenges to modern science.

Meaning in Decision-Making

Publication bias combined with the sheer volume of studies published today detracts from the meaning of the findings [23]. The preponderance of accessible studies meets statistical significance criteria simply by virtue of their publication, thus reducing the likelihood of drawing meaningful conclusions from statistical significance alone. While a number of efforts—including recommendations, databases for all trials and studies regardless of results, and even legislation—have been attempted to undercut the problem, there is still no effective solution to publication bias [7]. Given that physicians and their patients cannot change publication bias, they must learn to interpret meaning themselves.

Clearly, while hypothesis testing provides guidance as to whether an observed difference is statistically significant, it does not explain whether or not this difference has any meaning [24]. In a cautionary paper, dermatologic researchers provide a clear example of the distinction between statistical significance and clinical meaning. These authors reviewed a study that tested a topical treatment for early male pattern baldness [25]. Participants who received the treatment experienced a statistically significant higher hair count compared to the control participants (at a p-value of less than 0.05) [25]. Despite these results, however, the hair count improvement did not lead to any appreciably noticeable cosmetic improvement [25]. Without a meaningful subjective assessment showing improvement, statistically more hair strands was likely cold comfort to those men in the experimental group. In the academic field of research, statistical significance still reigns supreme. In the world of applied medicine, physicians must obtain an indication of clinical significance before incorporating research results into their practice.

Patients, too, should make their healthcare decisions based on meaningful findings, not simply statistically significant ones. Truly informed decision-making necessitates that patients are aware of what a finding says with regard to meaning, rather than significance alone. Statistically significant results should only be considered within the broader context of methodological procedures, other relevant statistical measures, and the preexisting literature [6].

Clinical Significance

While meaning is clearly subjective, the scientific process has attempted to codify
it. Statistical efforts to codify meaning result in the calculation of the magnitude
of the experimental effect [26]. These calculations are said to describe the impact
of an intervention, with impact acting as the statistical proxy for meaning. Even
when examining various impact indicators, physicians and patients alike should
continue to place a heavy emphasis on individual circumstances and common
sense.

Measures of meaning provide a more complete picture of what the data show
by including details such as the size of the difference and direction of the difference. The size of the difference matters from a practical standpoint. When
choosing whether or not to prescribe or undergo a treatment, the amount of
improvement, or the impact amount, is a crucial consideration. The direction of
the difference matters as well—if a treatment is statistically significantly different
from a placebo but the placebo performed better, than the treatment would not be
recommended.

Before exploring impact measures in depth, we should mention that measuring
impact is not the only method for assessing clinical significance. An examination
of the means and standard deviations for different groups is also more illuminating
than significance testing alone. Because these metrics provide such a clear picture,
they are actually called **descriptive statistics**. Many research articles provide relevant descriptive statistics in tables or figures within the text.

While examining the descriptive statistics illuminates clinical significance,
impact measurements provide an additional benefit supporting their use. Impact
indicators are standardized. This standardization helps researchers who perform
systematic reviews as well as individuals who may not be familiar with the variables used in a study.

Researchers who conduct systematic reviews and meta-analyses do so with
the aim of developing more sophisticated hypotheses and to provide the field
with comprehensive reviews [27]. Summarizing studies in these formats is
largely accepted for synthesizing previous work in a meaningful and helpful way.
Systematic reviews differ from basic literature reviews with narrative results in
that they explicitly define the scope of inquiry, the methods to determine which
studies are included in the review, the methods used to extract data, and the analysis thereof [27]. Some systematic reviews additionally include a meta-analysis
[27]. Meta-analyses gather any number of previous studies examining the same
hypothesis and pool their outcomes, provided the studies are similar enough [27].
If studies within the meta-analysis report impact, these impact results can be
pooled to gain a more comprehensive view of the benefit of the treatment [28].
This pooling is possible due to the standardization of effect sizes. For example,
pediatric oncologists may read about new treatments that show statistical significance. If the preponderance of these treatments produces only minimal evidence
of impact, optimism accompanying these new treatments should be tempered.

Standardization of impact measurements is also valuable for individuals reading results because studies report their outcomes using different scales [28]. For example, a review of studies testing a fever reduction agent may unearth some studies reporting outcomes in degrees Fahrenheit and others in Celsius. The standardization of impact measurements applies the same scale of meaning regardless of the original measurement used. In studies of less common concepts, the scales used are usually arcane to the lay reader. While an educated nonspecialist has some idea of what a decrease of a few degrees in Fahrenheit means, few outside the realm of specialized research would be able to interpret, for example, a drop in a few points on the Beck Anxiety Inventory. Standardization of meaning measurements ensures that lay readers need not first acquaint themselves with all of the variables in the study and their respective scales.

Indicators of Impact

Unlike the p-value, which is always presented as "p," the calculation of impact indicators depends on the original statistical test; impact indicators therefore have different names or symbols to identify them. Two broad categories of studies are those that test for differences (between groups) and those that examine relationships (between variables) [29]. In studies of difference, impact indicators provide guidance as to the magnitude and direction of the difference. In studies of relationship, impact indicators quantify the strength and direction of association.

For studies that examine differences between groups, popular indicators of impact attempt to estimate the differences between the groups or the amount of difference attributable to the intervention [30]. Studies might report the relative risk, odds ratio, standardized mean difference, probability of benefit, or number needed to treat [30]. Studies that examine relationships between variables use popular indicators of impact to quantify the strength of the association. These studies might report correlation or covariates to measure the strength and ascertain the direction of the relationship [31].

We are not reviewing indicators of effect in depth here. The U.S. Department of Education's Institute of Education Sciences' initiative, the What Works Clearinghouse, recommends that researchers provide an interpretation for readers of any reported impact measurements [29]. If interpretation is not provided within the paper, physicians can refer to a basic statistics book or online resource for guidance.

Underreported Impact—Caveat Emptor

One reason this book will not delineate different measurements of impact in detail is because popular media rarely report them. As such, most patients will not have access to impact indicators. Media outlets fail to report them, in no small part, because many published studies do not include them either. Journals pediatricians encounter are all but guaranteed to publish the statistical significance. However, it is still not assured that every study will report impact.

Without access to the original impact figures, patients rely on their physicians. The original online journal articles patients would like to know more about are often blocked to patients by pay walls. This is a barrier to informed consent that doctors, who may belong to medical associations or work for organizations that grant institutional access to the original text, can overcome on their patients' behalf. Patients who have considered a study and found it has merit according to funding, bias, methodological rigor, and statistical significance will still likely need their physicians' help to look for reported impact. If impact is reported for statistically significant findings, physicians should share the figures with their patients to help them to interpret the results. For example, consider a study finding that reading to children is statistically significantly correlated with later academic achievement. If the impact indicator is strong, the physician will want to impress upon the parent that not only are the variables correlated, they appear to be strongly associated.

If impact is not reported in the original research article, this is an indicator for physicians. As in our discussion of editors' and researchers' activities contributing to publication bias, inferring motives for not reporting impact indicators is an ambiguous task. One reason could be the pervasiveness of statistical significance, pushing the value of impact reporting to the side. Yet even with statistical significance's dominance, multiple scientific organizations have recommended for decades that impact be reported. To be unaware of the importance of impact reporting in research is a troubling indictor of the researcher's credentials.

Another reason for omitting impact results is that the researchers did not find a meaningful one in their study. Finding an effect size too small to be meaningful could prompt a researcher to leave out the information altogether. Unlike statistical significance, which is all but required for most study publications, many journals still print papers without impact results. Therefore, researchers dissatisfied with the size of their impact findings can omit it. Leaving out a small impact result in a research paper is analogous to omitting a short-lived job on a resume. The omission is not exactly a lie, but it indicates an underlying reluctance to provide the full picture for fear that it will dilute the case as a whole. Because strong impact scores seem impressive, researchers have every incentive to report them when they occur.

Conclusion

At this stage, we have fully reviewed the steps to research literacy that will assist patients in making fully informed consent. While we do not suggest all patients can take these actions on their own, physicians can help their patients with the steps along the way. By giving the correct terms to various research concepts as they explain them, doctors can increase their patients' literacy. As with other forms of literacy (financial, digital, cultural, etc.), fluency will not happen overnight. Building a comfort level with patients one step at a time increases their confidence and promotes a working relationship between physician and patient, which is key to effective patient-centered care.

References

1. Nuzzo R. Statistical errors. Nature. 2014;506(7487):150–2.
2. Head ML, Holman L, Lanfear R, Kahn AT, Jennions MD. The extent and consequences of P-hacking in science. PLoS Biol. 2015;13(3):e1002106.
3. Kahneman D. Thinking, fast and slow. Macmillan; 2011.
4. Motulsky HJ. Common misconceptions about data analysis and statistics. Br J Pharmacol. 2015;172(8):2126–32.
5. Caba J. Gum disease linked to breast cancer in postmenopausal women with a history of smoking. Medical Daily. http://www.medicaldaily.com/gum-disease-linked-breast-cancer-postmenopausal-women-history-smoking-366318 Accessed 21 Dec 2015.
6. Aarts S, Winkens B, van Den Akker M. The insignificance of statistical significance. Eur J Gen Pract. 2012;18(1):50–2.
7. Mayer M. A call to arms to help heal medicine's greatest ailment-publication bias and inadequate research transparency. F1000Research. 2015;4.
8. Masicampo EJ, Lalande DR. A peculiar prevalence of p values just below 05 Q J Exp Psychol. 2012;65 Suppl 11:2271–9.
9. Anonymous. How science goes wrong. The Economist. http://www.economist.com/news/leaders/21588069-scientific-research-has-changed-world-now-it-needs-change-itself-how-science-goes-wrong Accessed 19 Oct 2013.
10. Goodchild van Hilten L. Why it's time to publish research "failures." Elsevier. 2015. https://www.elsevier.com/connect/scientists-we-want-your-negative-results-too Accessed 6 Jan 2016.
11. Gill J. The insignificance of null hypothesis significance testing. Polit Res Q. 1999;52(3):647–74.
12. Taleb NM. Beware the big errors of 'big data." Wired. http://www.wired.com/2013/02/big-data-means-big-errors-people/ Accessed 08 Feb 2013.
13. Smith GD, Ebrahim S. Data dredging, bias, or confounding: they can all get you into the BMJ and the Friday papers. BMJ. Br Med J. 2002;325(7378):1437.
14. 2015 Journal Citation Reports. Philadelphia: Thomson Reuters; 2015. http://wokinfo.com/products_tools/analytical/jcr/ Accessed 6 Jan 2016.
15. Aschwanden C. Science isn't broken. FiveThirtyEight, 2015 http://fivethirtyeight.com/features/science-isnt-broken/.
16. Cipriani A, Barbui C. What is a clinical trial protocol? Epidemiol Psichiatr Soc. 2010;19(02):116–7.

17. Simmons JP, Nelson LD, Simonsohn U. A 21 word solution. Available at SSRN 2160588. Accessed 14 Oct 2012.
18. Bakker M, van Dijk A, Wicherts JM. The rules of the game called psychological science. Perspect Psychol Sci. 2012;7(6):543–54.
19. Begley CG, Ellis LM. Drug development: raise standards for preclinical cancer research. Nature. 2012;483(7391):531–3.
20. Prinz F, Schlange T, Asadullah K. Believe it or not: how much can we rely on published data on potential drug targets?. Nat Rev Drug Discovery. 2011;10 Suppl 9:712.
21. Carey B. Many psychology findings not as strong as claimed, study says. The New York Times. http://www.nytimes.com/2015/08/28/science/many-social-science-findings-not-as-strong-as-claimed-study-says.html Accessed 27 Aug 2015.
22. Insel T. Director's blog: P-hacking. The National Institute of Mental Health. http://www.nimh.nih.gov/about/director/2014/p-hacking.shtml Accessed 14 Nov 2014.
23. Peat G, Riley RD, Croft P, Morley KI, Kyzas PA, Moons KG, Perel P, Steyerberg EW, Schroter S, Altman DG, Hemingway H. Improving the transparency of prognosis research: the role of reporting, data sharing, registration, and protocols.
24. McCloskey D. The insignificance of statistical significance. Scientific American; 1995.
25. Bhardwaj SS, Camacho F, Derrow A, Fleischer AB, Feldman SR. Statistical significance and clinical relevance: the importance of power in clinical trials in dermatology. Arch Dermatol. 2004;140(12):1520–3.
26. Kazdin AE. The meanings and measurement of clinical significance.
27. Kirkwood BR, Sterne JAC. Essential medical statistics. 2nd ed. Massachusetts: Blackwell Science Ltd; 2003.
28. Lakens D. Calculating and reporting effect sizes to facilitate cumulative science: a practical primer for t-tests and ANOVAs. Front Psychol. 2013;4.
29. McMillan JH, Foley J. Reporting and discussing effect size: still the road less traveled. Pract Assess Res Eval. 2011;16(14):1–2.
30. Faraone SV. Interpreting estimates of treatment effects: implications for managed care. Pharm Ther. 2008;33(12):700.
31. Vacha-Haase T, Thompson B. How to estimate and interpret various effect sizes. J Couns Psychol. 2004;51(4):473.

Chapter 5
Incorporating Research into Healthcare Decisions

Overview

Researchers and physicians alike have long recognized that the conclusions of clinical research should have some practical applications. While basic science seeks to gain knowledge for its own sake, clinical research aims to contribute to improved wellbeing in individuals and populations. Still debated is the extent to which findings from research trials can be appropriately and feasibly applied in clinical settings [1]. Specific questions in this ongoing dialogue rest on the merits of particular findings, what information can be interpreted as evidentiary, and how that evidence is to be applied and integrated within existing practices [1].

Evidence-Based

The questions imply a distinction between treatments developed and tested in research studies and the practice of using research-backed therapies in clinical care. More than just a subtlety to be inferred, this distinction is a real one, marked by specific terminology. Within controlled research trials, the therapies, techniques, interventions, or medications that produced statistically and clinically significant changes are called **evidence-based treatments** (EBT) [1]. Alternatively, the broader clinical practice that maintains up-to-date knowledge of research findings and incorporates them into practice when deemed valuable within the context of individual patient needs, values, and clinical presentation is called **evidence-based practice** (EBP) [1]. Clinicians can engage in evidence-based practice without using a specific EBT. Consider a physician who keeps apprised of recent research developments in muscle hypotonia without prescribing a specific new EBT for a patient, who is already responding well to the current course

© Springer International Publishing AG 2017
C.A. Di Bartolo and M.K. Braun, *Pediatrician's Guide to Discussing Research with Patients*, DOI 10.1007/978-3-319-49547-7_5

of treatment. This clinician delivers evidence-based care by considering EBTs through the lens of a specific patient. Other doctors may want to deliver specific EBTs but cannot due to feasibility or logistical barriers.

On the other hand, clinicians may utilize an EBT without necessarily practicing in an evidence-based fashion. In this case, consider a physician who prescribes a new, evidence-based medication without considering whether or not the patient might achieve positive outcomes with a previously established treatment. Providing evidence-based practice requires that physicians make educated decisions, not simply dispense new treatments without question or at the urging of pharmaceutical representatives. Evidence, expertise, and patient characteristics are the hallmarks of evidence-based practice [1].

As a practice conceptualization, EBP began in the 1970s with British epidemiologist Archibald Cochrane [2]. He determined that women entering pre-term labor were not appropriately treated with corticosteroids because systemic reviews had not synthesized the results of research trials into meaningful clinical guidelines [2]. The needless and senseless deaths of thousands of premature babies spurred his creation of the Cochrane Collaboration in 1993 [2]. The collaboration's aim, from its inception to the present day, is to assist clinical decision-making by creating and updating publicly available systemic reviews of the latest and most reliable research findings for health practitioners [3]. This approach to intentionally remain abreast of research findings with the express purpose of delivering optimal care ushered in the era of evidence-based practice. Empirical support for evidence-based practice shows that clinical care incorporating treatments from rigorous studies improves patient outcomes by 28% compared to practices derived from tradition [2].

The past 20 years have shown the concept of evidence-based practice to be vastly influential in a number of areas [4]. A Medline search places the first usage of "evidence-based practice" in 1992, with 600 more appearances 5 years later [5]. The sharp increase continued, with over 1,000 results from 1995–2000 alone [5]. Clearly evidence-based practice gained traction and wide acceptance among those who publish—primarily, researchers. Impressions among practitioners are not as easy to quantify. Studies have found that positive impressions of utilizing research findings to inform on care have been widely adopted by practitioners and policymakers in the fields of medicine, nursing, psychology, and others [4]. Evidence also exists for a similarly positive impression in the field of pediatrics. One study of pediatricians and pediatric nurses found that these medical professionals displayed moderate to good scores with regard to their attitudes toward evidence-based practice [6].

When performed as intended, evidence-based practice bridges the gap between researchers and physicians. Researchers and doctors regularly observe the same phenomena, but their different perspectives quite frequently lead to misunderstanding and disagreement. Like the proverbial blind men examining parts of an elephant, those feeling the tail interpret a rope, those feeling the legs conclude a tree, and so on. Physicians criticize researchers for being out of touch with true clinical presentations, studying disease in a way that is not practically helpful, and producing treatments that cannot be delivered due to logistical constraints—time, money, apparatus, infrastructure, etc. Researchers voice exasperation when physicians continue to deliver ineffective care, as a result of entrenched practices, that lacks a basis in evidence.

While not completely unfounded, mutual critiques between the world of research and applied medicine drive a wedge between natural partners in the quest for better care. The magnitude of philosophical differences between researchers and physicians appears smaller when removed from the academic setting. Famous psychology researcher Alan Kazdin wryly notes that the personal lives of researchers and physicians show their tacit acknowledgement of the merits of their counterparts' approaches [1]. He points out that rarely would a researcher who has fallen ill eschew a treatment with insufficient evidence of efficacy, particularly if no evidence-based treatment exists for the ailment from which they suffer. Similarly, physicians who find themselves ill commonly begin researching their condition to learn more about possible treatment options, and their scientific backing, when approaching their own healing. Observed in this phenomenon are researchers and clinicians displaying significant agreement regarding evidence-based practice despite sometimes finding themselves at odds over the scientific method and specific EBTs.

Researchers and physicians both acknowledge individual variability in their work, albeit in different fashions. Researchers measure the extent to which a treatment works for participants of differing characteristics with **moderators**. Moderators are participants' characteristics that can be measured at the start of the study. After observing treatment effects, researchers review the moderator variables to assess whether or not they affected the treatment's impact on outcomes for participants with similar moderators. For example, a study may uncover that a sleep training intervention produces better outcomes for families reporting low levels of stress before implementing the intervention in their homes than it does for high-stress families. Without referring to them as moderators, physicians regularly address these same characteristics in their practice. Doctors consider clinical variables that they expect to either promote or hinder the effects of their prescribed treatment. In the sleep training example, a mother with concerns about her child's sleep asks her pediatrician for guidance. Before recommending sleep training, the pediatrician assesses conversationally whether the mother's stress levels will likely allow her to implement the procedure as designed. Comments indicative of high-stress guide the physician to conclude that the sleep training may not help the family in their current state and may in fact stress them further. The physician accordingly makes a different recommendation that is more likely to be successful in addressing the presenting problem.

Many clinical decision-making models involve a component of incorporating physician expertise and individual patient characteristics, such as clinical presentations, comorbidities, preferences, and values [2]. While these are important considerations, they are presumably employed in all manner of sensible healthcare decision-making. In this chapter, we focus on the considerations for decision-making more directly relevant to incorporating research findings into practice.

Specifically, this chapter addresses the practical and theoretical impediments to EBP as well as its facilitators. We will provide communication strategies for physicians to follow when holding discussions about research and EBP with patients.

Practical Impediments

Many physicians approve the concept of evidence-based practice in theory. Indeed, incorporating new knowledge into an already professionally established knowledge base of experience is one of the more interesting aspects of practicing medicine [7]. Despite theoretical acceptance, doctors encounter a number of factors impeding full implementation of evidence-based practice in reality.

Although the consideration of scientific evidence is a widely accepted practice, clinicians do not formulate their decisions on evidence alone. A deeply engrained method for decision-making relies on the consensuses that emerge within fields and communities of experts [7]. It is possible for a consensus view to form as a result of formal reviews of compilations of studies [7]. Practically, the constantly expanding body of knowledge hampers the integration of new knowledge into previous consensus decisions. As a result, real-world physicians rely on an informal network of other practicing clinicians to determine whether or not a consensus is building around a particular treatment [7]. This network effect is observed in the regional differences among malpractice litigation. Plaintiffs who experienced adverse outcomes are more likely to sue if they received procedures considered outside the standard of care. Comparing medical malpractice lawsuits across different regions shows how the standard of care varies from locale to locale, presumably driven by these networks [7]. Community standards on which physicians rely can be combined with a more systematic approach. However, this synthesis requires endeavors, such as journal clubs, that can only be created and sustained through physician time and effort [7]. While clinicians may want to practice evidence-based care, more easily accessible non-research sources of information often drive clinical decision-making.

Another practical factor deterring the implementation of evidence-based treatments in clinical settings is the lack of long-term follow-up results in many research studies. When safe and effective methods for treating an illness exist, a lack of evidence regarding long-term outcomes of newer methods means that the older treatment is more likely the safer one [7]. Balancing the interest and optimism in new treatments against reliable and established means of care presents an additional mental calculation for physicians who consider which treatment to prescribe. Ironically, the long-term outcomes of their own patients with the pre-established treatment are also typically not measured in a systematic way. Clinicians can collect data on their own patients (called an *n*-of-1 trial), but these efforts require a willing patient and physician to implement [7]. Given the wide body of expertise immediately accessible to a seasoned clinician on previously established treatments, evidence-based treatments are harder to learn about, and inherently riskier to implement.

Logistical barriers also hinder the integration of EBTs into existing clinical practice settings. Where administrative support is lacking, physicians encounter a more difficult time obtaining resources they may need to pursue evidence-based practice [2]. Insufficient mentors or advocates for EBP and inadequate knowledge circulation about EBP present key obstacles in light of the consensus-driven effect described above [2, 7]. Even when education and information are available to inform practicing doctors of new EBTs, it is often didactic in nature and resists uptake [2]. Worse, education for trainees in the area of EBP typically focuses on the research aspect without elaborating how to incorporate those research findings into practice [2].

Practical Facilitators

Despite practical hurdles to the implementation of evidence-based practice, there are facilitators for EBP as well. Some are positive opposites of the above barriers, including administrative support, EBP mentors or advocates, and a better connection between research and clinical practices within a region [2]. Other practical resources, such as time and money, also facilitate EBP [2]. Easily comprehensible and available writing on research also assists integration of EBTs into practice [2].

Theoretical Impediments

In addition to these practical challenges in EBP, there is a conceptual paradox inherent in utilizing evidence-based treatments to make decisions for an individual. Applying study findings to an individual has face validity, as decisions are often made for one person based on what is observed to happen for many people. For example, a traveler attempting to board a train in a foreign country might observe numerous people first going to a ticket window. The traveler can reasonably conclude that based on this observed sample, he as an individual ought to stop at the ticket window as well. Despite this intuitive sense that research results can be applied in a similar fashion, the goals of research and clinical care are vastly different. The goal of research is to acquire knowledge regarding phenomena. In service of this goal, research systematically gathers data on a number of individuals (the sample) to infer conclusions about the whole (the population) [4]. Notice there is no role of the individual in this process. Yet treating the individual is the goal of clinical care, and the paradox is formed.

EBP presents a special challenge for patient-centered care. First, clinical research studies tend to be disease-centered, not patient-centered [5]. For example, most recruitment efforts for clinical studies mention the disease of interest on the flyer, subway ad, or email blast. For example: "Does your child have difficulty breathing? If so, you may qualify for a clinical treatment study at our Asthma Center." Research does not recruit people, but rather samples of people who share a disease in common. This is because research commonly follows a biomedical approach, wherein a disease exists within a patient. Disease is considered an objective reality. By contrast, illness is a patient's subjective experience of feeling unwell. Patient-centered care focuses on patients experiencing illness within their specific psychological and social context [5]. Two individuals may suffer from the same disease, but one may consider himself ill while the other does not.

The distinction between disease and illness is made regularly clinically, but addressed rarely scientifically. Research studies seek to treat the disease, while a patient-centered physician seeks to cure the patient of illness. Evidence-based practice in its current format continues to draw from research studies' conclusions about diseases. Hence, the results are harder to situate within a patient-centered model.

Second, research studies often attempt to minimize differences between individuals [5]. As one example, the randomization process is intended to more equally distribute individual characteristics that may meaningfully interact with the treatment—whether positively or negatively—between the treatment and control conditions. Certain analyses after the data have been collected serve the same function: by covarying for specific baseline features, the analyses seek to show that the results would hold regardless of these individual characteristics. Patient-centered care takes the opposite approach, with individual characteristics often driving key treatment decisions [5]. If a child is sufficiently afraid of needles, his doctor may choose to administer the influenza vaccine via nasal spray rather than injection. The patient's characteristic drove the clinical choice irrespective of whatever the evidence may show regarding vaccine efficacy as a function of delivery method. This characteristic, in a research study, would be relegated to a discussion of moderator variables and might not even make the main outcomes paper. In clinical practice, this characteristic determined the clinical choice.

Theoretical Facilitators

The field at large can take actions to address the paradox of delivering evidence-based treatments to a sample size of one. Performing more meta-analyses observing clinical outcomes, particularly those examining effect sizes, provides a more complete picture as to clinical outcomes among different individuals [4, 5]. Researchers can also place more weight on individual variability, whether in the form of moderator results in research studies or a clinical appraisal of individual characteristics in a clinical setting [4]. Researchers can also plan their studies to incorporate patient preferences into the design [5]. In addition to the continued performance of randomized controlled trials, these kinds of designs would yield results that more closely reflect real-world outcomes, where patient preferences having some impact on treatment administration are the norm [5].

Physicians on an individual level can reduce the discrepancy between the two models of medicine through doctor–patient communication [5]. The relationship and information shared between doctor and patient serve as the true bridges connecting the gulf between the principles of EBP and patient-centered care [5]. A doctor's first question during an office visit is, "What brings you in today?" Taking care to listen to the specific answer is the first step to grounding the care that follows in the patient's needs. The goal is for the doctors to assess the patient's needs along two axes—disease versus illness, and control versus guidance. First of all, is the patient asking for a cure for a disease, or is the patient seeking relief from symptoms or functional impairment that promote illness? Second, does the patient want to remain in full control of the medical decisions, or is he asking for guidance from the doctor? In our discussion of patient-centered care in Chap. 1, we presented the evidence showing that not all patients are interested in making their healthcare decisions. Some prefer the paternalistic approach.

Once the doctor know where the patient's preferences fall along these two dimensions, the following discussion, treatments considered, and ultimate decision are grounded within the patient's needs regardless of whether or not evidence-based treatments are offered, considered, or chosen. Interactions in which the patient's preferences for conceptualizing their ailment and the level of control they prefer are rooted in patient-centeredness. This holds even in cases where the patient follows a biomedical approach and prefers that the doctor retain control over the clinical decision-making. This outcome may mimic the paternalistic view of medicine, but if it occurs as a result of patient preference, it remains patient-centered.

Initiation of Discussion of Research Findings

In the conversations about care, either party in the doctor–patient interaction can initiate discussion regarding research findings and clinical implications. Physicians may initiate a discussion of research findings because they have considered the statistical and clinical significance, the new intervention's anticipated effects compared to treatment-as-usual, possible side effects, and cost (both direct and indirect) [8]. The doctor's comfort level with trying a new treatment will moderate the likelihood of raising the discussion, and patient preferences will ultimately decide if the treatment is chosen [8].

While this rational approach is perfectly sensible, many clinicians will not necessarily make their decision to initiate discussion in such a structured fashion. When the information available is incomplete, as is often the case when initiating a conversation when the patient's preferences are unknown, clinical judgment typically takes precedence. Clinical judgment has been interpreted as the intuition of experts [9]. Much about the mechanisms of clinical intuition is still unknown [9].

However, reports of clinical intuition appear to reflect that it works via the rapid combination of (1) subconsciously accessing knowledge of past experiences; and (2) using this knowledge to fill in the gaps of information. While some clinicians may first analyze a research study before presenting an EBT to their patients, others may mention a recent finding based on an intuitive sense their patients would be open to hearing more.

Doctors also introduce new treatments when the older treatments or conceptualizations of a disease are outdated or are proven ineffective [7]. A rough guideline as to the pace of meaningful change in clinical interventions is that approximately every 5–10 years new evidence is sufficient to initiate a change in common practice [7]. We cautioned in Chap. 2 that some medical advances are developed and marketed aggressively despite the wide availability of already effective treatments. Without follow-up studies indicating that these new treatments do not pose a higher side effect or toxicity profile, clinicians who wait and continue to use the established treatment have superior patient outcomes, provided the established treatment is effective, safe, and reasonable [7]. When patients do not show sufficient response to an established treatment, then clinicians should seek out newer alternatives and initiate discussions if the evidence is strong.

Patients may initiate discussions about research findings due to curiosity, direct requests for certain interventions, or dissatisfaction with current treatment. The widespread availability of medical information and misinformation on the Internet has changed the way curious patients ask questions of their doctors and participate in decision-making. Surveys of patients accessing medical information on the Internet do not indicate they use this method of gathering information as a replacement for doctor visits [10]. Rather, patients indicate they access medical information online in advance of an office visit or after a visit to confirm the information their doctor provided and get more information. Many patients seek out websites intended for medical professionals, in part because these patients feel information for the lay public is too basic [10].

Now that an increasing amount of medical care is devoted to the treatment of chronic disease, many patients have ample time to live with and treat their condition. The extended time horizon of chronic illness permits patients to learn about their conditions and develop their own impressions [11]. In addition to the treatment of chronic conditions, pediatric practice is often characterized by preventative care or verification of healthy development. Parents of healthy children may not necessarily have the same motivation for seeking medical information online as their peers with unwell children. Those who seek out medical information for their healthy, typically developing children are clearly interested in learning, and have the time and access to information to prioritize this activity. As an implicit indicator of patient need, doctors should respond to this need of the parents of healthy children who seek information and initiate conversations based on their searches by participating in parent-initiated discussions.

Physicians with curious patients can take an open, collaborative approach to their patients' requests for further discussion [10]. Technologically savvy physicians might facilitate the patient's preference for information-gathering and "prescribe" specific trusted websites for patients to review [10]. This response is both patient-centered (addressing the patient's need to be informed) and also provides an opportunity for patients to access evidence-based information. Providing patients with the complex information they desire, but pre-screening it for accuracy, meets the needs of both patient and physician.

Responding to a request for discussion markedly differs from a patient's request for a specific treatment or test. Often interpreted as a response to pharmaceutical marketing's instructions to "Ask your doctor about" a given product or condition, patients are reportedly making more direct requests for specific treatments and tests [11]. An increasing number of patients are also observed in clinical practice requesting some kind of intervention based on research findings they see presented in the media. Doctors responding to direct or indirect patient requests for new treatments or tests often find themselves in a bind. While patient-centered care often follows the consumer approach of "the customer is always right," in medicine, the patient's impressions and understandings are not always accurate. The patient's request may not be beneficial or it may even be adverse to their desired outcome. Even in cases where a request is benign in terms of patient outcomes, physicians cannot always provide the service to appease the patient. Physicians feel pressure to keep costs low, so even when a particular test that poses no risk could be administered in response to a patient request, physicians are not in a position to be able to provide it without consequences to their practice [11].

Complicating doctor response to patient requests is the oblique manner in which many patients initiate these discussions. For example, researchers have found that rather than requesting antibiotics for their child's earache outright, parents make reference to an ear infection diagnosis during the presentation of symptoms. They also ask questions about antibiotics after receiving a prescription for a nonantibiotic intervention, thus suggesting that they consider the antibiotic a viable treatment that has not yet been offered [11]. The interactions between physician and patient in response to these patient initiations can feel like a negotiation [11]. While one study found the presence or absence of this negotiation did not affect patient satisfaction, it is hypothesized that the overall quality of this interaction does impact satisfaction [11].

Naturally, some patients do perform Internet searches of their conditions when they are dissatisfied with the information provided by their doctors [10]. Physicians threatened by this kind of patient participation in healthcare are more likely to shorten the evaluation and steer the patient toward the physician's treatment choice [10]. Assertive patients in these situations can be expected to seek corrective measures, such as non-adherence or switching doctors. Instead of responding defensively, physicians can take the patient's initiation as an opportunity to reassess patient needs, current treatment, and other available treatment options.

Communication Strategies

Clearly, regardless of initiator, effective communication between physician and patient is crucial to proper understanding and sharing of information. The appropriate strategy to be utilized is often a function of the goal of the communication. Here, we outline strategies for physicians as a function of their communication goals.

Ask, Listen, Elicit

We addressed how researchers often consider medical issues through the lens of disease, following a biomedical approach. In clinical practice, the actions of physicians imply that they too regularly focus on the disease first [12]. In an office visit, doctors ask questions regarding symptoms, examine medical history from the patient's chart, and gather objective assessments via physical examinations and laboratory tests, all with the aim of pinpointing the disease [12]. Meanwhile, patients may follow the disease or illness approach [12]. Patients in the doctor's office as part of chronic care might view their condition as a disease. When otherwise healthy patients decide to visit the doctor, they are usually prompted to do so by indicators of illness—symptoms that interfere either with their functioning (missed school days, inability to complete daily living tasks) or subjective wellbeing (feeling poorly enough to warrant seeking symptom reduction).

In order to assess if patients view their experience as a disease or an illness, physicians will want to first ask questions, listen to responses, and elicit clarifications. Medical anthropologist Arthur Kleinman established a number of questions that patients address when constructing a narrative around their experience [13]. He called this narrative the **explanatory model** (EM), which people rely on to understand their experience and generate ideas as to cause, treatment, and prognosis. Kleinman developed his questions for physicians to use for the purposes of uncovering their patients' explanatory models. Physicians who understand their patients' EMs can address illness from a biopsychosocial model [14]. For example, if a physician is aware that a patient's explanatory model of her daughter's middle ear infection as having been caused by swimming in a pool, this should prompt a corrected explanation before discussing treatment and future prevention. Kleinman's questions accommodate an interview format, as follows [13]:

- What do you call this problem?
- What do you believe is the cause of this problem?
- What course do you expect it to take? How serious is it?
- What do you think this problem does inside your body?
- How does it affect your body and your mind?
- What do you most fear about the treatment?

In the case of pediatrics, doctors learning about patients' EMs will have to decide whether to ask these questions of the parent only, both parent and children, or child only (in cases where the child in question is legally able to make health-care decisions). Parents with different EMs from their children could respond differently to treatment recommendations, as a function of how well the recommendation fits the EM. Given children's emerging cognitive development, many may not be able to comprehend the future-oriented questions (regarding course, fear, etc.) in a meaningful way. Their EMs will be accordingly incomplete.

This set of questions may prove too burdensome to ask in the course of the office visit. One doctor who utilizes the EM model to guide care reports asking minimally: "How is your health?" followed by "How do you know?" [15]. This streamlined format still addresses the patients' conceptions and their explanations for their impressions. We recommend revising the questions to reflect the age and cognitive abilities of the patient. Younger children may need the questions posed even more concretely, for example:

Pediatrician: How are you feeling?
Child: Bad.
Pediatrician: I'm sorry to hear that. What makes you say you're feeling bad?
Child: I have a really bad stomachache, and Mommy said we had to go to the doctor's.

Notice that from this relatively simple exchange, the child's EM is beginning to present itself. His response to the first question indicates that the child's subjective wellbeing has been compromised. In his response to the second question, we see the child has formed an illness conception of his difficulty. While he addresses a symptom (the stomachache) his illness is at least in part socially constructed based on his mother's reaction to his symptoms. The members of his social world are paying attention to his symptoms and reacting to address them. Observe how the questions might then be addressed to the parent, as follows:

Pediatrician: And Ms. Smith, how has his health been lately?
Parent: You know, he's been complaining about this stomachache every morning for a few weeks now. I just don't know.
Pediatrician: I see. You don't know how to explain what's been going on.

In this case, the parent is reluctant to offer an explanation as to her son's recent symptoms. The uncertainty may be a marker of ambivalence on the part of the parent to address whether it is an illness or a disease. It may also indicate a desire to avoid a feared outcome. Rather than push the parent to respond, the pediatrician reflects back what that parent reports to indicate understanding. The pediatrician can ask other EM questions to elicit further impressions from the parent.

Pediatrician: I see. You don't know how to explain what's been going on. Have you been trying to think of possible causes?
Parent: It's funny you should say that. I was wondering if it had anything to do with starting kindergarten. He started having the stomachaches right when school began.
Pediatrician: And when did school start?
Parent: Well, about three weeks ago. So then, I don't know, maybe that's not fair, because he could have picked up a bug from a classmate. I guess either one might make sense to me.

With the help of two more questions that elicit further information, we see that the parent is deciding between the illness model (anxiety about school manifesting as stomachache) or the disease model (viral transmission between classmates and her child). The physician also observes the parent's reluctance to give as much credence to an illness model of healthcare ("maybe that [the psychosomatic response explanation] is not fair") as she is to the disease model. This provides the physician with guidance that this parent is likely to prefer a biomedical approach to the interaction. Even if no specific disease can be found to explain the ailment, the doctor will take care to contextualize the visit as an approach to investigating (even if ultimately rejecting) a disease explanation for the health problem.

Kleinman's questions are both individualized and culturally sensitive. Here there is no paradox [16]. Contrary to common misconception, cultural competence is not synonymous with making assumptions about a patient's preferences or values based on some set of stereotypes of their ethnic, racial, religious, or national groups [16]. Each individual has a unique cultural identify that may contain all of these factors, and others besides [16]. Cultural competence requires the physician to ask specific questions of an individual so that the physician knows how that patient thinks and feels.

Pediatric care presents a particular obligation for assessing a patient's needs before proceeding too far into the visit. Preventative care is a common feature of pediatrics, in addition to responsive care. The American Academy of Pediatrics (AAP) recommends 18 well child visits as a matter of course between the ages of 1 month and 10 years [17]. Six visits are to occur prior to year one alone [17]. These well visits are focused on promoting wellbeing rather than decreasing illness. The academy recommends additional visits when growth and development is not meeting the expected trajectories. Further visits are also recommended for developmental, psychosocial, or disease chronicity. These recommendations exclude visits initiated by acute health concerns such as illness. Therefore, parents presenting in the pediatrician's office may initiate discussions of possible interventions that are preventative or designed to promote wellbeing as much as those that are responsive to an ailment. Even with ailments, the category is subdivided into acute and chronic care. As discussed, parents whose children have chronic conditions may have had more time to familiarize themselves with various treatment options through their own information searches.

Pediatricians' impressions of the facilitative effect the well child visits has on the therapeutic relationship illustrate the importance of asking questions of patients over time [18]. Doctors perceive these relationships to engender trust, mutual respect, and familiarity between the parties [18]. When physicians were more familiar with a parent and child, they reported an increase in delivery of tailored recommendations, an essential component to patient-centered care [18]. In fact, the pediatricians surveyed agreed that while they attempted to incorporate the AAP's recommendations for activities that should occur during well child visits, they prioritized the parents' concerns [18]. The number of recommended activities has increased past the bounds of what many physicians reported being able to complete in one visit. This overabundance of possible activities throws into sharp relief the need for physicians to feel comfortable in choosing what actions to take that fit the family's needs—something that can occur only when the doctor has sufficiently queried the family.

A final step in the process of asking patients about their healthcare ideas is to ascertain what actions the parent may already be taking in the child's care. This becomes especially important when some patient-initiated interventions have the potential to harmfully interact with a doctor-prescribed treatment. Given the wide array of health information available on the Internet, some parents initiate home remedies or over-the-counter treatments for their child without their doctor's direction. As patients often seek out health information on the Internet when they are dissatisfied with the options available to them from their doctors, the Internet is rife with information on Complementary and Alternative Medicine (CAM) [10]. Practices that fall under the CAM category fall outside the mainstream medical practices in Western countries [19]. Some are tested by research but the results remain inconclusive (e.g. acupuncture), others have been tested and found to be generally ineffective (e.g. oral administration of Vitamin C to reduce severity and duration of the common cold), and most troublingly, some have been shown to be ineffective and dangerous (e.g. chelation as a treatment for Autism Spectrum Disorder) [20–22]. In one study of parents of children with Autism Spectrum Disorder (a chronic and pervasive developmental condition that prompts many parents to seek help and support via the Internet), almost 95% reported using some complementary and alternative medicine (CAM) [23]. While some of the CAM therapies parents use may be relatively harmless even if ineffective, others pose risks to the child. For pediatricians to be aware if their patients are using CAM, eliciting this information becomes crucial. Physicians must inquire into the possible usage of CAM therapies in an open and nonjudgmental way to elicit this information from parents [23]. When parents disclose using CAM therapies, the physician response should be modulated to deliver the appropriate information in a way that continues to incentivize parents to be forthright in future visits [23].

Share, Inform, Explain

Physicians at times discuss research findings with patients with the purpose of sharing, informing, or explaining. This more didactic style of communication may result from a patient's explicit request for information or the physician's observations that an evidence-based treatment could be beneficial.

Physicians are often presented with patients who would like them to be able to respond to a particular piece of information the patient found prior to the visit [24]. The sheer number of websites with health information is too large for any one doctor to be fully familiar with, particularly when websites with poor credibility are included. Once other media (television, magazines, etc.) are added, the number is higher still. Physicians should not attempt to explain something the patient has read without being familiar with the original content. Attempts to do so will undermine the doctor's credibility. Fortunately, research shows patients do not respond unfavorably to hearing their doctors honestly acknowledge, "I don't know, but I will review the information and get back to you" [24]. In this case, the responsibility lies with the pediatrician to follow up with patient after reviewing the material. This follow up can occur over phone or at the next visit, depending on the complexity of the patient's original question and the physician's subsequent response.

If doctors prefer to address the question during the visit at least partially, we recommend that in doing so, they "show their work." That is, doctors should respond in a way that simultaneously increases their patient's research literacy skills *and* provides their reflections. This strategy should also begin with an explicit acknowledgement that the physician is not familiar with the precise study the patient is making inquiries about. Then, rather than giving an impression without facts, the doctor should guide the patient to the relevant information needed to generate an opinion. To begin, physicians can point out the importance of understanding researcher credentials and support: "Well, the first thing I'd want to know was who were these researchers who found that, and where did they get their funding. Do you remember reading anything about that?" Next, the doctor can highlight the importance of study design: "I would also want to find out how they designed the study—was this an animal study, or a study with humans? Did they say how many human participants were involved, and for how long they tracked outcomes? Speaking of outcomes, what did they use to measure that result?" Finally, the physician can educate the patient as to the difference between statistical and clinical significance as follows: "I know many studies are reported because their data show something called 'statistical significance.' Did what you hear any mention about clinical outcomes that were observed?" In asking these questions, the physician models for the patient how to review research findings for key information. By not attempting to draw conclusions before these questions have been answered, the doctor provides an example of how the patient should similarly approach interpreting research findings they encounter. Even if the patient cannot answer the questions, the doctor signals the importance of these questions before incorporating the findings into any clinical decisions.

In situations where the evidence base is clear and the physician wants to simply inform the patient of such, the goal becomes to make clear that there is one standard, recommended course of treatment. Communication can either serve or undermine this goal. For example, research shows that physician–parent communication is key to achieving appropriate vaccination rates among children [25]. One study observed two physician styles of communicating information about vaccines—one presumptive (e.g., "Alright, time for a shot"), the other participatory (e.g., "And what were you thinking you wanted to do about shots?") [25]. Vaccine-hesitant parents who were presented with the participatory statements were more likely to voice their resistance to the vaccine [25]. While the participatory presentation appears to align with patient-centered care, it is in fact misleading and detrimental to informed choice. Asking a question regarding patient preference when only one course of action is clearly scientifically backed implies that the preference should influence the decision. Parents have a choice of whether or not to vaccinate their child under the tenets of informed consent. But those who reject vaccinations should be aware that they are doing so based on their own feelings, and not because research has any indication that this is an efficacious medical choice. (We devote Chap. 6 entirely to the research on vaccine efficacy and safety.)

In their practice, doctors should make clear to their patients which recommendations are fully backed by research, making the clinical path obvious, and which present room for individual preference or decision-making metrics. Physicians should ask questions to assess patient preferences. When patients' answers to these questions demonstrate their hesitance for the evidence-based course of treatment, physicians can then use participatory statements to open the dialogue. In this way, doctors acknowledge the patient's preferences while explaining why the recommendation is being made. If the doctor instead used the presumptive style, the patient may feel uncomfortable with the recommendation but not feel comfortable enough to voice their concerns. The line between providing medically sound authority and disregarding a patient's concerns lies in the style of communication used.

Incorporating research findings into clinical decisions sometimes provides greater latitude for patient preference. The manner of presentation of this information also influences patient response. When presenting risk information, doctors can discuss risks of treatments qualitatively, quantitatively, or visually [26]. Qualitative presentations use general descriptions and common terms such as "frequently," "sometimes," and "rarely," to convey possible outcomes [26]. Quantitative presentations include facts and figures from third-party sources, such as systematic reviews [26]. Visual presentations, such as graphs or charts, show risk profiles comparing treatment(s) to no treatment [26]. One study of doctors and simulated patients compared the three presentation methods [26]. No clear consensus emerged as to the "best" presentation method; rather, each one had benefits and drawbacks.

Qualitative presentations were appreciated for their ease of delivery and comprehension [26]. The drawback in the qualitative presentation is implicit in the benefits of the quantitative method, in which the doctors appreciated having clear-cut facts to present (the qualitative presentation alone does not provide facts) [26]. Physicians reported feeling safest having actual numbers to present when patients were making the decision [26]. Meanwhile, the quantitative presentation at times seemed overwhelming to the patients, and concerns were raised as to the education level of the individual receiving the numerical information [26]. Receiving no information was deemed superior to receiving overwhelming information. Finally, the visual presentation simplified the quantitative information and presented absolute risk in addition to relative risk, all in one view [26]. However, not all patients find the visual depiction helpful to situating risk within a real-world context.

Further complicating matters of communication is that a particular treatment's possible outcomes and risks are subject to the **framing effect** [27]. If research indicates a treatment is 75% likely to be effective, it also has a 25% chance of being ineffective. Similar to a glass that is both half-full and half-empty, the framing effect influences people's decision-making as a function of how those options are presented, or framed. Both patients and physicians are influenced by the framing effect [27]. Overall, people are more likely to take risks when they perceive they may be able to avoid losses in doing so; they are less likely to be swayed by the ability to make gains [28]. Therefore, presenting an intervention in terms of its ability to avoid loss will make it more likely to be chosen than if it had been framed in terms of possible gains. Just as with any bias, the framing effect cannot be completely eliminated [27]. However, some communication strategies can help to uncover its effects. Placing the decision in terms of overall goals—is the patient more invested in achieving one outcome or avoiding another outcome—helps to clarify when the framing effect may be operating [28]. Additionally, asking patients to explain the reasons for their choice provides greater clarity and reduces the impact of the framing effect [28]. Given that physicians are similarly affected, before making recommendations, physicians can ask themselves these questions as well.

Correct Misconceptions

The final goal of physician–patient communication is to correct misconceptions that abound in the area of disseminated research findings. While estimates vary, one survey found that half of patients who had searched for health information online did not share this fact with their doctors [24]. The guidance patients receive during their office visits is often filtered through information they have already gathered themselves online [24]. While some is correct, the quality of health information available online is highly variable [24]. Some content is either misleading, easily misinterpreted, or outright fraud [24, 29]. Physicians find themselves in the precarious situation of addressing possible misinformation, oftentimes without having full knowledge of the misinformation patients have consumed.

Addressing misconceptions about health and the research (or lack thereof) supporting various treatment options is crucial to the delivery of evidence-based practice. Yet misconceptions are notoriously hard to fix once embedded. Patients who are simply ignorant are more easily able to learn accurate health information than misinformed patients [29]. For the ignorant patient, doctors need to only share, inform, or explain to provide an accurate and medically sound assessment of the patient's options and possible outcomes. Once a patient presents with misinformation, the physician's task is more challenging. Some methods are more likely to be successful at unseating misconceptions than others. Even when practitioners follow this guidance, it may still be impossible to correct certain misconceptions among select patients.

In attempting to correct a misconception, many physicians repeat the erroneous information in their clarification. While understandable, this is inadvisable. Any repetition of the false information strengthens the connection a patient has with the error. Due to the familiarity effect, the more a patient hears an incorrect statement (e.g., vaccines cause Autism) the more likely that patient is to continue to believe it, even when the false statement is provided within the context of the correction. Doctors should avoid restating the erroneous information and risk entrenching the misinformation further. If the myth must be stated, doctors should take care to always follow it with the correct information, a technique called **repeated retraction** [29]. If patients ask for an explanation as to why the misconception is false, doctors should refute with one simple explanation, even when multiple explanations exist. People prefer simple information and are more likely to remember and incorporate it, even when complex information is more accurate.

Rather than restating the myth, physicians should focus on presenting the correct explanation. The correct information should tell a coherent story—if it leaves a gap in the narrative, then patients are more likely to hold on to the wrong information because it more satisfyingly provides a complete explanation [29]. This is particularly challenging in the field of research, where information gaps are the norm. If researchers have not yet uncovered the correct explanation, physicians should acknowledge for the patient that it is hard not to have all the information.

Affirming patients' worldviews is strongly recommended before providing information about why their current views are false and correcting them [29]. Physicians should first endorse the values of the patient that led them to incorporate this erroneous information into their explanatory model. The patient might have a deep love and caring for their child, strong intellectual curiosity, tenacity for not settling for incomplete information, a desire for fairness and balance that drives them to seek understanding in multiple viewpoints, etc. With the worldview in mind, doctors can then link the new information back to the admirable patient quality that drove them to seek an explanation.

Finally, physicians can help prevent further misconceptions from forming by providing reliable sources of information for their patients to access. A list of credible sources is as follows:

NOAH-Health.org: http://www.noah-health.org/
National Institutes of Health: http://www.nih.gov
MedlinePlus: https://www.nlm.nih.gov/medlineplus/
Cochrane: www.Cochrane.org
Centers for Disease Control and Prevention: www.cdc.gov.

References

1. Kazdin AE. Evidence-based treatment and practice: new opportunities to bridge clinical research and practice, enhance the knowledge base, and improve patient care. Am Psychol. 2008;63(3):146.
2. Fineout-Overholt E, Melnyk BM, Schultz A. Transforming health care from the inside out: advancing evidence-based practice in the 21st century. J Prof Nurs. 2005;21(6):335–44.
3. Cochrane.org. About us | Cochrane. http://www.cochrane.org/about-us (2016). Accessed 15 January 2016.

4. Bouffard M, Reid G. The good, the bad, and the ugly of evidence-based practice. Adap Phys Act Quart. 2012;29(1):1–24.
5. Bensing J. Bridging the gap.: the separate worlds of evidence-based medicine and patient-centered medicine. Patient Educ Couns. 2000;39(1):17–25.
6. Maaskant JM, Knops AM, Ubbink DT, Vermeulen H. Evidence-based practice: a survey among pediatric nurses and pediatricians. J Pediatr Nurs. 2013;28(2):150–7.
7. Larson EB. How can clinicians incorporate research advances into practice? J Gen Intern Med. 1997;12(s2):20–4.
8. Mariani AW, Pêgo-Fernandes PM. Statistical significance and clinical significance. Sao Paulo Med J. 2014;132(2):71–2.
9. Cioffi J. Heuristics, servants to intuition, in clinical decision-making. J Adv Nurs. 1997;26:203–8.
10. McMullan M. Patients using the Internet to obtain health information: how this affects the patient–health professional relationship. Patient Educ Couns. 2006;63(1):24–8.
11. Teas Gill V. Patient "demand" for medical interventions: exerting pressure for an offer in a primary care clinic visit. Res Lang Soc Inter. 2005;38(4):451–79.
12. Siminoff LA. Incorporating patient and family preferences into evidence-based medicine. BMC Med Inform Decis Mak. 2013;13(Suppl 3):S6.
13. Kleinman A. The illness narratives: Suffering, healing, and the human condition. Basic books; 1988.
14. Fox N, Ward K, O'Rourke A. Pro-anorexia, weight-loss drugs and the Internet: an 'anti-recovery'explanatory model of anorexia. Sociol Health Illn. 2005;27(7):944–71.
15. Kandula N. The patient explanatory mode. The Health Care Blog. http://www.northwestern.edu/newscenter/stories/2013/06/opinion-health-blog-kandula-.html (2013). Accessed 8 Jan 2016.
16. Kleinman A, Benson P. Anthropology in the clinic: the problem of cultural competency and how to fix it. PLoS Med. 2006;3(10):e294.
17. Bright Futures/American Academy of Pediatrics [Internet]. [Place unknown]: Recommendations for preventative pediatric health care; 2016. https://www.aap.org/en-us/Documents/Periodicity Schedule2015_Visionscreening.pdf.
18. Tanner JL, Stein MT, Olson LM, Frintner MP, Radecki L. Reflections on well-child care practice: a national study of pediatric clinicians. Pediatrics. 2009;124(3):849–57.
19. Nlm.nih.gov. Complementary and Integrative Medicine: MedlinePlus. https://www.nlm.nih.gov/medlineplus/complementaryandintegrativemedicine.html#summary (2016). Accessed 16 January 2016.
20. NCCIH. | NCCIH. https://nccih.nih.gov/health/acupuncture/introduction#hed3 (2008). Accessed 18 January 2016.
21. Mayoclinic.org. Vitamin C (ascorbic acid) Evidence—Mayo Clinic. http://www.mayoclinic.org/drugs-supplements/vitamin-c/evidence/hrb-20060322 (2016). Accessed 18 January 2016.
22. Mayoclinic.org. Autism treatment: Can chelation therapy help?—Mayo Clinic. http://www.mayoclinic.org/diseases-conditions/autism-spectrum-disorder/expert-answers/autism-treatment/faq-20057933 (2016). Accessed 18 January 2016.
23. Harrington JW, Rosen L, Garnecho A, Patrick PA. Parental perceptions and use of complementary and alternative medicine practices for children with autistic spectrum disorders in private practice. J Dev Behav Pediatr. 2006;27(2):S156–61.
24. Wald HS, Dube CE, Anthony DC. Untangling the Web—The impact of Internet use on health care and the physician–patient relationship. Patient Educ Couns. 2007;68(3):218–24.
25. Opel DJ, Heritage J, Taylor JA, Mangione-Smith R, Salas HS, DeVere V, Zhou C, Robinson JD. The architecture of provider-parent vaccine discussions at health supervision visits. Pediatrics. 2013;132(6):1037–46.
26. Edwards A, Elwyn G, Gwyn R. General practice registrar responses to the use of different risk communication tools in simulated consultations: a focus group study. BMJ. 1999;319(7212):749–52.

27. Marteau TM. Framing of information: Its influence upon decisions of doctors and patients. Br J Soc Psychol. 1989;28(1):89–94.
28. Levin IP, Schneider SL, Gaeth GJ. All frames are not created equal: A typology and critical analysis of framing effects. Organ Behav Hum Decis Process. 1998;76(2):149–88.
29. Lewandowsky S, Ecker UK, Seifert CM, Schwarz N, Cook J. Misinformation and its correction continued influence and successful debiasing. Psychol Sci Pub Interest. 2012;13(3):106–31.

Part II
Special Topics

Chapter 6
Vaccines

Overview

The advent of vaccinations for the prevention of dangerous infectious diseases is largely considered one of the greatest scientific advances in modern medicine [1]. In 1954 the United States government, researchers, and physicians strongly encouraged uptake of the polio vaccine. In the effects observed after wide adoption, the vaccine's efficacy and safety would seem irrefutable. Subsequently, scientists were perplexed to find that despite the strong evidence in favor of the polio vaccine, a considerable amount of parents were still hesitant to vaccinate their children. This hesitancy is credited with causing a resurgence of polio just 4 years later. Faced with the fact a psychological factor appeared to inhibit implementation of this evidence-based treatment, researchers began exploring the reasons for parental hesitancy around vaccines [2].

Vaccine hesitancy is characterized by a wide range of beliefs and subsequent behaviors about the safety, efficacy, and/or need for vaccination [3]. The term vaccine hesitancy is suggested to decrease the polarization created by the more static terms "pro-vaccine" and "anti-vaccine" [4]. It also more accurately describes the diverse psychological landscape of those with concerns about vaccines. Vaccine hesitant parents (VHP) are a heterogeneous group, defined by a multitude of characteristics influenced by local and global contexts [4]. The reasons for parents' hesitancy about vaccines are similarly complex, stemming from various reasons, and influenced by social factors [4].

Despite national and international research on vaccine hesitancy, the field still lacks a clear model to comprehensively explain parental views and resulting actions [2, 4]. For example, some parents who ask questions about vaccines are not displaying hesitancy in the traditional sense of the word [1]. Their questions may indicate healthy parental interest in medical practices and general regard for their children's health [1]. Many parents consider their vaccine inquiries a form of advocacy for their children [3]. Parental advocacy has a hypothesized connection with parental self-efficacy, the sense of feeling competent and confident in being able to achieve desired outcomes through effort and action on the part of the individual [3, 5]. In turn, parental self-efficacy has been linked with higher vaccination rates [6]. Without a viable explanatory model for VHP, most recommendations to physicians for responding to vaccine inquiries are not backed by evidence [2, 4].

Just as the reasons for vaccine hesitancy are varied, the behaviors resulting from vaccine hesitancy are similarly diverse. VHPs may vaccinate their children but express reticence or resentment, accept some vaccines but refuse others, delay vaccine administration creating an alternate schedule based on preference instead of evidence, refuse vaccines outright, or delay and then ultimately refuse [2, 4]. Researchers directly observe the distinction between beliefs and actions by asking parents what they think and measuring what they do. When a traditional healthcare provider was involved in their decision-making process, rates of on-time vaccination remain high even in populations with a high proportion of VHPs [2, 7]. The Centers for Disease Control and Prevention track vaccination rates on an ongoing basis to monitor if population herd immunity (defined as at least 90% vaccination) is being maintained [1]. The CDC reports that in 2014, less than 1% of children 19–35 months received no vaccinations at all [8]. The center estimated that the 90% target coverage rate met for at least three doses of the polio vaccine, at least one dose of measles, mumps, and rubella vaccine, at least three doses of hepatitis B vaccine, and at least one dose of the varicella vaccine [8].

Concerns regarding vaccines have been present since their introduction to the public, but modern factors mark the current climate of vaccine hesitancy. The unique characteristics of twenty-first century vaccine hesitancy can perhaps guide specific recommendations for response.

Ubiquitous information technology is an oft-cited reason for modern vaccine hesitancy. The rise of easily disseminated, accessible, unreliable information through the Internet and social media is a potential source for misinformation that subsequently drives vaccine hesitancy [1, 9, 10]. It is unclear whether or not patients can, independently, distinguish accurate sources of information from the boundless misinformation available [3]. One study found that parents who had not followed the recommended vaccine schedule were more likely to have reported that their most trusted source of information about vaccines came from an Internet health information site than parents who did follow the schedule [11]. Although this statistic is discouraging, the overall proportion of parents who reported placing the most trust in the Internet for their health care information was low. Even among parents who did not follow the recommended schedule, only 7.7% reported placing most trust in the Internet [11]. This chapter outlines how to discuss false material posted online that patients have encountered.

The twenty-first century has also seen a rise of influential individuals with no medical background, such as celebrities, disseminating their personal, unscientific views to a wide audience [2]. Beyond simply stating their own unproven or blatantly false views, some individuals carry their influence further: They urge parents to refuse or delay vaccinations for their children, making a general recommendation despite their lack of medical training and pediatric healthcare knowledge [2]. Although misguided, these celebrities' pleas to avoid vaccination typically arise from painful personal experiences with their own children's health that they attribute to vaccines [12]. Personal entreaties are uniquely suited to persuade others in their decision-making. This chapter explores how the power of the personal can be used to convey accurate information rather than false information.

Finally, the increasing number of vaccinations, which has crowded the vaccination schedule, has raised parental confusion and concern [9, 13]. As medicine advances, more vaccines are recommended, and they can be administered in varying combinations [4]. Researchers acknowledge that the new vaccination schedule is "more crowded and confusing" than ever [9]. For example, the recommended immunization schedule now includes protection for infants from rotavirus and for adolescents from meningitis [1]. Today's parents did not receive these vaccines themselves as children and most are unfamiliar with them [1]. The addition of the annual influenza vaccination is another new recommended vaccine for parents to question every year [1]. The current schedule has prompted some parents who are not otherwise against vaccines to balk at the number of vaccines recommended, the number that are administered within one visit, and the frequency of vaccinations [1]. Rather than assume these parents are globally negative about vaccines and interact with them according to this false presumption, this chapter provides recommendations for responding to parents' specific concerns (Table 6.1).

Common Misconceptions

Vaccine hesitancy is due to underestimating the severity of the diseases the vaccines prevent, particularly because these diseases and their effects have been out of the general population's experience for a generation

This explanation for vaccine hesitancy is widely posited [1, 10]. Despite its popularity, the data do not support this explanation as the exclusive reason for vaccine hesitancy. In one survey of 376 parents, only 11% expressed concern that children are given vaccines for diseases they are unlikely to get, and 8% believed that vaccines are given for diseases that are not serious [1].

As far as diseases whose effects have been forgotten by the collective public memory, the vaccine with the weakest tie to this argument is influenza. Influenza kills an estimated 36,000 Americans per year and hospitalizes approximately 200,000 [10]. Even with these high rates, in a survey of 1,500 parents, respondents reported refusing the influenza vaccine most frequently [11]. The most common reason parents cited for refusal was that the vaccine was not necessary [11]. In another study that specifically outlined the dangers of influenza, no change was seen among participants in terms of their belief about the severity of the flu or

Table 6.1 Common parental concerns

Concern	Response
Too many vaccines can "overload" a young immune system [1, 2, 9, 10, 13–16]	Babies' immune systems encounter trillions of bacteria, each of which has between 2,000 and 6,000 immunological components. Today's vaccines contain 150 immunological components [13]. Babies' immune systems respond to many more germs in their day to day lives than they do when they get vaccines.
Vaccines contain harmful ingredients [1, 3, 14, 17]	All ingredients in vaccines are safe [17]. Vaccines are made of: *antigens*—the thing that shows the body how to respond to specific viruses and bacteria—the representative of the virus or bacteria *adjuvants*—make vaccines work better than they used to. Ingredients added to vaccines to make them work *preservatives*—keep vaccines free of germs *additives*—keep vaccines effective when not used right away *residuals*—needed to make the vaccines; largely filtered out, but tiny amounts remain
Vaccines contain mercury [14, 16–18]	Some vaccines, including the influenza vaccine, do contain trace amounts of mercury [16]. The kind of mercury in vaccines is also found in water, air, soil, and breast milk [18]. Infants who breast-feed receive 15 times the amount of mercury found in one influenza vaccine from their mothers' milk. The less safe form of mercury is found in fish [18].
Vaccines contain Thimerosal [9, 10, 15, 16, 18]	Thimerosal is a residual in the influenza vaccine, and it does contain small amounts of safe mercury [18]. Thimerosal used to be in more vaccines [16]. Despite having no evidence it was unsafe, the AAP and Public Health Service asked for its removal [16]. Parents are now subsequently skeptical that it is safe, because it has been removed from so many vaccines.
Vaccines contain formaldehyde [14, 16, 17]	Formaldehyde is a residual in the polio, Hepatitis A, diphtheria, and tetanus vaccines [17]. Formaldehyde is also found in paper towels, mascara, carpet, and human blood. Human blood contains ten times the amount of formaldehyde than is in any vaccine [16].
Vaccines contain aluminum [14, 16, 17]	Aluminum is in vaccines because it makes them work better [16]. Aluminum is in air, water, food (including breast milk), and human blood. Researchers tested babies' blood after receiving a vaccine to see if the normal aluminum level (5 billionths of a gram per milliliter of blood) increases after getting a vaccine. It does not.
Vaccines contain gelatin [16, 17]	Gelatin is an additive in vaccines [16]. It is safe and found in many dietary products. Because gelatin comes from skin or hooves of pigs, some people are uncomfortable with it and some religions prohibit consumption of pig byproducts. Gelatin in vaccines is purified and broken down by water, so it resembles nothing like skin or hooves. Religious leaders have spoken out in favor of vaccines with gelatin because: the component has been broken down, the amount of gelatin in vaccines is smaller than any amount found in nature, it is not ingested, and encountering gelatin in this format is unimportant when weighed against saving the lives of children.
Vaccines contain antifreeze [14, 17]	Vaccines do not contain antifreeze (ethylene glycol, which is unsafe). They do contain polyethylene glycol, which is safe. Polyethylene glycol is also found in toothpaste [17].

(continued)

Table 6.1 (continued)

Concern	Response
Vaccines cause allergic reactions [3, 14, 16, 17]	Vaccines either contain or are packaged in four things that can cause allergic reactions in individuals with these allergies: gelatin, antibiotics, egg protein, and latex (packaging). Doctors ask about these allergies before administering vaccines that contain these ingredients. Children with these allergies cannot receive all their vaccinations, so they depend on children who can to protect them via herd immunity [16].
It is more "natural" for children to get diseases than receive the vaccine [3, 14]	Vaccines do not protect children from disease; they alert children's bodies to make antibodies to the disease. Children's bodies create these antibodies in the same fashion whether prompted to by a vaccine or contracting the illness [14]. On a broader note, everyone engages in "unnatural" activities every day, such as washing hands, using electricity, and sleeping on mattresses. Natural is not necessarily safer or better.
Vaccines can cause long-term complications [1, 9, 14]	Vaccines have been used in the United State since 1954 [2]. If there were long-term complications, they would be ubiquitous and well known [14]. There are no plausible explanations as to how vaccines could cause long-term side effects.
Vaccines cause short-term effects such as pain, crying, and stress [1, 9, 13]	Babies do experience distress associated with vaccines, such as pain and stress, which lead to crying. To find out if multiple vaccines given at once caused babies more stress than one, researchers looked at their levels of cortisol (a marker of stress) in their saliva. Babies who received two shots were not more stressed than those receiving one [13].
Vaccines give children the disease [10, 14]	Only one vaccine might give a child the disease: the oral polio vaccine, which is no longer administered in the United States [14]. No other vaccine gives the child the disease. In some cases, the child's body may show it is making antibodies in response to the vaccine [14]. These indicators appear like minor aspects of the disease, such as a small rash [14].
Vaccines cause autism [1, 9, 10, 15, 17–19]	That vaccines cause autism is a myth based on the activities of one fraudulent researcher. This researcher received payments from lawyers of parents who were suing companies who made vaccines [20]. The researcher manipulated his selection of 12 children (some of whom were parties in the lawsuit), to publish a paper suggesting there may be a link between the MMR vaccine and autism [20].
Vaccines are unnecessary because they prevent diseases that are not common [1–3, 9–11, 14]	Vaccination is just one of many modern practices performed to protect against unlikely but grave events. Another example is wearing seatbelts. Some of the diseases vaccines protect against are rare. But vaccination is recommended for two reasons: to protect the vaccinated child and to protect other children who are medically vulnerable and cannot be vaccinated [14].
Vaccines are unnecessary because they prevent diseases that are not serious [1, 9–11]	Many diseases that parents may have lived through (chickenpox, influenza) are dangerous because of their potential for devastating complications [14]. True influenza kills 36,000 Americans per year, and children are particularly vulnerable [14]. Before the varicella vaccine, chicken pox used to kill 1 child per week in the United States [14]. These deaths stemmed from complications such as infections of the brain, flesh-eating strep, toxic shock syndrome, hepatitis, and pneumonia [14].

(continued)

Table 6.1 (continued)

Concern	Response
Vaccines are recommended because pharmaceutical companies profit from them [3, 9]	Pharmaceutical companies would not be as rich as they are if they relied on vaccinations for their profits. Vaccines make up a very slim proportion of overall sales [21]. This figure is reduced further after factoring in the costs of an average of 15 years' worth of research and development per vaccine, only 10% of which ultimately enter the market [21, 22].
More testing is needed to show that vaccines are safe and effective [1, 3, 13]	Vaccines have been extensively tested, and each time a new vaccine combination is recommended, it is tested in **concomitant use studies**. These studies determine that not only is the vaccine safe, but that it is safe to be given with the other vaccines administered at the same time [13].
Laws requiring vaccination for certain activities disregard individual rights [1, 10, 14]	True. Many laws disregard the rights of the individual, such as laws requiring motorists to have car insurance, drivers to stop at red traffic lights, or people not to murder one another. That is because some actions are recognized as crucial to saving lives, but they require the cooperation of many to be effective [14].

their intention to vaccinate [23]. The study authors concluded that the dangers of the illness were already widely accepted, so providing further information was not effective in increasing intent to vaccinate [23]. This stands in contrast to MMR, which protects against less prevalent diseases. In this case, the same 1,500 parents surveyed reported hesitancy due to a concern of serious side effects from the vaccine rather than lack of concern about disease severity or likelihood [11].

The World Health Organization SAGE working group created the "Three C model" to explain the reasons parents show vaccine hesitancy [24]; *complacency*, *convenience*, and *confidence* [24]. Subsequent researchers examining the behavioral aspects of VHP added in a fourth—*calculation*—that involves the calculation of expected utility that parents conduct when deciding whether or not to vaccinate [25]. Calculation appears to have an overarching effect on hesitancy regardless of whether the parent is complacent, barred by inconvenience, or concerned. The process of calculating the cost versus benefit of engaging in any medical intervention lies at the heart of informed consent. Rather than assume ignorance on the part of parents, it is more prudent to determine which of the "Cs" are driving their hesitancy [25]. In our recommendations section, we outline the three unique Cs and suggested responses.

Parents who ask questions about vaccines do not trust their physicians

Approximately 30% of sampled doctors report dissatisfaction in their practice when parents express concerns around vaccines [9]. Among this group, 29% interpreted the parents' questions as a lack of trust in their experience and respect for their judgment [9]. Yet patients consistently identify physicians as their most trusted source of vaccination information [9, 11, 26–28].

Initially hesitant parents who changed their minds about vaccinating their children reported largely doing so as a result of their trusted physician providing them with assurance as to the decision to vaccinate [9, 29]. This effect of physician influence held for both parents who wanted to delay vaccinations and those who initially refused vaccinations outright [9]. One study of 122 VHP participants found that approximately 87% reported their physician was their trustworthy source for information on vaccines [3]. When creating a measure to quantify parents' levels of vaccine hesitancy, the developers had to remove the item about trusting one's doctors because the responses they received on preliminary versions of the measure were too positively skewed to provide any meaningful input into the score [3].

Parents also identify friends (26%), family (25%), and the Internet (39%) as sources of reliable health information [3]. Aware that their patients also seek out other sources of information, physicians may misattribute these conversations or searches to a lack of trust in their opinion. While this may be true for certain patients, others consider researching vaccines as part of their role as health advocate for their children [3]. Rather than avoid the opinions of friends and family, physicians can directly ask their patients to share what their social group thinks. In this way, the physician validates the parents' social support group and information-seeking behaviors. If friends and family have communicated any misinformation, the doctor can address it in the same manner as if the patient had arrived at that incorrect information on their own—nonjudgmentally and nondefensively.

With the Internet available to many parents at almost all hours of the day, it is not surprising that some will research vaccine information online. Evidence shows that many parents access this kind of information. In one survey of 376 parents, 60% reported searching the Internet for either "some" or "a lot" of vaccine information [1]. Fortunately, accurate information from reliable sources regarding vaccines is widely available to both parents and doctors. The AAP, CDC, and the Vaccine Education Center at the Children's Hospital of Pennsylvania provide detailed information sheets specifically addressing common parental concerns regarding vaccination [3]. These organizations provide online information sheets and toolkits [3]. In their practices, however, few physicians make use of these resources [9]. Only 28% of physicians in one study were observed to distribute such information sheets to their patients [9]. Given that many parents report searching for this information, collaborating with patients in their searches guides them to more accurate sources. Embracing the new learning and advocacy styles of parents includes showing them reliable sources of information and teaching them to remain skeptical of ambiguous sources.

There is not enough time in a typical office visit to discuss vaccines to patients' satisfaction

A large number of physicians are concerned about the amount of time needed to effectively discuss vaccines with parents, particularly VHP. In one study, 62% of clinicians reported that time was at least somewhat a barrier to these discussions, if not a major barrier [9]. Yet studies indicate that patients do not require longer visits to experience an increase in satisfaction and adherence with their physicians' recommendations [1]. In fact, both patients and physicians rate shorter interactions as more positive, indicating goal alignment [1]. It has been found that the length of discussions with VHP could reach 19 minutes, with 92% of physicians reporting discussions this length or shorter [9]. Specifically, 53% spent between 10 and 19 minutes on these conversations, and 36% spent between 5 and 9 minutes [9]. Addressing patient concerns rather than pursuing physician agenda was also rated as more positive by patients [1]. Recommendations to tailor information to the parent's specific concerns will help to keep the discussions short and the visit patient-centered.

Current Research

Many rigorous research studies show that most of the parental concerns (Table 6.1) are either completely unfounded or only marginally founded in scientific evidence. There is a seeming contradiction in parents who take their children to pediatricians but state skepticism of the results of the scientific process. Western medicine in general is founded on scientific principles. Even treatments that were originally uncovered through nonscientific means (tree bark for the treatment of pain, for example), have been subsequently proven through the scientific method [30]. Parents who visit pediatricians show an implicit trust and respect for the scientific method. Why then, when presented with research disputing false claims about vaccines, do they remain skeptical?

At least part of the answer lies in the precision with which the scientific method operates and the limitations it places on itself. Results that are conclusive from a research standpoint appear inconclusive when relayed to individuals who do not understand how research studies and statistical analyses are performed. The root cause of the confusion can be traced back to the null hypothesis, discussed in Chap. 2. As cautioned then, the null hypothesis—that A does not cause B—cannot be proven in the scientific method. Unfortunately, many parental concerns stem from whether A did cause B. While parents are concerned that vaccines cause any number of adverse outcomes, the scientific process can only conclude when A *does* cause B. Science cannot provide conclusive assurance that A did not cause B, which is exactly what parents are asking it to when they explain their vaccine hesitancy [19]. These parents insist that they will only be reassured when a study proves, for example, that the MMR vaccine does not cause autism. Scientists remaining faithful to their method and its limitations cannot provide false reassurance [19].

Researchers usually cannot definitively state findings, even when there is overwhelming evidence to support them, which can lead to confusion for parents and in the media [19]. Meanwhile, anti-vaccine advocates will stress that science still has not performed a study conclusively proving vaccines do not cause autism. What they fail to acknowledge is that science cannot do this. Even if a double-blind, randomized controlled study were performed where in some children received vaccines and others did not (an unethical study that would never be conducted), there would still be an element of statistical doubt. Clearly, clarification of the scientific process is needed in these cases.

To Explain to a Patient

I understand why many intelligent people say that, until a study is done proving vaccines do not cause autism, scientists are still unsure of the answer. When a committee performs an extensive review of the research literature showing a multitude of evidence that vaccines do not cause ill effects and then says things like, "its conclusion does not exclude the possibility that MMR vaccine could contribute to ASD in a small number of children" [31] it sounds like scientists still have no idea.

But really, they do. You know how in a court of law in the United States, an accused person is said to be presumed innocent unless proven guilty? That means that people do not have to prove their innocence to be set free; they simply have to not be proven guilty. Science is like that. Science cannot prove something like vaccine's innocence even if it wanted to. All it can do is fail over and over again, in many repeated trials, to find it guilty beyond a reasonable doubt. Science is only ever the legal team for the prosecution, never the defense. Asking science to provide vaccine don't have ill effects is like asking the prosecution to go work for the defense. It can't.

Imagine you were on trial for a crime you didn't commit. How many times would you be able to sit through trials, each time with the verdict coming back "Not guilty" until you would demand to be set free? Vaccines have been through many such trials, and each time the verdict is "not guilty beyond a reasonable doubt." I know finding proof that vaccines are innocent of the crimes they've been accused of would feel better, but the way the scientific method is set up, it just cannot do that.

(An explanation such as this does two things. First, it validates the confusion that arises when only one side of an issue can be proven. Second, it highlights that things other than just medicine can only operate when a certain amount of uncertainty is involved.)

Current Research

Research is still ongoing as to the optimal way to discuss vaccines with VHP [11]. Here, however, are some recommendations that are founded on the research on VHP that has conducted so far.

Listen to Parent Concerns First [10]

This recommendation appears first because it should occur first in the consultation. Without initially familiarizing themselves with a patient's specific concerns, physicians cannot root the subsequent discussion in patient-centeredness. Pediatricians should identify the specific concerns parents have by asking open-ended questions. Some parents may not have specific concerns, but instead say they are generally worried. Doctors who ask these parents what they are worried might happen if they vaccinate their children will have a better sense of what the specific concern is, even if the parent cannot articulate it directly.

Empathize and Reflect Back Concerns [2]

At this point, we integrate the research showing that physicians' personal guidance is rated as most helpful to patients. Physicians can introduce their own impressions into the consultation at the point of discussing concerns. Pediatricians are well equipped to handle parents' emotions. Here, they can empathize with the feeling of fear or worry without acknowledging those feelings to be founded in true risk. Statements such as, "I feel concerned about medical procedures until I learn more about them, too," validate the patient's feelings, bring the physician into the conversation in an authentic way, and do not erroneously give the impression that the specific fear is well-founded. Then, to acknowledge that the parent's specific concerns have been heard, the physician can reflect it back in an emotionally neutral fashion, "It sounds like one thing you want to learn more about is potential side effects of this vaccine."

Determine Which Cs Are Driving the Hesitancy [25]

- **Complacency**: Parents who are complacent do not have particularly strong feelings for or against vaccines [25]. Therefore, asking them for their concerns about vaccines is unlikely to be a fruitful effort. These parents are also more likely to perceive that the risks of contracting a vaccine-preventable illness are low, making engagement in protective action a low priority [25]. To identify complacent parents, doctors can listen for comments that indicate a non-committal attitude and a lack of concern.

Complacent parents would benefit from hearing risk information about the diseases vaccines protect against, hearing about social motives to vaccinate so that they feel more comfortable with the decision to vaccinate, and strong recommendations from their physicians [25].

- **Convenience**: Parents who are vaccine hesitant due to convenience factors also do not have strong feelings about vaccines [25]. Therefore, other life needs will come between them and vaccination. To identify parents with convenience concerns, pediatricians can listen for statements about the family's functioning and identify missed appointments or scheduling difficulties. Structural barriers impede vaccination but are unlikely to be truly preventing them if the parent is already in the physician's office.

  Physicians can take steps to reduce the barriers for the patients' next appointments, such as asking parents to explicitly state their intentions to continue the vaccinations as scheduled, scheduling the next appointment during the current one, and asking office staff to place repeated phone calls and reminders for upcoming appointments. Similar to recommendations for complacent parents, pediatricians with parents affected by convenience should provide risk information about the diseases vaccines prevent, discuss social motives to vaccinate, and provide strong recommendations.

- **Confidence**: Parents struggling with confidence do not have sufficient trust in either the efficacy or safety of the vaccines themselves, the system of vaccine delivery, and/or the motivations of those who make vaccination recommendations [24]. Unlike parents who are either complacent or affected by convenience, parents with concern do show strong feelings about vaccines in general [25]. Their knowledge of vaccines is more likely to be inaccurate rather than absent [25]. Concerned parents are more likely to identify as someone who is anti-vaccine or associate with social groups who identify as such [25]. To determine VHP with concerns, pediatricians will want to listen to the concerns parents provide. Concerns of these parents are likely to reflect a lack of trust (in "Big Pharma," the government, etc.) or a misplaced trust in incorrect information about vaccines that have already been debunked in mainstream literature and media.

Strategies to reduce hesitancy in concerned parents differ from the recommendations for complacent or inconvenienced parents. The main strategy proposed by researchers is to debunk the myths that cause their concerns. Doctors would do well to follow Lewandowsky's process for debunking myths [32], discussed in Chap. 5. Attempts to debunk myths that do not follow his procedures can backfire, making the parent believe the myth even more. Providing an alternative explanation to supplant the parent's misinformation is strongly recommended. Without an alternative explanation, the parent is left with a gap in their mind that they must fill with something [32]. Individuals who fill these gaps with conspiracy theories have also been found to be more likely to reject mainstream scientific evidence [33–35].

Research on VHP discourages attempting to provide a social context to concerned parents. These parents likely already identify as outside the social norm [25]. Their affiliation with a smaller, anti-vaccine social context is likely to become further entrenched if they perceive it as being directly attacked [25].

Also discouraged is delivering risk information in extremes, particularly when parents already lack trust in the source of information [36]. Parents with low trust are more likely to reject information about risk that claims that vaccines have no risk than they are a tempered statement about risk [36]. If parents are wary of pharmaceutical companies, provide information from alternative sources. For example, parents with strong conviction in complementary and alternative medicine (CAM) are more likely to incorporate accurate information about vaccines if it comes from a website devoted to CAM practices.

Address Only Stated Concerns [1, 11]

This recommendation is based on three pieces of evidence. First, this suggestion tailors the information provided to the individual patient's needs [1, 11]. While the first recommendations set up the physician to provide a patient-centered experience, this recommendation is the necessary follow-through.

Second, research shows that neither patients nor physicians garner more satisfaction from longer discussions, which indicates that briefer discussions are preferable. Brevity, however, cannot be the ultimate goal, because all the concerns the patient raises need to be addressed. The goal is to address all concern efficiently. The greatest efficiency is achieved by providing only the information parents will need to put their concerns to rest.

Third, research shows that providing information that is not connected to a given patient's concerns can backfire [23]. In particular, providing accurate information about the side effects of both the MMR and influenza vaccines to parents with high levels of concern about side effects backfired [23, 37]. While providing the information did result in an increase in parental knowledge, intentions to vaccinate their children actually decreased among the parents with high levels of initial concern [23].

Remain Open and Non-Coercive [2]

During the discussion, parents may say things that are inaccurate because they either do not have all the information or have been misinformed. Neither of these situations ensure that they will refuse vaccines, and neither of these necessarily mean that they do not trust their doctors. Yet, as often observed in the political realm, when people's views are threatened, they tend to dig in their heels further [38]. Researchers found artifacts of a similar effect when presenting parents with corrective information about vaccine side effects [23, 27]. Certain parents actually reduced their intentions to vaccinate after learning about the real, lower risk of side effects than they originally believed in [23, 37]. The researchers inferred that those respondents must have had additional concerns that they were attempting to preserve, and therefore held on more tightly to their decision not to vaccinate even after the side effect information was appropriately conveyed [23]. Physicians who are coercive are not following a patient-centered approach. Physicians who remain open, ask questions, and provide information, without pressuring, when patients ask, have a better chance of their patients arriving at the medically indicated conclusion.

Exercise Caution When Asking Parents to Sign the Refusal to Vaccinate Form [10]

To dissuade parents from settling into static stances or roles, physicians should remain flexible about parents' decisions to withhold or delay vaccines at any given visit. As we have seen, parents can have specific views or concerns without letting those thoughts affect their ultimate choice in behavior. This is because views need not equate to identity. However, parents who take on an identity as an "anti-vaccine" parent will be much less likely to change their views in future. Therefore, the AAP recommendation that pediatricians ask parents to sign a Refusal to Vaccinate form should be followed carefully. Physicians can explain that a signature on the form is for the physician to be clear about the parent's choice that day. They can also explain that this form serves as a reminder to the physician to follow up at the next visit to reconsider vaccination at that time. In this way, the doctor plays a key role in helping parents to see their decision as one choice made at a specific point in time, and not as part of their identity.

Conclusion

Hand in hand with these recommendations is a reminder that while many parents show concerns about vaccines, most still choose to vaccinate their children anyway [14]. This framework guides recommendations in two ways. The first is to keep any pressure or coercion out of the process. In all likelihood, parents asking these questions will vaccinate their children. The second is to manage parents' ideas and feelings more than to focus on their resulting behavior. Clearly, some parents are vaccinating their children without confidence or satisfaction in their choice to do so. Some parents will vaccinate but feel afraid when doing so. Other parents will vaccinate but feel resentful when doing so. Resentment is particularly implied when parents vaccinate due to regulations requiring them for admission to schools or day care. These regulations can lead parents to feel coerced or that their rights as a parent have been disregarded [1, 14]. In addition to helping parents achieve adequate vaccination for their children, pediatricians are in a unique position to also reassure parents as to their decision.

Delivery of patient-centered care is uniquely challenging when there is only one medically indicated choice, but the decision itself is value-laden [26]. Vaccines fit the criterion of having one clear medical prescription. Barring religious objections, which have largely been addressed by spiritual leaders recommending their followers vaccinate their children, there is no remaining value prohibiting parents from accepting vaccines [16]. Skepticism, misunderstanding, and fear are not values. To treat them as such fuels the view that patients are not capable of incorporating new knowledge into their frameworks, and thus learning and overcoming their fears. Such a conception of patients' capabilities is a decidedly paternalistic one. Addressing a specific patient's questions and concerns in an approach tailored to meet their needs while ultimately recommending the evidence-based intervention meets the standard for patient-centered care.

References

1. Kennedy A, LaVail K, Nowak G, Basket M, Landry S. Confidence about vaccines in the United States: understanding parents' perceptions. Health Aff. 2011;30(6):1151–9.
2. Smith PJ, Humiston SG, Marcuse EK, Zhao Z, Dorell CG, Howes C, Hibbs B. Parental delay or refusal of vaccine doses, childhood vaccination coverage at 24 months of age, and the Health Belief Model. Public Health Rep. 2011;126(Suppl 2):135.
3. Opel DJ, Mangione-Smith R, Taylor JA, Korfiatis C, Wiese C, Catz S, Martin DP. Development of a survey to identify vaccine-hesitant parents: the parent attitudes about childhood vaccines survey. Human vaccines. 2011;7(4):419–25.
4. Larson HJ, Jarrett C, Eckersberger E, Smith DM, Paterson P. Understanding vaccine hesitancy around vaccines and vaccination from a global perspective: a systematic review of published literature, 2007–2012. Vaccine. 2014;32(19):2150–9.
5. Bandura A. Self-efficacy: toward a unifying theory of behavioral change. Psychol Rev. 1977;84(2):191–215.
6. Taylor JA, Cufley D. The association between parental health beliefs and immunization status among children followed by private pediatricians. Clin Pediatr. 1996;35(1):18–22.
7. Williams SE, Rothman RL, Offit PA, Schaffner W, Sullivan M, Edwards KM. A randomized trial to increase acceptance of childhood vaccines by vaccine-hesitant parents: a pilot study. Acad Pediatr. 2013;13(5):475–80.
8. Cdc.gov. National, State, and Selected Local Area Vaccination Coverage Among Children Aged 19–35 Months—United States, 2014. 2016 http://www.cdc.gov/mmwr/preview/mmwrhtml/mm6433a1.htm Accessed 26 Jan 2016.
9. Kempe A, Daley MF, McCauley MM, Crane LA, Suh CA, Kennedy AM, Basket MM, Stokley SK, Dong F, Babbel CI, Seewald LA. Prevalence of parental concerns about childhood vaccines: the experience of primary care physicians. Am J Prev Med. 2011;40(5):548–55.
10. American Academy of Pediatrics. Immunization Resources Addressing Common Concerns of Vaccine-Hesitant Parents. 2016 https://www.aap.org/en-us/Documents/immunization_vaccine-hesitant%20parent_final.pdf Accessed 19 Jan 2016.
11. McCauley MM, Kennedy A, Basket M, Sheedy K. Exploring the choice to refuse or delay vaccines: a national survey of parents of 6-through 23-month-olds. Acad Pediatr. 2012;12(5):375–83.

12. Rapp ID, Braasch JL, Ecker UK, Swire B, Lewandowsky S. Correcting Misinformation—A Challenge for Education and Cognitive Science.
13. Chop.edu. Too Many Vaccines? What you should know. 2016. http://www.butlercountyo-hio.org/health/content/documents/Can%20We%20Get%20Too%20Many%20Vaccines.pdf Accessed 19 Jan 2016.
14. U.S. Department of Health and Human Services. Parent's Guide to Childhood Immunizations. 2016. http://www.cdc.gov/vaccines/pubs/parents-guide/downloads/parents-guide-508.pdf Accessed 19 Jan 2016.
15. Chop.edu. Vaccines and Autism: What you should know. 2016. http://www.immune.org.nz/sites/default/files/resources/ConcernVaccinesAutismChop2012.pdf Accessed 19 Jan 2016.
16. Chop.edu. Vaccine Ingredients: What you should know. 2016. https://vec.chop.edu/export/download/pdfs/articles/vaccine-education-center/vaccine-ingredients.pdf Accessed 19 Jan 2016.
17. HealthyChildren.org. Vaccine Ingredients: Frequently Asked Questions. 2016. https://www.healthychildren.org/English/safety-prevention/immunizations/Pages/Vaccine-Ingredients-Frequently-Asked-Questions.aspx Accessed 19 Jan 2016.
18. Chop.edu. Vaccine Ingredients – Thimerosall The Children's Hospital of Philadelphia. 2016. http://www.chop.edu/centers-programs/vaccine-education-center/vaccine-ingredients/thimer-osal#.Vp6cdk-bGNl Accessed 19 Jan 2016.
19. Offit PA, Coffin SE. Communicating science to the public: MMR vaccine and autism. Vaccine. 2003;22(1):1–6.
20. Rao TS, Andrade C. The MMR vaccine and autism: sensation, refutation, retraction, and fraud. Indian J Psychiatry. 2011;53(2):95.
21. Offit PA. Why are pharmaceutical companies gradually abandoning vaccines? Health Aff. 2005;24(3):622–30.
22. Lam B. Vaccines Are Profitable, So What? The Atlantic. 2015. http://www.theatlantic.com/business/archive/2015/02/vaccines-are-profitable-so-what/385214/ Accessed 31 Jan 2016.
23. Nyhan B, Reifler J. Does correcting myths about the flu vaccine work? an experimental evaluation of the effects of corrective information. Vaccine. 2015;33(3):459–64.
24. MacDonald NE. Vaccine hesitancy: definition, scope and determinants. Vaccine. 2015 Apr 17.
25. Betsch C, Böhm R, Chapman GB. Using behavioral insights to increase vaccination policy effectiveness. Policy Insights from the Behav Brain Sci. 2015;2(1):61–73.
26. Opel DJ, Heritage J, Taylor JA, Mangione-Smith R, Salas HS, DeVere V, Zhou C, Robinson JD. The architecture of provider-parent vaccine discussions at health supervision visits. Pediatrics. 2013;132(6):1037–46.
27. Freed GL, Clark SJ, Butchart AT, Singer DC, Davis MM. Parental vaccine safety concerns in 2009. Pediatrics. 2010;125(4):654–9.
28. Gellin BG, Maibach EW, Marcuse EK. Do parents understand immunizations? A national telephone survey. Pediatrics. 2000;106(5):1097–1102.
29. Gust DA, Darling N, Kennedy A, Schwartz B. Parents with doubts about vaccines: which vaccines and reasons why. Pediatrics. 2008;122(4):718–25.
30. Mahdi JG, Mahdi AJ, Bowen ID. The historical analysis of aspirin discovery, its relation to the willow tree and antiproliferative and anticancer potential. Cell Prolif. 2006;39(2):147–55.
31. Stratton K, Gable A, Shetty P, McCormick M, editors. Institute of Medicine. Immunization safety review: measles-mumps-rubella vaccine and autism. Washington, DC: National Academy Press. 2001.
32. Lewandowsky S, Ecker UK, Seifert CM, Schwarz N, Cook J. Misinformation and its correction continued influence and successful debiasing. Psychol Sci Public Interest. 2012;13(3):106–31.
33. Lewandowsky S, Gignac GE, Oberauer K. The role of conspiracist ideation and worldviews in predicting rejection of science. PLoS ONE. 2013;8(10):e75637.
34. Lewandowsky S, Gignac GE, Oberauer K. The robust relationship between conspiracism and denial of (climate) science. Psychol Sci. 2015;26(5):667–70.

35. Lewandowsky S, Oberauer K, Gignac GE. NASA faked the moon landing—therefore, (climate) science is a hoax an anatomy of the motivated rejection of science. Psychol Sci. 2013;24(5):622–33.
36. Betsch C, Sachse K. Debunking vaccination myths: strong risk negations can increase perceived vaccination risks. Health Psychol. 2013;32(2):146.
37. Nyhan B, Reifler J, Richey S, Freed GL. Effective messages in vaccine promotion: a randomized trial. Pediatrics. 2014;133(4):e835–42.
38. Nyhan B, Reifler J. When corrections fail: the persistence of political misperceptions. Polit Behav. 2010;32(2):303–30.

Chapter 7
Diet

Overview

On the whole, parents report that providing their children with a healthy diet is one of their highest priorities [1, 2]. Parents correctly perceive the importance of their role in their children's nutrition; they are the primary "gatekeepers" of their children's diet up to the age of approximately 6 years old [1]. Despite parents' stated investment in this goal, they often fall short. Parents find that feeding their children a nutritious, well-balanced diet is one of their most stressful parenting tasks [1]. According to one hypothesis, this frustration originates, in part, from the drastic difference between feeding practices in early human history and the environment in which parents currently find themselves [3]. Specifically, most of human evolution occurred in the context of food scarcity and high levels of activity required to obtain sufficient food [3]. As such, humans are biologically conditioned to seek out calorie-dense foods to offset the influences of limited food and great energy expenditure [3]. Today's landscape for most people living in developed nations includes an abundance of foods, eliminating energy acquisition as a problem [3]. However, sufficient nutrition intake remains a challenge. Coupled with the lack of energy expenditure in common society, the consumption of high-energy, low-nutrition foods has given rise to obesity [4].

Obesity, a so-called "disease of affluence," has struck children as well as adults in the United States [5]. Owing to under-consumption of key food groups, such as vegetables and fruits, children often do not receive the recommended amount of many key nutrients. In addition, children are eating too many low-nutrient, high-energy foods [5]. Eating patterns established in childhood persist well into adulthood, making the goal of providing a healthy diet all the more important [6]. Given the discrepancy between parents' stated goals and actual goal attainment, researchers have begun investigating the possible reasons parents have been unable to achieve a healthy diet for their children [1]. In addition to exploring the

© Springer International Publishing AG 2017
C.A. Di Bartolo and M.K. Braun, *Pediatrician's Guide to Discussing Research with Patients*, DOI 10.1007/978-3-319-49547-7_7

mechanisms that obstruct healthy eating, the second purpose of this research is to develop effective interventions [1]. To date, there are few effective interventions that target the individual parent-child dyad [7].

A simple proposed theory as to why parents do not provide healthy diets for their children despite their intentions is that parents do not have the requisite nutrition knowledge to do so. Theories focusing on lack of parental knowledge naturally recommend distributing more information to parents [8]. According to this model, information should include what constitutes a healthy weight in addition to the components of a healthy diet. Without awareness that their children's diet is inappropriate, it is presumed parents cannot be motivated to improve it [9].

It appears, however, that dissemination interventions must include more than simply passing along needed knowledge. The information must be provided at the correct time to be useful. One such example is the timing of sharing information about breastfeeding. During pre-natal appointments with their physicians, women are widely informed about the benefits of breastfeeding for at least 1 year [8]. This is in contrast to the recommendation to delay the introduction of solid foods until a child is 6 months old, which is less known. Many parents introduce solid food before the recommended age [8]. Consequently, the 6 month visit is too late for a pediatrician to discuss the guideline with families. It becomes clear that knowledge alone is not sufficient, but that the information must be given when parents can make use of it.

Parents' perception of the field of nutrition research appears negative. Contradictory information from various sources, such as advertisers, media, and academic sources, undermine parents' ability to parse out which source is providing reliable information [9]. Questionable motives come into play, as advertisers' main goal is to sell a product [9]. The widely touted health claims advertisers make serve to undermine the information parents hear from more impartial sources, which leads to confusion [9]. The academic field contributes to the conflicting array of knowledge, as new developments in research require revisions of previous hypotheses. These revisions lead to an impression among parents that advice is constantly changing [9]. Out of frustration with the steady stream of corrections and updates, some parents become apathetic and begin ignoring information altogether [9].

Strategies for improving diet that target individual factors have shown limited efficacy [10, 11]. In addition to acquiring basic nutritional knowledge, changes in diet require concerted changes in behavior. The Theory of Planned Behavior provides a possible explanation for the struggles parents encounter when attempting to change their children's diet [12]. This theory posits that individuals require three conditions to change their behavior: 1) a positive attitude regarding the change (i.e., believe the change is important and that positive outcomes would ensue as a result of the change); 2) a perception that the norm in their social group includes the new behavior (and motivation to fit with their social group); and 3) a perception of control over whether or not the change happens [12]. Individuals with a positive attitude towards the change, a social norm that includes the new behavior, and a sense of control are thought to be more likely to establish an intention to change their behavior [12]. Some researchers hypothesize that this framework may explain the psychological barriers parents encounter when attempting to form an intention to improve their children's diet [1]. Their qualitative review of parents' statements in the three areas indicates that this theory may explain some of the discrepancy between parents' goals and their behaviors [1].

In addition to presenting individual psychological factors that may impede efforts to provide a healthy diet, parents in the Theory of Planned Behavior study were also heavily concerned about factors outside their control [1]. The parents' concerns mirror the investigative avenues of researchers who study the numerous external factors that influence children's diets [4]. While individual factors clearly impact children's diets, social, physical, and macro-environmental factors are observed to interact with outcomes as well [4]. Parents report many challenges and outright barriers in their attempts to provide a healthy diet for their children. They notice the influence advertising has on their media-consuming children [1]. Once children enter daycare or school, peers also begin to influence the foods children will try and prefer. Structural barriers such as lack of parental time to procure, prepare, and clean up after meals made of healthy foods is a commonly cited impediment. Parents also endure their children's food selectivity traits, which can range from normative to mild to extreme, but all of levels of which pose some challenge to feeding and can create a great source of frustration [1].

Finally, one of the most notable and consistent findings in feeding research is an influence not tied to parents' knowledge or external barriers. As we explore in this chapter, parenting styles—that is, not what children are fed but how parents feed their children—exert considerable sway over diet. A highly recommended parenting style is seen to reduce the influence of normative food selectivity that children begin to display around 2 years of age. This parenting style is also associated with an increased amount of nutrient-dense food consumption, along with a reduction in the amount of low-nutrient, high-energy food intake. Finally, the recommended parenting style reduces conflict between parent and child without sacrificing parental expectations for appropriate food consumption.

Despite the accurate nutrition information pediatricians have to impart, many parents do not ask their health care practitioner feeding questions [13]. Instead, parents commonly report that they ask their social group for assistance [13]. This can, unfortunately, compound the challenge of maintaining a healthy diet and healthy weight because the parents' peers may not prove to be accurate sources of information. Parents experience a spectrum of feeding problems, ranging from misperceived feeding problems, to mild feeding problems, to feeding disorders [14]. When a feeding problem rises to a meaningful level of concern for a parent, she or he may then opt to bring it up with a physician rather than rely on peers [14]. Physicians, however, need not wait until a parent raises a concern before sharing information. Parents can overestimate their knowledge of dietary recommendations, or may not realize there are errors in their knowledge that require correction [1]; a physician who proactively provides accurate information may prevent or correct problems that the parent has not even addressed. This chapter covers topics physicians can discuss with any parent, irrespective of their particular feeding concerns. Much of this information can be given preemptively, before issues arise.

Common Parental Concerns

What is Considered Healthy?

Parents consistently endorse that a nutritious diet is crucial for their child's medical, social, and educational development [1]. Despite this, 31.8% of American children and adolescents from 2009–2010 were either overweight or obese [5]. The first step in addressing the discrepancy is often to examine parental knowledge of nutrition and health. Children are unlikely to receive adequate nutrition when their parents act on knowledge that is incompatible with recommended dietary guidelines. These same children are also more likely to ingest an excess of energy compared to expenditure.

Parents have variable knowledge in both the areas of nutrition and health. On the one hand, parents feel that health information is relatively straightforward [13]. A high number of parents report they are interested in food labels so that they can compare their knowledge with the food they are considering for purchase [15]. When examining health claims on food packaging, parents consider certain foods to be either "good" or "bad" [15]. Foods that are "bad" include fat, salt, sugar, and energy (i.e., calories) [15]. Aspects of foods that parents also consider but do not necessarily disqualify the food from purchase include vitamins, minerals, cholesterol, carbohydrates, protein, fiber, saturated fats, and unsaturated fats [15].

On the other hand, parents demonstrate confusion about the specifics of nutritional knowledge [13]. We will address the source of some of the confusion in our final section regarding the overall state of nutritional research. When they have questions about diet or feeding, parents access information from the Internet, their friends and family, and their pediatricians [13]. Where parents look for information depends on the nature of their question. In one study, parents unanimously reported visiting Internet sites as their primary source of information [13]. While a preferred method, parents also report that the amount of information on the Internet feels overwhelming [13]. Parents also display concern for the authenticity of the information they find on the Internet [13]. In one study, parents reported an awareness that some level of critical thinking was required to determine accurate sources of information from inaccurate sources [13]. However, the propagation of false dietary information on social media implies that many parents are either unaware of the need for critical appraisal or require more assistance in accomplishing that task successfully.

Friends and family are sought out when parents think their social contacts have prior experience with the situation they currently face and can consequently offer insight [13]. In one study, parents reported that they asked their children's doctors for answers to their dietary questions only as a last resort [13]. These parents explained that before speaking with their doctor, their question had to have risen to a level they felt was of clinical significance [13]. Thus, we can infer that patient-initiated discussions of diets mainly occur when parents have already identified the gap in their own knowledge.

Realistically, parents may not always know when a situation is out of their depth. One study of Australian parents revealed that among their sample, even parents who reported a strong investment in a nutritious diet were unable to name a heavily promoted government public health message as to the number of recommended daily servings of fruits and vegetables [1]. Parents in that study also reported that they were feeding their children more healthfully than their peers, thus reducing the likelihood of changing their feeding practices even when they fell below recommended dietary guidelines [1]. In the United States, data from the Third National Health and Nutrition Examination Survey uncovered that nearly one third of mothers with overweight children did not consider their children to be overweight [16]. Among low-income families, seventy to 80% of mothers of overweight children thought their children were a healthy weight or even underweight [17]. This gap in recognition may be partially explained by the perception of some parents that a heavy child is a healthy child [2]. These parents believe that a heavy child is a sign of good parenting [2]. Given that most parents report accessing information from the Internet, they may be further unaware of the influence of misinformation. Increasing amounts of non-clinical dietary recommendations (such as "clean eating") have infiltrated the popular consciousness without needed checks on accuracy. Therefore, pediatricians should consider dietary discussions with parents without waiting for parents to raise the issue. Because habits established when children are young linger into adulthood, conversations held during the pre-school years are most likely to have a meaningful, lasting impact [2].

We make a distinction between parental knowledge of nutrition and knowledge of feeding practices. For example, one study showed that the children of parents with higher nutrition knowledge less likely to eat fat in the home [18]. Greater general nutrition knowledge was associated with higher consumption of fruits and vegetables [18]. The association between general nutrition knowledge and parenting style found that parents' knowledge of nutrition alone neither predicted nor mediated outcomes in their children's diets [18]. Only in cases where the parenting style was already optimal was increased nutrition knowledge observed to have a small impact on children's consumption of non-core (i.e., not fruits or vegetables) foods [18]. While this study supports interventions designed to increase parental nutritional knowledge, clearly parental knowledge is a necessary but not sufficient component of a healthy diet for children [18]. Therefore, conversations with parents to increase their knowledge should not focus solely on nutritional content; they should also mention the research presented below on parenting styles, the overall state of nutrition research, and address any parents who may be following diets not currently established in the research base as effective.

Influence of Advertisers

A common parental complaint about their efforts to provide their children with a healthy diet is the nature of advertising [19]. Advertising in the media is a significant challenge, with children between the ages of 8–18 spending on average more time on media consumption daily than any activity other than sleeping [9]. In addition to advertisements, many products aimed at children's palates use packaging featuring promotional characters; such characters are used predominantly to promote less-healthy foods [20]. A qualitative survey of 124 children in three schools in Australia (selected to include low-, medium-, and high-economic status school districts) found that both parents and children widely discussed advertisements [4]. Parents commented that the intensity of advertising was correlated with specific food properties, such that the most advertisements seen were for foods highest in fat, salt, and/or sugar [4]. Their observations were consistent with content analysis studies that have quantified the amount of advertising spent based on food type [21]. Nearly all of the advertisements aired during children's television shows promote foods that are low in nutrients and high in fat, sodium, and added sugars [22]. It would be barely an exaggeration to state that if a child is viewing the ad, the product marketed is automatically low in nutritional value and high in energy.

The strategies employed by most advertisements follow principles of classical conditioning [23]. Commercials widely pair images of children who are happy, popular, loved, and/or having fun with the advertised product [4]. After repeated viewings, children begin to associate the food product with the desirable social and emotional characteristics of the children in the advertisements. This same strategy is used when marketing food to parents; however, the emotions and behaviors paired with the food differ markedly from the child versions. In one study, researchers coded food commercials that aired during children's television programming based on intended audience: parent or child [24]. Parents were coded as the audience when the commercials sent messages of family bonding and love, contrasted with messages highlighting fun when children are the audience [24]. These content analysis findings were consistent with the reports of the Australian parents and their children who described similar themes in commercials [1].

After children receive these messages from advertisements, they are likely to bother their parents until they obtain the desired food [4]. Parents in one small focus group study stated that dealing with the effects advertising had on their children felt like a "battle" [13]. Their impressions are borne out in observational research. Both academic and consumer research reveals that young children who accompany their parents during grocery shopping indeed influence their parents' food purchases [9]. While parents' engagement with their children about these messages can mitigate the advertisements' influence, the messages remain persistent enough to continue to exert influence over children's preferences [25]. Given the sums food companies spend on advertising annually, we assume that directly marketing to children has an appreciable effect on sales.

Social learning theory proposes one mechanism by which commercials exert influence on children [26]. According to this theory, children learn by observing the social world around them and incorporating the behaviors and beliefs they observe into their operational framework [26]. Yet young children are thought not to understand that the social world displayed in commercials is influenced by a specific point of view, that is, with the aim of selling a product [26]. The distinction between objective and subjective information needed to parse out this motive is typically not appreciated until children are 9 years old [26]. By this age, children have already been exposed to countless advertisements, which have contributed to the formation of their thinking and behavior [26]. Thus, children are particularly susceptible to accepting marketers' messages [26].

Many parents report awareness of the influence advertisements exert over their children, but it is not clear how parents understand their own perceptions of advertisements and front-of-packaging health claims. Current regulations permit food producers to post nutrition- or health-related (NH) claims on their packaging, provided the claim is not misleading [27]. To this end, the Food and Drug Administration regulates the types of NH claims products can make in accordance with the scientific evidence available [27]. Claims range from merely providing content (e.g., "Contains fiber") to asserting health claims (e.g. "Reduces risk of heart disease") [27]. Despite regulators' careful attention to these distinctions, research shows that adults considering these claims largely do not distinguish between the types of claims [27]. In particular, a **halo effect**, in which people attribute many positive qualities to a product based on only one narrow claim, is consistently observed [27, 28]. The halo effect is an example of overgeneralization, which leads parents to assume the non-featured ingredients in the product are just as healthy or beneficial as the featured ones [27]. A strong example of overgeneralization is seen in the purchase of artificially low-fat or low-sugar products. Products low in fat often compensate for lack of flavor by increasing the amount of sugar, salt, or other ingredients [29]. Products marketed as low in sugar often use sugar substitutes that are sweeter than natural sugar, adjusting the taste preferences of the consumer to desire even more sugary substances [29]. Preliminary studies with humans suggest that a preference for sweet foods established in childhood may last well into adulthood [29]. So while one aspect of the food may appear healthy (e.g., low-fat or low-sugar) the product as a whole is not healthy.

While parents typically report negative opinions of giving their children foods with artificial sweeteners, parents often select these foods for purchase [29]. The discrepancy between belief and action implies parents may not understand the information they are presented with when purchasing food for their children [29]. As is true in all advertising, the marketer will present the information desirable to parents and withhold the information that would dissuade them from purchasing.

Influence of Peers

While parents remain the primary gatekeepers of young children's food, once they start school (or daycare) other individuals play a prominent role in children's lives. Peer impressions of foods begin to factor into children's social worlds. In one study, when teachers enthusiastically ate a novel food, children were more likely to eat it [30]. However, if their classmates showed an aversion to the food the teacher was eating, children were more likely to reject it themselves [30].

Peers (particularly those from school) provide a reference point for foods consumption patterns other than those children experience in their family of origin [13]. Armed with the knowledge that other children who are like themselves in many respects eat certain foods, children are known to then bother their parents to purchase those same foods [13]. In particular, heavily advertised foods are also perceived as high-status among the peer group [4]. This provides a double challenge for parents in responding to requests for foods high in fat, added sugars, or sodium, and low in nutritional value. Parents report submitting to such entreaties particularly when tired, stressed, or emotionally vulnerable (e.g., feeling guilty for lack of time spent with child or for not being able to provide other, more expensive, high-status items) [13]. Peers' impressions of the food children eat strike at a core aspect of human connection—the need to belong. Parents are reluctant to enforce food choices that complicate their children's assimilation into their peer group [4]. In fact, when faced with conflicting priorities about food, parents in one study reported regularly prioritizing psychosocial factors such as belongingness over nutrition, reports that are borne out by direct researcher observations [4]. While parents in this study acknowledged the importance of providing their children with a nutritious diet, they stated their overall goal was to provide food their children would enjoy and that their peers would consider appropriate [4].

Costs of Nutrition

The costs of providing nutritious food can be measured in terms of dollars and time [2]. With regard to money, parents show a higher concern for relative value over absolute cost. While parents understand the importance of vegetables and fruits in a meal, they report being dissuaded by a perception of higher cost [9, 13]. When specifically comparing these costs against less nutritious foods, parents consider how much of the food they buy that their children will eat [13]. Therefore, while the cost of vegetables may not be higher than fast food, parents avoid spending money on foods they predict their children will be more likely to reject, seeing it as a waste of their money [9, 13]. While some parents state that fast food is a money-saver, they simultaneously acknowledge the presumed profitability of fast food based on aggressive advertising [13]. Fast foods are less expensive than healthy foods using a price per calorie reference [31]. However, when comparing their price per edible gram and price per portion, healthy foods are the less expensive option [31].

The cost of time is a hypothesized constraint for parents as well [9]. Single-parent households rely heavily on rapid food preparation techniques, such as microwaving nutrient-poor convenience foods [32]. Among two-parent households, the cultural and economic shift towards dual-incomes has also increased parental reporting of challenges in preparing meals that are healthy and an increased reliance on convenience foods containing higher levels of fat, sodium, and energy [9]. Children's entrance to school often coincides with a parental return to work, thus presenting a confluence of factors around increased peer influence, access to foods outside the home, and limited parental time and energy for preparing meals after a day of work [4].

Rather than assume parents lack knowledge about nutritious foods, pediatricians can directly address their concerns pertaining to the financial and time costs associated with healthy eating. If parents cite cost as a concern, physicians can ask what they have tried so far to overcome these barriers. Inquiring about past efforts validates the parents' challenges and shows empathy for difficult situations. Assessing prior attempts also minimizes the chance that the physician will provide advice the parent has already heard and discarded for being infeasible. Parents concerned about the short-term cost of throwing away rejected nutritious foods should be oriented to the framework of comparing short-term waste (vegetables in the trash) to long-term waste (non-nutritive foods in their children's bodies). Rather than focus on filling their children's stomachs, doctors can reorient parents to the idea of filling their children's nutritional needs. In this framework, fast foods that are low in nutrition and high in energy are wasteful, because they cost money without providing any assistance towards the nutritional goal.

Addressing parental concerns regarding lack of time should be handled with a similar level of respect for the challenges the parents face and efforts they have already made to find solutions. Simply recommending that parents seek out recipes that are easy to make does not diminish the influence of limited time. In fact, this approach exacerbates the short-term time burden further by placing an expectation that parents first research and learn new recipes. Instead, physicians who provide direct sources for such recipes impose no additional initial time burden on parents. Culturally significant types of foods are passed from generation to generation. Rather than attempt to influence flavor profiles, recommendations for recipes should focus on methods of cooking that are simple, rapid, and can be applied to any types of food. Examples include slow cooker recipes, "one-pot" recipes, stir-fries, or baked casserole dishes, made from whatever ingredients are familiar to the parent.

Common Misconceptions

The child is a picky eater, thus, the parent has no control over the child's diet

There is a widespread perception among parents that their children are more selective than other children about what they eat. This phenomenon of children refusing wide swaths of food is colloquially called **picky eating** [14]. Picky eating is not a medically recognized feeding disorder (a feeding disorder is a diagnosis stemming from severe feeding problems resulting in functional consequences) [14]. Instead, picky eating is used indiscriminately to describe children who are fussy, have low appetites, or dislike particular taste or texture sensations [14]. As we will outline in the next section, difficult parent-child interactions around food have lasting consequences. Even though picky eating is not a medical diagnosis, parents who complain their children are picky eaters require a response from their primary care physicians [14].

Dealing with their children's food selectivity is one of the highest reported frustrations of parents [14]. Most pediatricians will encounter this complaint, as over 50% of parents report that at least one of their children is a picky eater [33–35]. While this percentage appears high, many of these parents may be responding to emerging **neophobia** [14]. Neophobia is a developmental phase that typically occurs around the age of 1.5–2 years when children display hesitancy about ingesting unknown foods [8]. This response is thought to be evolutionarily adaptive, with children most commonly rejecting foods that are bitter or sour, tastes associated with spoiled or poisonous foods [8]. This phenomenon is not unique to humans; it appears in all omnivores [14]. There is evidence that one's level of neophobia is at least partially determined by heredity [36]. Two studies found that genetic factors may explain 69–78% of the variance between reported neophobic behaviors in twins [36]. One review study found strong-to-moderate influence of heritability on children's taste and food preferences [37]. Genetics have also been implicated in children's tendencies to eat when they are not hungry and in their overall daily intake patterns [36]. However, children's experiences of neophobia are not completely determined by forces outside of parents' control. For example, selective children were more likely to try new foods if their parents offer a variety of foods in the home and if they witnessed their parents trying new foods [9, 36].

While neophobia is a normative stage, many parents are still dismayed to find their children rejecting foods they ate easily just a few weeks before [8]. Faced with new resistance, parents who are unaware that this is a phase may attribute the new challenges to a permanent characteristic of their child's personality [8]. Parents with a static view of their children's food selectivity may begin to feel hopeless about their ability to influence their children's diets [9]. Correcting the misperception for parents is key to reducing this frustration as well as suggesting strategies that help to decrease a child's selectivity [14].

Fortunately, neophobia can be overcome by repeated exposures to the novel food [14]. While parents are aware of the need for repeated exposures, most parents drastically underestimate the number of exposures needed to overcome neophobia. On average, research shows that parents present a novel food no more than 5 times before being convinced that their child does not like it and giving up [38–40]. In reality, conquering neophobia requires that the same food be presented, without pressure to eat, between 8 and 15 times [33]. When parents do not persist in re-exposing their children to the food, they compensate with other behaviors [9]. For example, some parents allow their children to consume only preferred foods, so that the child at least eats [9]. Parents of children passing through the neophobic stage could benefit from reassurance that the stage is transient and that their concerted efforts are only required while their children are in the phase [14].

Some proportion of children are not passing through neophobia, but instead present with inappropriate selectivity [14]. Among children with mild food selectivity, toddlers were found to try as many new foods as their peers, but they simply liked fewer of them [14]. While children with mild selectivity alarm their parents, they typically grow and develop along normal trajectories [14]. Their energy and nutrient intakes are similarly average [14]. The challenge among true picky eaters is parents' response to their selectivity [14]. In response, parents provide alternative foods that their children do accept, thus reinforcing the children's impressions that the non-preferred food is to be avoided [9]. As a result, many parents find themselves creating different meal options for various family members. As parents already report a lack of time for healthy meal preparation, creating separate dietary options creates an additional burden.

There is a final subset of children who have severe selectivity, defined as eating no more than 10–15 foods [14]. These children tend to reject entire food groups based on categorical dislike of particular flavor profiles, textures, or smells [41]. If parents report this level of selectivity, a referral to a specialist is required to provide more intensive interventions [14].

Because children initially do not like the taste of vegetables, parents should disguise them in more palatable foods so that their children receive the needed nutrients

When parents want their children to consume healthy foods but are exhausted by battles, they may conclude that disguising healthy food in their children's preferred food is an appropriate option. Research has shown that disguising foods in this manner does lead to an increased intake of vegetables [42]. In this manner, disguising food achieves a short-term goal of nutrient intake. However, it is not a recommended strategy [2]. One small study interviewed two groups of parents arranged according to the healthfulness of their children's diets [2]. The study uncovered that children with unhealthy diets were more likely to have parents who engaged in disguising healthy foods than children with healthy diets [2]. By disguising the food, children are not able to build an appreciation for the food's flavor through the repeated exposures necessary to integrate the food into their diets [2]. This strategy also reinforces the concept that unhealthy foods are undesirable and consequently works against the long-term goal of allowing children to learn to appreciate and enjoy high nutrient foods in addition to those higher in salt, fat, and sugar [2].

Parents should use preferred foods as a reward for eating non-preferred foods

To facilitate their children eating non-preferred foods (typically healthy ones), parents often resort to using a preferred food (typically less healthy) as a reward [2]. This strategy results in the same paradoxical conundrum as disguising food. By making the eating of healthy food the task to be completed in service of a larger goal (e.g., enjoying dessert or another preferred food), parents continue to reinforce the idea that healthy foods cannot be enjoyed in and of themselves [8]. Indeed, children whose parents use preferred food as a reward begin to grant the preferred food an even higher status [8]. Children who have been trained to highly covet preferred foods in this manner are more likely to eat them to excess when the foods are not under their parents' control (such as when at a birthday party or when sharing food in the school cafeteria) [8]. For this reason, using food as a reward (either for eating a certain amount of food or for eating a non-preferred food first) is not recommended.

Current Research

While misguided, these common misconceptions illuminate parents' desires to provide healthy diets for their children in the context of suboptimal conditions. Some factors are outside of parents' immediate control, but others are not. Parents want to know what they can do. The more time and energy parents spend on ineffectual or even counter-productive practices, the fewer mental and practical resources they will have left for evidence-based strategies. Therefore, parents and their children's diets benefit from knowing the most robust developments in nutrition research.

Parenting Styles

One finding regarding parental actions repeatedly shown to be associated with child diet quality is parenting style. There are four widely recognized parenting styles, each derived from considering parental engagement with children along two axes: demandingness and responsiveness [43]. Parental style is assessed by determining where a parent's behaviors lie along these two dimensions [43]. Parents with high levels of demandingness exert control over their children's actions [43]. Parents with low levels of demandingness make few efforts to dictate their children's behavior. Parents high in responsiveness show support by engaging with their children verbally and nonverbally in a warm manner [43]. Parents low in responsiveness show less frequent engagement with their children or understanding of their children's needs [43]. As parents can be either low or high on each of the two dimensions, four parenting styles result.

Traditionally called "strict," parents high in demandingness and low in responsiveness are said to use an **authoritarian** parenting style [43]. These parents have clear goals for their children's behavior, and they do not tend to adjust those expectations in response to children's preferences or individual characteristics. These parents are typically seen as opposites of the lax parenting style, called **permissive**. While permissive parents are highly responsive to their children's preferences, they do not use this information in service of ensuring that their children behave in a particular way. Instead, because their level of demandingness is low, they allow their children's preferences to dictate behavioral outcomes. The balance between these two styles is the **authoritative** parenting style. Authoritative parents exert control over their children's behavior in order to ensure desirable outcomes. However, they modify how these outcomes are achieved in response to their children's needs, thus maintaining a warm and supportive relationship with their children [43]. The fourth parenting style is fortunately the least common, as these parents are low in their demands but also low in responsiveness. This style is officially termed **neglectful** or **uninvolved** [43].

With regard to diet, researchers have observed many ties to parenting style. Authoritarian parents are more likely to use coercive feedings practices, such as demanding children eat a set amount of food irrespective of the child's appetite and using certain foods as contingent rewards for engaging in other behaviors [44]. When authoritarian parents exert this level of control over their children's feeding habits, children are subsequently not as easily able to establish their own control over their feeding [45]. For example, placing a "forbidden" food within a child's sight but out of reach decreases the child's ability to practice exerting self-control [46]. Children need self-control as they age and become responsible for knowing how much to eat in the absence of their parents [45]. On the other side, permissive parenting has been tied to providing only preferred foods to children 20–36 months in order to avoid conflict [44]; lower intake of fruits and vegetables in 2–5 year-olds [18]; higher child Body Mass Index (a rough but often-used measure of relative weight) in 3–8 year-olds [47]; and increased consumption of fat, snacks, and sweet foods in adolescents [48].

Authoritative parenting has been shown to be consistent with healthy diets. Parents of children whose diets were rated as healthy were more likely to engage in authoritative practices such as setting consistent, firm limits while allowing the child some autonomy within those boundaries [2]. Children of authoritative parents establish healthier diets [49] and consume more fruits and vegetables [50]. The nature of the association between the authoritative parenting style and healthy diets is not fully understood [8]. It may be possible that children naturally predisposed towards eating healthy foods reduce stress for their parents [8]. In turn, their parents need not begin attempting the suboptimal strategies used by authoritarian or permissive parents (e.g., exerting tighter and tighter control; giving up control entirely) [8]. Despite not being able to definitely state that authoritative parenting causes healthy diets, feeding practices that align with the authoritative parenting style are recommended [3]. The authoritative parenting style balances parental expectations and child autonomy within pre-defined, consistent, and parent-enforced limits [3].

Nutrition Claims

Emerging research should also be considered when parents present with an interest in nutritional claims that are untrue or unfounded. For example, some parents of children with Autism Spectrum Disorders have placed faith in the concept of providing a gluten- and casein-free diet despite evidence showing it is ineffective in reducing problematic behaviors [51, 52]. There has also been debate regarding the relative safety of genetically modified (or engineered) foods, typically called GMOs in the United States [53]. Extensive research on genetically modified crops has yielded no evidence that these foods are unsafe [53]. Other parents may be interested in nutritional terms that are too ambiguous to be meaningful. Specifically, food producers, aware that consumers are interested in health products that taste good, use the public concern over nutrition to their advantage when marketing highly processed foods [54]. They commonly use "buzzwords" that connote health without actually imparting additional nutrients or reduction in calories [54]. Such buzzwords that parents should be cautioned to remain skeptical about include "all natural," "organic," and "whole grain" [54]. While these words were originally used to describe healthy foods such as vegetables and whole-wheat grains, creators of processed foods now use them to describe all manner of foods [54]. For example, makers of Chef Boyardee Beefaroni pasta touted a full serving of vegetables in their product [54]. When researchers examined the nutritional label, only two vegetables were listed: tomato puree and carrots (the content of the latter was so small that it appeared after salt in the listing). The researchers concluded that while this nutritional claim may have been factually accurate, it provided a greater impression of the overall health of the product than was warranted [54]. One need only peruse the snack food aisles of high-end grocery stores to see the propagation of seeming paradoxes, such as "all natural" candies and chips. Consumers who equate "natural" with healthy may be misled by these labels and assume that these foods will convey some benefit to their children's diets. This is not, however, always the case. For example, the recent trend to avoid refined and manufactured forms of sugar has resulted in a plethora of "natural" sugar options, such as agave syrup, "raw" sugar, and stevia extract. To the chagrin of those attempting to reduce the overall impact of sugar consumption in their children's diets, consuming less traditional forms of sugar is unlikely to yield major health benefits. While the body metabolizes refined sugars more rapidly than those found naturally occurring in fruits and dairy (leading to a temporary rapid increase in insulin and blood sugar levels), all forms of sugar have the same effect on the metabolic system after passing through the stomach. While high amounts of refined and manufactured sugar are detrimental to a balanced diet, overconsumption of natural sugars is also linked to most indicators of metabolic syndrome in humans [55].

Researchers have observed parents' struggles in interpreting nutritional science [1]. On the one hand, parents feel that nutritional guidelines are plain and straightforward [1]. On the other hand, parents feel as though they cannot keep up with the steady stream of new information as science evolves and upends old recommendations [1]. Unfortunately due to cost and feasibility, most of the studies performed in nutrition research are not randomized controlled trials [56]. Nutrition claims tend to come from large epidemiology data sets, whereby many statistically significant conclusions can be found through chance alone [56]. Those that are randomized and controlled have other steep limitations, such as extremely few participants, insufficient control over participant intakes, brief intervention time frames, or outcomes tracked for a very limited amount of time [56].

Conclusion

The role of the pediatrician in assisting parents in providing their children with a healthy diet is an important, albeit limited one. Structural barriers outside physician and parent control limit the amount of influence parents have on their children's diets. Despite these limitations, parents still have more influence over their children's diets than any other person or factor. Providing parents with accurate knowledge is crucial and must be undertaken even when parents are unaware of the gaps in their understanding. Even when parents do have questions, many do not ask their physicians for assistance. Accordingly, doctors should consider providing information before parents ask.

Specifically, physicians can encourage parents to focus on the methods they use to encourage their children to eat healthfully. An authoritative parenting style is associated with children's development of life-long skills in appetite regulation and self-control. With regard to specific foods or nutrients, doctors can encourage parents to think of their child's diet as a whole, rather than focus on certain "good" or "bad" foods. Parents who show an interest in either including or excluding specialized foods from their children's diets for having specific functional capabilities despite lacking evidence can be encouraged to focus on the known properties of foods rather than spend limited resources on unproven foods.

References

1. Duncanson K, Burrows T, Holman B, Collins C. Parents' perceptions of child feeding: a qualitative study based on the theory of planned behavior. J Dev Behav Pediatr. 2013;34(4):227–36.
2. Peters J, Parletta N, Lynch J, Campbell K. A comparison of parental views of their pre-school children's 'healthy' versus 'unhealthy' diets. Qual Study Appetite. 2014;1(76):129–36.
3. Savage JS, Fisher JO, Birch LL. Parental influence on eating behavior: conception to adolescence. J Law, Med Ethics. 2007;35(1):22–34.
4. Roberts M, Pettigrew S. Psychosocial influences on children's food consumption. Psychol Mark. 2013;30(2):103–20.
5. Ogden CL, Carroll MD, Kit BK, Flegal KM. Prevalence of obesity and trends in body mass index among US children and adolescents, 1999–2010. JAMA. 2012;307(5):483–90.

6.   Kelder SH, Perry CL, Klepp KI, Lytle LL. Longitudinal tracking of adolescent smoking, physical activity, and food choice behaviors. Am J Public Health. 1994;84(7):1121–6.

7.   Bluford DA, Sherry B, Scanlon KS. Interventions to prevent or treat obesity in preschool children: a review of evaluated programs. Obesity. 2007;15(6):1356–72.

8.   Mitchell GL, Farrow C, Haycraft E, Meyer C. Parental influences on children's eating behaviour and characteristics of successful parent-focussed interventions. Appetite. 2013;1(60):85–94.

9.   Adamo KB, Brett KE. Parental perceptions and childhood dietary quality. Matern Child Health J. 2014;18(4):978–95.

10.   Kamath CC, Vickers KS, Ehrlich A, McGovern L, Johnson J, Singhal V, Paulo R, Hettinger A, Erwin PJ, Montori VM. Behavioral interventions to prevent childhood obesity: a systematic review and metaanalyses of randomized trials. J Clin Endocrinol Metab. 2008;93(12):4606–15.

11.   McGovern L, Johnson JN, Paulo R, Hettinger A, Singhal V, Kamath C, Erwin PJ, Montori VM. Treatment of pediatric obesity: a systematic review and meta-analysis of randomized trials. J Clin Endocrinol Metab. 2008;93(12):4600–5.

12.   Ajzen I. The theory of planned behavior. Organ Behav Hum Decis Process. 1991;50(2):179–211.

13.   Velardo S, Drummond M. Understanding parental health literacy and food related parenting practices. Health Sociol Rev. 2013;22(2):137–50.

14.   Kerzner B, Milano K, MacLean WC, Berall G, Stuart S, Chatoor I. A practical approach to classifying and managing feeding difficulties. Pediatrics. 2015;135(2):344–53.

15.   Hoefkens C, Verbeke W, Van Camp J. European consumers' perceived importance of qualifying and disqualifying nutrients in food choices. Food Qual Prefer. 2011;22(6):550–8.

16.   Maynard LM, Galuska DA, Blanck HM, Serdula MK. Maternal perceptions of weight status of children. Pediatrics. 2003;111(Supplement 1):1226–31.

17.   Baughcum AE, Chamberlin LA, Deeks CM, Powers SW, Whitaker RC. Maternal perceptions of overweight preschool children. Pediatrics. 2000;106(6):1380–6.

18.   Peters J, Dollman J, Petkov J, Parletta N. Associations between parenting styles and nutrition knowledge and 2–5 year-old children's fruit, vegetable and non-core food consumption. Public Health Nutr. 2013;16(11):1979–87.

19.   Morley B, Chapman K, Mehta K, King L, Swinburn B, Wakefield M. Parental awareness and attitudes about food advertising to children on Australian television. Aust N Z J Public Health. 2008;32(4):341–7.

20.   Hebden L, King L, Kelly B, Chapman K, Innes-Hughes C. A menagerie of promotional characters: promoting food to children through food packaging. J Nutr Educ Behav. 2011;43(5):349–55.

21.   Cairns G, Angus K, Hastings G. The extent, nature and effects of food promotion to children: a review of the evidence to December 2008. Geneva: World Health Organization; 2009.

22.   Stitt C, Kunkel D. Food advertising during children's television programming on broadcast and cable channels. Health Commun. 2008;23(6):573–84.

23.   Cohen J, Pham M, Andrade E. The nature and role of affect in consumer behavior. In: Haugtvedt C, Herr P, Kardes F, editors. by. 1st ed. Mahwah: Lawrence Erlbaum; 2016. p. 297–348.

24.   Emond, JA, Smith, ME, Mathur, SJ, Sargent, JD, Gilbert-Diamond D. Children's food and beverage promotion on television to parents. Pediatrics:peds, 2015.

25.   Ferguson CJ, Muñoz ME, Medrano MR. Advertising influences on young children's food choices and parental influence. J pediatr. 2012;160(3):452–5.

26.   LoDolce ME, Harris JL, Schwartz MB. Sugar as part of a balanced breakfast? What cereal advertisements teach children about healthy eating. J Health Commun. 2013;18(11):1293–309.

27. Van Trijp HC, Van der Lans IA. Consumer perceptions of nutrition and health claims. Appetite. 2007;48(3):305–24.
28. Roe B, Levy AS, Derby BM. The impact of health claims on consumer search and product evaluation outcomes: results from FDA experimental data. J Public Policy Mark. 1999;1:89–105.
29. Sylvetsky AC, Dietz WH. Nutrient-content claims—guidance or cause for confusion? N Engl J Med. 2014;371(3):195–8.
30. Hendy HM, Raudenbush B. Effectiveness of teacher modeling to encourage food acceptance in preschool children. Appetite. 2000;34(1):61–76.
31. Carlson A, Frazão E. Are healthy foods really more expensive? It depends on how you measure the price. It depends on how you measure the price. USDA-ERS economic information bulletin. 2012; 96.
32. Stewart SD, Menning CL. Family structure, nonresident father involvement, and adolescent eating patterns. J Adolesc Health. 2009;45(2):193–201.
33. Carruth BR, Ziegler PJ, Gordon A, Barr SI. Prevalence of picky eaters among infants and toddlers and their caregivers' decisions about offering a new food. J Am Diet Assoc. 2004;31(104):57–64.
34. Jacobi C, Agras WS, Bryson S, Hammer LD. Behavioral validation, precursors, and concomitants of picky eating in childhood. J Am Acad Child Adolesc Psychiatry. 2003;42(1):76–84.
35. Saarilehto S, Lapinleimu H, Keskinen S, Helenius H, Talvia S, Simell O. Growth, energy intake, and meal pattern in five-year-old children considered as poor eaters. J Pediatr. 2004;144(3):363–7.
36. Faith MS, Heo M, Keller KL, Pietrobelli A. Child food neophobia is heritable, associated with less compliant eating, and moderates familial resemblance for BMI. Obesity. 2013;21(8):1650–5.
37. Harris G. Development of taste and food preferences in children. Curr Opin Clin Nutr Metab Care. 2008;11(3):315–9.
38. Aldridge V, Dovey TM, Halford JC. The role of familiarity in dietary development. Dev Rev. 2009;29(1):32–44.
39. Cashdan E. A sensitive period for learning about food. Human Nat. 1994;5(3):279–91.
40. Zajonc RB. Attitudinal effects of mere exposure. J Pers Soc psychol. 1968. 9(2p2):1.
41. Chatoor I. Diagnosis and treatment of feeding disorders in infants, toddlers, and young children. Zero to three. 2009.
42. Spill MK, Birch LL, Roe LS, Rolls BJ. Hiding vegetables to reduce energy density: an effective strategy to increase children's vegetable intake and reduce energy intake. Am J Clin Nutr. 2011;94(3):735–41.
43. Maccoby EE, Martin JA. Socialization in the context of the family:parent-child interaction. Handbook of child psychology: formerly Carmichael's Manual of child psychology/Paul H. Mussen, ed. 1983.
44. Rigal N, Chabanet C, Issanchou S, Monnery-Patris S. Links between maternal feeding practices and children's eating difficulties. Valid Fr Tools. Appetite. 2012;58(2):629–37.
45. Birch LL, Fisher JO. Development of eating behaviors among children and adolescents. Pediatrics. 1998;101(Supplement 2):539–49.
46. Mischel W, Shoda Y, Rodriguez MI. Delay of gratification in children. Science. 1989;244(4907):933–8.
47. Olvera N, Power TG. Brief report: parenting styles and obesity in Mexican American children: a longitudinal study. J Pediatr Psychol. 2010;35(3):243–9.
48. De Bourdeaudhuij I. Family food rules and healthy eating in adolescents. J Health Psychol. 1997;2(1):45–56.
49. Ventura AK, Birch LL. Does parenting affect children's eating and weight status? Int J Behav Nutr Phys Act. 2008;5(1):15.

50. Blissett J, Haycraft E. Are parenting style and controlling feeding practices related? Appetite. 2008;50(2):477–85.

51. Hurwitz S. The Gluten-free, Casein-free Diet and Autism: limited return on family investment. J Early Interv. 2013;9:1053815113484807.

52. Bauset SM, Zazpe I, Mari-Sanchis A, Llopis-Gonzalez A, Morales-Suarez-Varela, M. Evidence of the gluten free and casein free diet in autism spectrum disorders (ASDs): a systematic review.

53. Nicolia A, Manzo A, Veronesi F, Rosellini D. An overview of the last 10 years of genetically engineered crop safety research. Crit Rev Biotechnol. 2014;34(1):77–88.

54. Northup T. Truth, lies, and packaging: how food marketing creates a false sense of health. Food Studies. 2014:9.

55. Kelishadi R, Mansourian M, Heidari-Beni M. Association of fructose consumption and components of metabolic syndrome in human studies: a systematic review and meta-analysis. Nutrition. 2014;30(5):503–10.

56. Carroll A. Unexpected honey study shows woes of nutrition research [Internet]. Nytimes. com. 2016 [cited 1 February 2016]. Available from: http://www.nytimes.com/2015/10/27/upshot/surprising-honey-study-shows-woes-of-nutrition-research.html?_r=0.

Chapter 8
Food Allergies

Overview

Food allergies among children are a prevalent issue in the United States. It is estimated that between 2 and 8% of children are affected [1]. Prevalence rates vary according to the food in question, the method of survey, region, and time period studied [2, 3]. The range in prevalence rates is just one example reflecting the field's overall state. Research and clinical practice in food allergies are marked by ambiguity in definitions, variability of individual symptoms, lack of consensus as to testing thresholds for diagnostic clarity, and ambiguity as to preferred testing methods, all leading to a great deal of uncertainty in the field [4]. Even taking these uncertainties into account, data from the National Health Survey indicate that prevalence rates in the United States appear to be increasing [5].

The nine foods most commonly reported as producing allergic reactions in children are egg, fish (fin), milk, peanut, sesame, shellfish, soy, tree nuts, and wheat [6]. There are still no preventative treatments or permanent cures for food allergies [7]. Therefore, the commonly prescribed action is food avoidance and response to allergic reactions with appropriate treatment [7]. Complying with food avoidance and responding to accidental ingestion requires a number of activities, such as monitoring food intake, reading labels, monitoring for reactions, determining severity of reactions, and taking appropriate medication in response [8]. For younger children, parents largely assume these responsibilities [8, 9]. It is crucial that parents understand their children's food allergies so that they may respond with the appropriate level of intervention.

The symptoms of food allergies can range from mild to life-threatening [7]. The range of possible symptoms may implicate the skin, gastrointestinal system, and/or respiratory system [7]. Mild symptoms include itchy mouth, a few hives or mild itching on skin, and mild nausea and discomfort [10]. Mild symptoms are typically treated using over-the-counter antihistamines [10]. Severe symptoms

© Springer International Publishing AG 2017
C.A. Di Bartolo and M.K. Braun, *Pediatrician's Guide to Discussing Research with Patients*, DOI 10.1007/978-3-319-49547-7_8

include shortness of breath, wheezing, repetitive cough, pale or blue skin, dizziness, confusion, faintness, weak pulse, tight or hoarse throat, trouble breathing or swallowing, and swollen tongue or lips [10]. A combination of more mild symptoms can be classified as a severe reaction when the symptoms affect different bodily systems [10]. For example, a child who presents with hives, itchy rashes, or swelling, along with gastrointestinal symptoms like vomiting, diarrhea, or cramps, would be said to be experiencing severe symptoms [10].

The primary life-threatening response to food allergies is anaphylaxis [7]. Anaphylaxis is characterized as a severe, life-threatening response to consuming an allergen that results in simultaneous impairment in more than one organ system [10]. Just as in more mild allergic reactions, the combination of symptoms that constitute anaphylaxis can vary by individual [11]. As such, there is no specific threshold for determining the severity of an anaphylactic reaction [11]. The indicated treatment for anaphylaxis is a dose of epinephrine, administered via injection in the outside thigh using an adrenaline auto-injector [10]. More severe reactions or anaphylaxis that presents in two waves may require more than one dose [12].

Parents become concerned about food allergies in various stages of their children's development, such as *in utero*, during infancy, and throughout childhood, and concern can be seen as either preemptive or reactive. Mothers who are concerned about food allergies due to genetic load may ask questions or consider avoiding potentially allergenic foods even during pregnancy. The genetic influence of food allergies is challenging to study definitively due to individual variability in diagnosis [4]. However, there are indicators that allergies are at least partly determined by genetics. For example, children are seven times more likely to develop a peanut allergy if they have either a parent or a sibling with peanut allergy [13]. Monozygotic twin studies illuminate a strong genetic component, with children having a 64% increased risk of developing a food allergy if their identical twin has such an allergy [14]. These same mothers whose children can be classified as high-risk for developing food allergies may also be reluctant to eat highly allergenic foods during breastfeeding. Previously, mothers of high-risk infants were encouraged to avoid allergens while breastfeeding [15]. New evidence, however, which we will review, suggests that not only is maternal avoidance of allergens during breastfeeding not helpful, it may have deleterious effects on children's development of immunities [4]. There were also similarly premature recommendations from the World Health Organization for parents to delay exposing high-risk children to allergens [4]. Another set of parents may not be preemptively concerned, but instead react to their children's onset of allergies. Parental anxiety understandably increases when children have experienced anaphylaxis, as reported by young adults reflecting on memories of their parents' overprotectiveness following such dramatic incidents [16].

We will review common parental concerns specific to food allergies pertaining to Quality of Life and child growth. Misconceptions about food allergies and methods to mitigate their effects abound. This chapter will review common misconceptions that cause parents to expend energy in likely unfruitful endeavors, or worse, may worsen their children's allergies or place them at higher risk of serious adverse events. Finally, research about food allergies is still inconclusive in a number of areas. We will outline current findings in food allergy prevention and treatment research.

Common Parental Concerns

General

Clinicians frequently encounter parents who are concerned about food allergies. Compared to other health concerns, a 2012 survey of 1,119 parents indicated that allergies (including food allergies) captured the concerns of the highest percentage of parents [17]. Allergies were a significant concern for 69% of parents, with 38% of these reporting it as a medium problem and another 31% reporting it as large [17]. When examined according to child age group, the issues common to all ages were mental health, healthy nutrition, healthy growth and development, and safety [17]. A quick review of these concerns reveals that all of these are implicated in a food allergy [17]. This section will review findings in parental concerns regarding Quality of Life and child growth.

Quality of Life

Robust research shows that food allergies directly affect Quality of Life [18, 19]. When related to health, Quality of Life typically refers to the effects of an illness and the treatment of the illness on the patient [20]. Patient perception of the impact of the illness on his or her life also affects Quality of Life [20]. With regard to food allergies, we can include the impact of efforts to prevent an allergic response within this definition. Mild allergic responses are bothersome, and severe reactions are frightening and life-threatening [7]. In addition to the temporary incidents associated with allergic reactions, quality of life in between such incidents is affected by the vigilance required by parents and children [20]. Parents of young children, for whom accidental ingestion is common, show considerable vigilance [20]. At the same time, research shows that having a child with a food allergy has a detrimental effect of on family quality of life [21].

In their vigilance, parents engage in many behaviors to prevent or reduce their children's ingestion of the offending food. Behaviors include reading labels, paying attention to methods of food preparation, providing alternative food options outside the home (e.g., at school, during play dates, on trips), educating key adults in their children's life who also assume some responsibility for feeding (e.g., teachers, grandparents, parents of child's friends), and making needed preparations for emergency responses [9]. Given that children must eat multiple times a day, it is not surprising that among one sample of 221 parents, most reported thinking about their children's food allergy on a daily basis [9].

Well-documented food allergy anxiety is clearly helpful for initiating and maintaining the vigilance needed to implement avoidance successfully [22]. In the same sample of 221 parents of children with food allergies, more than half reported frequently feeling fearful for their children's safety [9]. Parents of children who suffered anaphylaxis or who have allergies to more than one food reported higher levels of fear than other parents of food allergic children [9]. Very high levels of anxiety are associated with initial diagnosis, prior to the establishment of familiarity with symptom prevention and management [22]. Fortunately, parents' fear tends to decrease as their children's age increases [9]. Similarly, there is not current evidence of clinically meaningful differences in anxiety among teenagers with food allergies compared to their nonallergic peers [23].

Extra counseling is recommended in cases where parents' or children's levels of anxiety do not remit [22]. Among a sample of Italian families with a food allergic child, four categories of problems that led families to seek additional counseling for living with food allergies were: (1) social/emotional functioning, (2) managing the allergy, (3) eating, and (4) behavior [22]. Of those who sought additional counseling, 36% were referred by clinicians such as allergists, pediatricians, or dieticians [22]. That fully one-third of families obtained help after referrals emphasizes the need for primary care physicians to make referrals when they perceive a family struggling with any of those four issues.

Models of health promotion have hypothesized that increased knowledge regarding food allergies would lead to increased sense of self-efficacy, the sense that people are able to achieve a specific outcome through their own behaviors [24, 25]. However, the research does not support this theory. Research instead indicates that the more knowledge parents have about food allergy, the lower their quality of life [18]. For example, one study of nearly 300 parents of food allergic children from the Netherlands found that while they had less knowledge about allergies than their American counterparts, they were also more optimistic about their children's condition [8]. To explain the finding, study authors proposed that as parents learn about their children's illness and the possible symptoms, their anxiety about potential outcomes and their frustration about their ability to keep their children safe increase [8]. Increased negative emotions such as anxiety and frustration could easily affect quality of life.

Another study examined differences between maternal and paternal quality of life in relation to their sense of competence and knowledge about food allergies [24]. As fathers spend more time with their children than in previous generations, they also take on increasing responsibility for management of their children's chronic health conditions [26]. Despite fathers' increased involvement, it appears the primary burden for education, competence, and management of allergies still falls on mothers [24]. Mothers reported statistically higher levels of competence in dealing with their children's food allergies than fathers and at the same time reported a lower quality of life [24]. In this case, the proposed mechanism explaining the results is that mothers' higher involvement in the daily management of their children's allergies simultaneously improves their personal competence in this area and decreases their quality of life [24]. Put another way, parental empowerment was not associated with increases in quality of life [24]. Study authors suggest that parents with greater knowledge of food allergies are more aware that most fatal reactions occur outside of the home, where parental competence cannot mitigate risk [24].

Knowledge may be more positively linked to quality of life when the knowledge is delivered at clinically relevant times and in formats that parents find useful [27–30]. Parents who accessed information subsequent to their children's diagnosis felt higher competence than they did at the time of diagnosis [9]. Many parents already seek out the information they feel they need to help their food allergic children, with most parents in one sample reporting that they frequently seek out information about allergies [9]. When properly educated, parents improve their skills in food avoidance, identifying reactions, and administering emergency treatment [31, 32]. A randomized controlled trial of distributing a parent handbook found that parent satisfaction with information is attainable [33]. Among 87 parents who received a handbook (most of whom reported spending one to 2 h reading it) significantly improved their knowledge and confidence ratings from baseline to post, in contrast with the control group, who reported no such improvement in confidence [33].

Growth

Most food allergies appear in the first 2 years of life, coinciding with a critical growth period in child development [34]. When children avoid foods due to allergy, their intake of macronutrients, such as protein, carbohydrates, and fat is affected [35]. These children are also at risk of not receiving the micronutrients needed for appropriate growth, such as vitamins, minerals, and trace elements [35]. Children with allergies to foods common to a healthy diet, such as milk, eggs, or wheat, are most at risk of retarded growth [35]. Children with more than one allergy have diets that are further restricted, impacting the ability of their parents to provide them with a sufficiently nutrient-dense diet. Fortunately, most children are allergic to no more than two food allergens [36, 37]. Regardless, macro- and micronutrients found in allergy-producing foods must be supplemented elsewhere in diets of food allergic children [35].

Case studies have found that parental misconceptions or misunderstandings about their children's adverse reactions to food, if not properly checked with a physician's expertise, can lead to severe elimination diets [38–40]. These diets have resulted in instances of vitamin and mineral inadequacies [38], kwashiorkor [39], and failure to thrive [40]. Most of the research on growth in children with food allergies focuses on cow's milk [41]. One longitudinal study found that children who developed an allergy to cow's milk experienced a slowing in their growth after their diagnosis, and their height and weight had not normalized by 2 years of age [42]. Other studies found that children with milk allergy had a lower height-to-age ratio than their unaffected peers [43, 44]. One study, while small (197 children, 98 of whom had at least one food allergy), assessed food allergies more broadly (i.e., not just milk) [41]. This study found that while 16% of children with one allergy were in the twenty-fifth percentile of height-for-age, 35% of children with more than one food allergy fell into the lowest quartile [41]. While height-for-age was normally distributed across children with food allergies, more children with food allergies were in the lowest quartile than children without [41]. Accordingly, the NIAID Food Allergy Guidelines recommends food counseling for all parents of children with food allergies to facilitate appropriate substitutions to compensate for removal of key foods from children's diets [10]. An annual nutritional assessment for children with food allergies has also been recommended to assess whether their growth is on track and that they are consuming adequate nutrients [41].

Common Misconceptions

Food sensitivities are the same as food allergies

A number of different adverse reactions to food can occur, which are classified differently according to symptom presentation and—when known—underlying causal mechanism [45]. Confusion can occur when parents are not aware of the symptomatic differences between food allergies and other food reactions, when similar symptoms present for different underlying reasons, and when they misattribute their children's symptoms as caused by consumption of a food. Allergies are specific to an immunologic process by which the body misidentifies proteins found in food as foreign and reacts with initiation of an immunologic response [45]. Adverse reactions to foods not caused by this immunologic response to proteins include lactose intolerance, celiac disease, and reactions that are toxic, metabolic, infectious, or pharmacologic [45]. One commonly cited misconception is that lactose intolerance is the same as a dairy allergy. In the case of lactose intolerance, the body does not produce a sufficient amount of the enzyme needed to break down sugars within milk [45]. Symptoms of lactose intolerance result from the excess gas that is produced as a result, such as cramps, bloating, flatulence, and diarrhea [45]. This is in contrast to a milk allergy, in which the protein in milk is perceived as a direct threat to the body due to insufficient barriers in the gut that, when functioning correctly, cause antigens found in food to be admitted safely in the body [45]. Symptoms of a milk allergy include systems other than the digestive tract (as in lactose intolerance), such as skin and respiratory reactions [7].

Some portion of parental confusion about their children's diagnostic status may stem from incomplete or incorrect diagnoses made in doctors' offices. One survey of 2,355 parents of children with reported food allergies found that approximately 32% of children did not obtain a diagnostic test (skin test, blood test, or oral challenge) [6]. In this sample, only one of every five reported allergy diagnoses were supported with collateral results of an oral challenge [6]. Children with the most severe reactions were more likely to receive a diagnosis from a physician [6]. Children with peanut, milk, and tree nut allergies were the most likely to have received a diagnosis from their physician [6]. Shellfish diagnoses were significantly less likely to be diagnosed or assessed with blood or skin testing [6].

The study authors hypothesized a few mechanisms by which parents might report their children have food allergies without diagnosis from a physician, as occurred in one third of their sample [6]. They propose that once parents suspect a food allergy, they may begin to eliminate that food from their children's diets without consulting their physician [6]. Even once parents seek medical support, diagnosis of food allergies is difficult due to the wide range of symptoms, differential symptom presentation based on individual characteristics (of the child and the food), and the changing reaction severity over repeated exposures [6]. The level of diagnostic testing indicated depends on the symptom presentation, family history, and age of child [7]. Some allergic reactions are life-threatening, and the average time between referral to allergist and visit to allergist is 4 months [7]. Accordingly, primary care physicians who suspect food allergy based on reports of severe reactions should refer an allergist immediately and prescribe epinephrine, antihistamines, and counsel parents about food management for the interim [7].

Parents who observe their children experiencing reactions to foods should simply remove that food from their children's diet, as there is no cure for food allergies, anyway

Similar to the above misconception wherein parents attempt to diagnose a food allergy without medical expertise, parents who initiate treatment for their children's perceived food allergies without consulting their physician are similarly placing their children at risk. While there is still no established definitive mode for food allergy testing, physicians can clarify further for parents the level of caution they should take in response to an observed reaction. For example, if children show an allergic response to one food, a comprehensive skin prick battery should still not be performed in absence of clinical history for other food allergies [7, 45]. While some parents may want a battery performed, skin prick testing produces many false positives [7, 45]. Skin prick tests can be further misleading to parents because the magnitude of response during testing (i.e., size of skin reaction to the prick) is not associated with severity of response [46]. In fact, the size of the skin reaction is connected to the likelihood that the food indeed caused the reaction [46]. Blood tests can provide further diagnostic clarity, but primary care physicians have varying levels of confidence in interpreting laboratory results [7]. Oral food challenge—the most labor-intensive method for assessing food allergy—should be performed by only an allergist due to the potential for severe reactions during the test [7]. Oral food challenge consists of the child consuming the suspected allergen in gradually increasing amounts under close supervision from a professional equipped to respond to possible severe reactions [47].

Without a formal diagnosis, parents take the chance that they will eliminate foods from their children's diets that are not true allergic offenders [6]. Removing the incorrect food is problematic for three reasons. First, because removing common foods diminishes quality of life, unnecessary elimination should be avoided [6]. Second, removing the incorrect food fails to identify the true cause of the child's adverse reaction to the food [6]. If the observed reaction was due to a food allergy, the child remains at risk for ingestion of the true offender [6]. Third, parents who choose to manage their children's allergies via elimination without consulting with a physician may miss crucial information about food allergies, such as that previous reaction history does not accurately predict severity of future reactions [6]. Instead, parents who confer with pediatricians about a suspected allergy before attempting elimination receive counseling and education about label reading and emergency response. Education about label reading is recommended because food manufacturers commonly utilize several allergy-producing foods in one product, increasing the risk of accidental ingestion [41]. After consulting with a physician, parents can also obtain life-saving injectable epinephrine in case of accidental ingestion if their child's allergy warrants [6].

Young children are most at risk for suffering severe reactions to food allergies

Certainly quality of life and accidental ingestion are legitimate concerns for parents of young children with food allergies. However, the quality of life concerns regarding food avoidance and accidental ingestion that affect young children also present in adolescents [23]. An elevated number of psychiatric symptoms were observed in food allergic adolescents (ages 10–15) compared to nonallergic peers [23]. The observed increase in symptoms was not clinically meaningful—on average, food allergic adolescents displayed one additional psychiatric symptom [23]. Study authors proposed the possibility that these additional symptoms did not reflect true psychiatric concerns, but rather were thoughts or behaviors associated with the tasks needed to avoid certain foods [23]. For example, preoccupying thoughts about food that may indicate an eating disorder in a nonallergic adolescent reflect appropriate thought patterns needed to sufficiently avoid the offending foods in allergic teens [23].

While adolescents' quality of life appears to be influenced in a way similar to that of young children, differences emerge between children and adolescents in the realm of anaphylaxis [48, 49]. Fatal allergic reactions disproportionately affect adolescents [48, 49]. Adolescents engage in risk-taking behaviors when managing their food allergies, such as not carrying their AAIs, consuming foods they know themselves to be allergic to, or eating foods with a "may contain" label [11]. Adolescent risk-taking behavior is commonly misunderstood as a lack of appreciation for the risks of their actions. Consequently, interventions for teenagers often focus on providing information about allergies [50]. These narrow interventions must be limited, because knowledge alone does not address the psychosocial concerns teenagers face when managing their food allergies.

Adolescents present unique psychosocial profiles that make adherence to safety protocols challenging [22]. By around age 8 years old, children begin demonstrating awareness that their allergies set them apart from their peers [51]. Allergic teenagers report feeling misunderstood and insecure [52]. Many teens also report being teased or bullied by peers as a consequence of their food allergies [11, 51, 53–55]. Many adolescents come to understand having an allergy as a way of life [51, 52]. The constant vigilance needed to remain safe is a source of frustration for many teens [22]. Concurrently, the developmental stage of adolescence promotes increasing independence and autonomy from parents. Food allergic teens are attempting to separate and individuate from their parents, which requires assuming increasing responsibility for managing their condition. This transfer of responsibility occurs in the context of anxiety from parents and sometimes the teens themselves [22]. Subsequently, the emphasis on simply informing teenagers about the risks of food allergies oversimplifies adolescents' reasons for not engaging in strategies to stay safe from their food allergy [11]. The simplistic understanding neglects to view the teenager as a whole person with other factors to consider in decision-making than just their food allergy [11].

Surveys have found no association between factual knowledge of risk and risk-taking behaviors [56]. The higher risk-taking teenagers actually had more accurate knowledge of the risks, whereas the lower risk-taking teens overestimated the risks [56]. There are many reported reasons why teenagers might choose to consume foods they know to be dangerous to them, or to fail to carry their prescribed epinephrine pen. Some reasons pertain to knowledge. For example, food allergic subjects have indicated that they do not always know how to identify their own anaphylactic symptoms or when the severity is of a magnitude that requires intervention [57]. Adolescents may also not understand the appropriate treatment for anaphylaxis; subsequently treat their symptoms inappropriately with antihistamines or their asthma medication [57]. Other reasons are more psychological in nature. Perception of importance for carrying an epinephrine pen is linked to personal experience. Specifically, the longer it has been since patients suffered anaphylaxis, the less likely they are to carry emergency medication [58]. Adolescents weigh various considerations as to whether or not they should carry epinephrine with them, such as how different it makes them feel from their peers [51, 53] and if they are in a familiar environment where they feel confident they will be able to sufficiently avoid their allergen [53, 59]. Adolescents also weigh relative risk when deciding whether to avoid a food or not [11]. They may consider prior experience with eating food products with labels such as "may contain," and use that prior experience to determine present risk of consumption [59]. What these adolescents may not realize is that food manufacturers can change their processes over time, and past experiences do not accurately and confidently predict future outcomes [11]. Paradoxically, adolescents also consider whether or not their epinephrine is close by when deciding whether or not to try to eat an allergen [53, 59]. The presence of epinephrine would seem to reduce the perception of risk of ingesting a food.

Generally speaking, adolescents will interpret a didactic format for discussing allergies as paternalistic and antithetical to their emerging independence and competence [11]. Adolescents may benefit more from a dialogue in which their physician solicits their impressions, joins them in their feelings of frustration or anxiety, and asks them questions. Any discussions with teenagers to help them increase avoiding allergens and carrying their epinephrine must be focused on the individual adolescent's concerns [11]. Health care providers who wish to discuss the teenagers' true concerns about avoiding food and carrying epinephrine should consider whether the conversation is more likely to be honest and open without the teenagers' parents in the consulting room [11].

There is not yet sufficiently rigorous evidence for specific modes of interacting with teens in a way that addresses their psychological, social, and emotional concerns about their food allergies [11]. Past research initially examined which psychological models might account best for teens' allergy management [11]. While not yet tested in a trial, some allergists hypothesize that exposing teenagers to oral food challenge testing provides a more salient understanding of their allergy and responses than the skin prick test [11]. Preliminary examinations of cognitive adjunctive therapy to address teenagers' behaviors are underway [11]. A possible area for future research could seek to understand if the severity of adolescents' previous allergic reactions affects their prevention and treatment response behaviors [11].

Because peanut allergies can cause anaphylaxis, schools should ban children from bringing in peanuts or peanut products

The practice of schools imposing bans on peanuts is increasing, yet not without controversy [60]. Peanut bans are universally applied, often without regard for the affected children's true severity of allergic reaction [60]. While eight foods cause 90% of food allergies, schools have singled out peanuts for banning over other more common allergens [12, 60, 61]. It is supposed that schools only ban peanuts because to ban all common allergens is simply too impractical a response to food allergies [60]. Criticisms of bans include that they transfer responsibility for keeping a child safe from parents to institutions; that they require monitoring of unaffected peers; and that they overburden teachers and other educational staff with medical directives that they may not be prepared to implement [60]. Despite these criticisms, if the practice of banning foods had established evidence for saving lives, an argument could be made for its merit. Similar to public health efforts to reduce smoking in shared spaces, the bans on peanuts often assume a moral tone, implying that banning foods is the right thing to do regardless of whether it is medically or scientifically indicated [60]. Whereas smoking bans can be justified because smoking and secondhand smoke are objectively deleterious to all individuals, bans on foods that are otherwise safe and healthy for the great majority of people, due to their effect on specific students, are an overgeneralization of community health efforts [60].

There is no current evidence base suggesting that school bans reduce allergic reactions in schools [12]. Given the lack of scientific evidence supporting school-wide peanut bans, schools that implement bans must be responding to a different impetus. Should severe allergic reactions happen on school grounds, schools face possibly litigious parents [60]. The perception that schools should treat their students as parents treat their children is underpinned by the legal mandate "in loco parentis," which delineates the responsibility schools have to children in their parents' absence [60]. As a defensive strategy, many schools implement bans for the entire school rather than follow recommended guidelines for addressing a student with a food allergy [60]. Responding to parents' fears rather than science, results in bans that are more stringent than necessary. For example, there is a misconception that severe allergic reactions can occur from inhaling properties of the food [12]. In reality, room temperature peanut vapors contain no protein (the agent that causes the immunologic response) from the peanut [62]. Yet parents who believe vapors can cause a severe reaction may push schools to remove them completely, effectively asking schools to prevent an incident that the evidence indicates does not occur.

To Explain to a Patient

Many events that humans fear are either extremely unlikely or not possible at all. While there have been case reports of children having reactions to peanut vapors, a study that attempted to confirm this found no evidence of reaction due to inhalation [63]. Scientists have also examined vapors emanating from peanuts, and the proteins that cause peanut allergies are not present in room temperature vapors [62]. Therefore, any attempts to prevent allergic response to inhalation will look like they are "working." In reality, that event was not going to happen, anyway.

If you bought elephant repellant and sprayed it on yourself every morning, you could easily conclude that the elephant repellent is keeping elephants away from you. But you know that this doesn't make sense—there are no elephants anywhere near your home. You would correctly identify someone who took "precautions" such as spraying the repellent to be engaging in unnecessary behavior.

You may think, "What's the harm? If elephants are dangerous and spraying the repellent is such a minor task, why not just do it?" In preventing and responding to severe allergic reactions, there is always trade-offs. Time spent enforcing unneeded peanut bans in schools is time not spent training staff to use epinephrine injectors, not spent teaching about how children with unidentified food allergies my need help, not spent learning how to identify allergic reactions, and so on. Bans give a false sense of safety, which reduces the urgency felt to remain vigilant about food allergies.

Recommendations endorsed by the National School Board Association, the Food Allergy and Anaphylaxis Network, the National Association of School Nurses, and the National Association of School Principals are considerably more modest than outright bans of foods that apply to entire schools [12]. Recommendations are based on current knowledge of how anaphylaxis is most likely to occur and refrains from making recommendations based on as-of-yet unknown information [12]. Judicious schools take into account the age of children (presuming the younger to be more likely to accidentally ingest) and number of children to monitor at once in their efforts [12]. Schools should not focus solely on cafeterias, as only 12% of anaphylactic reactions occur there [64]. Rather, children touching products such as peanut butter during craft activities in the classroom were more likely to have a reaction [64]. Anaphylaxis has not been shown to occur due to inhalation, therefore there are no recommendations to monitor foods in ways that seek to minimize airborne allergens [12]. Because 25% of anaphylactic reactions occur in students with no previously known food allergies, schools should have extra epinephrine on hand [12].

Current Research

In the area of food allergies, research has produced extensive questions. A systematic review of the food allergy literature could not identify a consensus definition of the condition [65]. Researchers cannot always employ the most rigorous methodology, a randomized controlled trial, due to feasibility and/or ethical reasons [65]. Elimination diets, the mainstay treatment of food allergies, have only been examined in one study that measured antibodies in 86 children with atopic dermatitis as a result of food allergies [65, 66]. Despite the lack of evidence-based answers, parents attempt various unproven methods to either prevent or cure their children's allergies. Below we review the research available on the prevention and treatment during various stages in a child's life.

Prevention

Due to the genetic component of food allergies, women are characterized as high-risk of giving birth to a child with food allergy if either of the children's parents or a sibling have such an allergy [67]. Maternal antigens have been observed to cross into the placenta, prompting researchers to conclude that maternal diet during prenatal development may influence the unborn child's allergic profile [68]. A review of the limited work in this area to date found no evidence in favor of mothers avoiding common allergens during pregnancy [67]. While various studies have suggested some possible influence of maternal consumption of allergens on child allergy development once born, others directly refute these findings [69]. When differences between children whose mothers avoided allergens and mothers who did not were noted, they were typically small and in favor of non-avoidance [67]. Lower gestational weight gain in mothers who avoided allergens, higher risk of preterm birth (difference not reaching statistical significance), and lower birth weight (again, not statistically significant) were observed in the avoidance mothers [67]. The studies that found positive benefits to avoidance were small [70] or did not confirm children's allergies with food challenges [71]. A review of all the studies performed to date indicates that there is not sufficient evidence to recommend that women avoid common allergens when pregnant, even mothers of high-risk children [69].

Breastfeeding

To date, a very limited number of studies have examined maternal diet during breastfeeding to determine if avoiding common allergens helped reduce emergence of childhood allergies [65]. Previous recommendations for avoidance of allergens during lactation were based on an early study that examined various avoidance methods in infants already at risk of developing allergies [72, 73]. The methodology of the study included a number of other avoidance interventions, including a staggered introduction of foods and significant supplementation of breast milk with an extensively hydrolyzed formula [73]. While the results of the study indicated some reduction in food-associated skin reactions and stomach problems among treated children, the use of extensively hydrolyzed formula is a significant confounder, limiting the generalizability of the findings [73]. The modest changes seen in the avoidance group cannot be definitively attributed to maternal diet during breastfeeding [73]. Similar to maternal avoidance of common allergens during pregnancy, the data on avoidance during breastfeeding continue to be conflicting [69]. At this time, the only avoidance of food in maternal diet recommended during breastfeeding is when a breastfeeding child shows symptoms of allergic reaction in response to breast milk [69]. Due to the crucial nutritive and caloric needs of infants, nutritionists should closely supervise mothers who avoid foods during lactation to ensure that growth is not adversely affected [69].

Food Delay

Out of concern that children's immune systems cannot process proteins found in common allergens, some parents delay introducing such foods into their children's diets. There may be some benefit associated with allergen avoidance in very young children, but it appears limited to infants between 3 and 4 months old [73]. Restricting children's exposure after 4 months may detrimentally effect allergy prevention [73]. A study of 856 children found a negative association between the diversity of foods children ate in their first year of life and subsequent development of food allergies by up to 6 years old [74]. That is, the more kinds of foods children ate in their first year, the fewer allergies were observed at 6 years old. It should be cautioned that this is a correlational finding, and causation is not implied. Study authors could not conclude a causal mechanism because children who show early symptoms and parents with food allergy are both conditions that are more likely to lead to a delay in the introduction of complementary foods to the child's diet [74]. Therefore, the lack of food diversity observed in the first year may reflect an early prevention or response to the allergy that is already predetermined to emerge by 6 years. These results lend support to the hypothesis that providing children's bodies an opportunity to develop a healthy response to the antigens found in allergens may assist the maturational process of their immune systems [74]. Researchers refer to a so-called "critical early window" between 4 and 6 months, in which children should be introduced to solid foods as complimentary in their diet to continued breastfeeding [73]. Consequently, current guidelines recommend that foods should be introduced into a breastfeeding child's diet no earlier than 4 months but certainly by 6 months [15, 73, 75].

Treatment

As previously stated, there are currently no established treatments for food allergies. There is an emerging body of research on immunotherapy, that is, introducing the allergen gradually in a highly regulated environment (due to the risk of anaphylaxis) in order to build desensitization or possibly tolerance [76]. Desensitization is the body's ability to tolerate small amounts of the food, with frequently repeated exposures required to maintain the remittance of symptoms [76]. Tolerance, on the other hand, is a relatively longer-lasting state in which the body continues to maintain the effects of treatment while requiring only periodic reintroduction to the allergens [76]. There are different procedures for introducing the allergen during the process, such as eating the food directly or placing the allergen under the tongue [76]. Immunotherapy is an extensive process, requires direct supervised care, has risks associated with poor reactions, and the effects are typically sufficient only to allow for possible accidental ingestion [76]. The goal of immunotherapy is for children to be able to tolerate a small amount of the allergen in the event of accidental ingestion [76]. It is not designed to permit children to consume copious amounts of the allergen. Immunotherapy has been tested for some allergens, but not others [76]. The long-term outcomes of immunotherapy are still unknown [7]. Despite showing promise, immunotherapy is not approved by the Food and Drug Administration and is therefore not available in clinic settings [76].

Studies examining the possibility of an herbal remedy are currently under way [7]. A 9-herb formulation, called FAHF2 (for food allergy herbal formula) has been shown to suppress an allergic response in mice [77]. As the formula did not produce any side effects in preliminary human trials, further human trials are currently underway [7].

Conclusion

With regard to food allergies, research is unlikely to provide concerned parents with satisfactory responses due to the large amount of unanswered questions. Healthcare practitioners should continue to keep lines of communication open with their patients concerned about food allergies. Quality of life and nutrition in the face of avoidance diets are two areas that require specific attention. Parents of adolescents may require support in the gradual transfer of food allergy management in a way that acknowledges the teens' experience while still emphasizing safety. As no treatment currently exists for food allergies, parents benefit from support in managing the chronic condition.

References

1. Gupta RS, Springston EE, Warrier MR, Smith B, Kumar R, Pongracic J, Holl JL. The prevalence, severity, and distribution of childhood food allergy in the United States. Pediatrics. 2011;128(1):e9–17.
2. Venter C, Arshad SH. Epidemiology of food allergy. Pediatr Clin North Am. 2011;58(2):327–49.
3. Kuehn BM. Food allergies becoming more common. JAMA. 2008;300(20):2358.
4. Lack G. Epidemiologic risks for food allergy. J Allergy Clin Immunol. 2008;121(6):1331–6.
5. Branum AM, Lukacs SL. Food allergy among children in the United States. Pediatrics. 2009;124(6):1549–55.
6. Gupta RS, Springston EE, Smith B, Pongracic J, Holl JL, Warrier MR. Parent report of physician diagnosis in pediatric food allergy. J Allergy Clin Immunol. 2013;131(1):150–6.
7. Gupta RS, Dyer AA, Jain N, Greenhawt MJ. Childhood food allergies: current diagnosis, treatment, and management strategies. InMayo Clinic Proceedings 2013 May 31 (Vol. 88, No. 5, p. 512–26). Elsevier.
8. Goossens NJ, Flokstra-de Blok BM, Meulen GN, Botjes E, Burgerhof HG, Gupta RS, Springston EE, Smith B, Duiverman EJ, Dubois AE. Food allergy knowledge of parents–is ignorance bliss? Pediatr Allergy Immunol 2013;24(6):567–73
9. LeBovidge JS, Stone KD, Twarog FJ, Raiselis SW, Kalish LA, Bailey EP, Schneider LC. Development of a preliminary questionnaire to assess parental response to children's food allergies. Ann Allergy Asthma Immunol. 2006;96(3):472–7.
10. Boyce JA, Assa'ad A, Burks AW, Jones SM, Sampson HA, Wood RA, Plaut M, Cooper SF, Fenton MJ, Arshad SH, Bahna SL. Guidelines for the diagnosis and management of food allergy in the United States: report of the NIAID-sponsored expert panel. J Allergy Clin Immunol 2010;126(6 0):S1.
11. Marrs T, Lack G. Why do few food-allergic adolescents treat anaphylaxis with adrenaline?–reviewing a pressing issue. Pediatr Allergy Immunol. 2013;24(3):222–9.
12. Young MC, Muñoz-Furlong A, Sicherer SH. Management of food allergies in schools: a perspective for allergists. J Allergy Clin Immunol. 2009;124(2):175–82.
13. Hourihane JO, Dean TP, Warner JO. Peanut allergy in relation to heredity, maternal diet, and other atopic diseases: results of a questionnaire survey, skin prick testing, and food challenges. BMJ. 1996;313(7056):518–21.
14. Sicherer SH, Furlong TJ, Maes HH, Desnick RJ, Sampson HA, Gelb BD. Genetics of peanut allergy: a twin study. J Allergy Clin Immunol. 2000;106(1):53–6.

15. Greer FR, Sicherer SH, Burks AW. Effects of early nutritional interventions on the development of atopic disease in infants and children: the role of maternal dietary restriction, breastfeeding, timing of introduction of complementary foods, and hydrolyzed formulas. Pediatrics. 2008;121(1):183–91.

16. Herbert LJ, Dahlquist LM. Perceived history of anaphylaxis and parental overprotection, autonomy, anxiety, and depression in food allergic young adults. J Clin Psychol Med Settings. 2008;15(4):261–9.

17. Garbutt JM, Leege E, Sterkel R, Gentry S, Wallendorf M, Strunk RC. What are parents worried about? Health problems and health concerns for children. Clin Pediatr. 2012;51(9):840–7.

18. Springston EE, Smith B, Shulruff J, Pongracic J, Holl J, Gupta RS. Variations in quality of life among caregivers of food allergic children. Ann Allergy Asthma Immunol. 2010;105(4):287–94.

19. Cohen BL, Noone S, Muñoz-Furlong A, Sicherer SH. Development of a questionnaire to measure quality of life in families with a child with food allergy. J Allergy Clin Immunol. 2004;114(5):1159–63.

20. Cummings AJ, Knibb RC, King RM, Lucas JS. The psychosocial impact of food allergy and food hypersensitivity in children, adolescents and their families: a review. Allergy. 2010;65(8):933–45.

21. Sicherer SH, Noone SA, Muñoz-Furlong A. The impact of childhood food allergy on quality of life. Ann Allergy Asthma Immunol. 2001;87(6):461–4.

22. Polloni L, Lazzarotto F, Bonaguro R, Toniolo A, Celegato N, Muraro A. Psychological care of food-allergic children and their families: an exploratory analysis. Pediatr Allergy Immunol. 2015;26(1):87–90.

23. Shanahan L, Zucker N, Copeland WE, Costello EJ, Angold A. Are children and adolescents with food allergies at increased risk for psychopathology? J Psychosom Res. 2014;77(6):468–73.

24. Warren CM, Gupta RS, Sohn MW, Oh EH, Lal N, Garfield CF, Caruso D, Wang X, Pongracic JA. Differences in empowerment and quality of life among parents of children with food allergy. Ann Allergy Asthma Immunol. 2015;114(2):117–25.

25. Bandura A (1977) Self-efficacy: Toward a unifying theory of behavioral change. Psychol Rev 1977;84(2): 191–215.

26. Parker K, Wang W. Modern parenthood: Roles of moms and dads converge as they balance work and family. Pew Research Center; 2013.

27. Vargas PA, Sicherer SH, Christie L, Keaveny M, Noone S, Watkins D, Carlisle SK, Jones SM. Developing a food allergy curriculum for parents. Pediatr Allergy Immunol. 2011;22(6):575–82.

28. Hu W, Grbich C, Kemp A. Parental food allergy information needs: a qualitative study. Arch Dis Child. 2007;92(9):771–5.

29. Abdurrahman ZB, Kastner M, Wurman C, Harada L, Bantock L, Cruickshank H, Waserman S. Experiencing a first food allergic reaction: a survey of parent and caregiver perspectives. Allergy Asthma Clin Immunol. 2013;9(18):1492–9.

30. Gillespie CA, Woodgate RL, Chalmers KI, Watson WT. "Living with risk": mothering a child with food-induced anaphylaxis. J Pediatr Nurs. 2007;22(1):30–42.

31. Kapoor S, Roberts G, Bynoe Y, Gaughan M, Habibi P, Lack G. Influence of a multidisciplinary paediatric allergy clinic on parental knowledge and rate of subsequent allergic reactions. Allergy. 2004;59(2):185–91.

32. Arkwright PD, Farragher AJ. Factors determining the ability of parents to effectively administer intramuscular adrenaline to food allergic children. Pediatr Allergy Immunol. 2006;17(3):227–9.

33. LeBovidge JS, Michaud A, Deleon A, Harada L, Waserman S, Schneider L. Evaluating a handbook for parents of children with food allergy: a randomized clinical trial. Ann Allergy Asthma Immunol 2016.

34. Bock SA. Prospective appraisal of complaints of adverse reactions to foods in children during the first 3 years of life. Pediatrics. 1987;79(5):683–8.
35. Mehta H, Groetch M, Wang J. Growth and nutritional concerns in children with food allergy. Curr Opin Allergy Clin Immunol. 2013 Jun;13(3):275.
36. Burks AW, James JM, Hiegel A, Wilson G, Wheeler JG, Jones SM, Zuerlein N. Atopic dermatitis and food hypersensitivity reactions. J Pediatr. 1998;132(1):132–6.
37. Sampson HA, McCaskill CC. Food hypersensitivity and atopic dermatitis: evaluation of 113 patients. J Pediatr. 1985;107(5):669–75.
38. Bierman CW, Shapiro GG, Christie DL, VanArsdel PP, Furukawa CT, Ward BH. Eczema, rickets, and food allergy. J Allergy Clin Immunol. 1978;61(2):119–27.
39. Liu T, Howard RM, Mancini AJ, Weston WL, Paller AS, Drolet BA, Esterly NB, Levy ML, Schachner L, Frieden IJ. Kwashiorkor in the United States: fad diets, perceived and true milk allergy, and nutritional ignorance. Arch Dermatol. 2001;137(5):630–6.
40. Tarnow-Mordi WO, Moss C, Ross K. Failure to thrive owing to inappropriate diet free of gluten and cows' milk. British Med J (Clinical research ed.). 1984;289(6452):1113.
41. Christie L, Hine RJ, Parker JG, Burks W. Food allergies in children affect nutrient intake and growth. J Am Diet Assoc. 2002;102(11):1648–51.
42. Isolauri E, Sütas Y, Salo MK, Isosomppi R, Kaila M. Elimination diet in cow's milk allergy: risk for impaired growth in young children. J Pediatr. 1998;132(6):1004–9.
43. Paganus A, Juntunen-Backman K, Savilahti E. Follow-up of nutritional status and dietary survey in children with cow's milk allergy. Acta Paediatr. 1992;81(6–7):518–21.
44. Tiainen JM, Nuutinen OM, Kalavainen MP. Diet and nutritional status in children with cow's milk allergy. Eur J Clin Nutr. 1995;49(8):605–12.
45. Forbes LR, Saltzman RW, Spergel JM. Food allergies and atopic dermatitis: differentiating myth from reality. Pediatr Ann. 2009;38(2).
46. Sampson HA. Update on food allergy. J Allergy Clin Immunol. 2004;113(5):805–19.
47. Sicherer SH. Food allergy: when and how to perform oral food challenges. Pediatr Allergy Immunol. 1999;10(4):226–34.
48. Pumphrey RS, Gowland MH. Further fatal allergic reactions to food in the United Kingdom, 1999-2006. J Allergy Clin Immunol. 2007;119(4):1018–9.
49. Bock SA, Muñoz-Furlong A, Sampson HA. Further fatalities caused by anaphylactic reactions to food, 2001–2006. J Allergy Clin Immunol. 2007;119(4):1016–8.
50. Ewan PW, Clark AT. Long-term prospective observational study of patients with peanut and nut allergy after participation in a management plan. Lancet. 2001;357(9250):111–5.
51. Akeson N, Worth A, Sheikh A. The psychosocial impact of anaphylaxis on young people and their parents. Clin Exp Allergy. 2007;37(8):1213–20.
52. MacKenzie H, Roberts G, Van Laar D, Dean T. Teenagers' experiences of living with food hypersensitivity: a qualitative study. Pediatr Allergy Immunol. 2010;21(4p1):595–602.
53. Macadam C, Barnett J, Roberts G, Stiefel G, King R, Erlewyn-Lajeunesse M, Holloway JA, Lucas JS. What factors affect the carriage of epinephrine auto-injectors by teenagers. Clin Transl Allergy. 2012;2(1):3.
54. Sampson MA, Muñoz-Furlong A, Sicherer SH. Risk-taking and coping strategies of adolescents and young adults with food allergy. J Allergy Clin Immunol. 2006;117(6):1440–5.
55. Singh J, Aszkenasy OM. Prescription of adrenaline auto-injectors for potential anaphylaxis—a population survey. Public Health. 2003;117(4):256–9.
56. Uguz A, Lack G, Pumphrey R, Ewan P, Warner J, Dick J, Briggs D, Clarke S, Reading D, Hourihane J. Allergic reactions in the community: a questionnaire survey of members of the anaphylaxis campaign. Clin Exp Allergy. 2005;35(6):746–50.
57. Simons FE, Clark S, Camargo CA. Anaphylaxis in the community: learning from the survivors. J Allergy Clin Immunol. 2009;124(2):301–6.
58. Mullins RJ. Anaphylaxis: risk factors for recurrence. Clin Exp Allergy. 2003;33(8):1033–40.
59. Monks H, Gowland MH, MacKenzie H, Erlewyn-Lajeunesse M, King R, Lucas JS, Roberts G. How do teenagers manage their food allergies? Clin Exp Allergy. 2010;40(10):1533–40.

60. Rous T, Hunt A. Governing peanuts: the regulation of the social bodies of children and the risks of food allergies. Soc Sci Med. 2004;58(4):825–36.
61. Waggoner MR. Parsing the peanut panic: the social life of a contested food allergy epidemic. Soc Sci Med. 2013;31(90):49–55.
62. Perry TT, Conover-Walker MK, Pomés A, Chapman MD, Wood RA. Distribution of peanut allergen in the environment. J Allergy Clin Immunol. 2004;113(5):973–6.
63. Simonte SJ, Ma S, Mofidi S, Sicherer SH. Relevance of casual contact with peanut butter in children with peanut allergy. J Allergy Clin Immunol. 2003;112(1):180–2.
64. Sicherer SH, Furlong TJ, DeSimone J, Sampson HA. The US peanut and tree nut allergy registry: characteristics of reactions in schools and day care. J Pediatr. 2001;138(4):560–5.
65. Chafen JJ, Newberry SJ, Riedl MA, Bravata DM, Maglione M, Suttorp MJ, Sundaram V, Paige NM, Towfigh A, Hulley BJ, Shekelle PG. Diagnosing and managing common food allergies: a systematic review. JAMA. 2010;303(18):1848–56.
66. Agata H, Kondo N, Fukutomi O, Shinoda S, Orii T. Effect of elimination diets on food-specific IgE antibodies and lymphocyte proliferative responses to food antigens in atopic dermatitis patients exhibiting sensitivity to food allergens. J Allergy Clin Immunol. 1993;91(2):668–79.
67. Kramer MS, Kakuma R. Maternal dietary antigen avoidance during pregnancy or lactation, or both, for preventing or treating atopic disease in the child. Evidence-Based Child Health: A Cochrane Rev J. 2014;9(2):447–83.
68. Loibichler C, Pichler J, Gerstmayr M, Bohle B, Kiss H, Urbanek R, Szepfalusi Z. Materno–fetal passage of nutritive and inhalant allergens across placentas of term and pre-term deliveries perfused in vitro. Clin Exp Allergy. 2002;32(11):1546–51.
69. Fleischer DM, Spergel JM, Assa'ad AH, Pongracic JA. Primary prevention of allergic disease through nutritional interventions. J Allergy Clin Immunol In Practice. 2013;1(1):29–36.
70. Frank L, Marian A, Visser M, Weinberg E, Potter PC. Exposure to peanuts in utero and in infancy and the development of sensitization to peanut allergens in young children. Pediatr Allergy Immunol. 1999;10(1):27–32.
71. Sicherer SH, Wood RA, Stablein D, Lindblad R, Burks AW, Liu AH, Jones SM, Fleischer DM, Leung DY, Sampson HA. Maternal consumption of peanut during pregnancy is associated with peanut sensitization in atopic infants. J Allergy Clin Immunol. 2010;126(6):1191–7.
72. Zeiger RS, Heller S. The development and prediction of atopy in high-risk children: follow-up at age seven years in a prospective randomized study of combined maternal and infant food allergen avoidance. J Allergy Clin Immunol. 1995;95(6):1179–90.
73. Prescott SL, Smith P, Tang M, Palmer DJ, Sinn J, Huntley SJ, Cormack B, Heine RG, Gibson RA, Makrides M. The importance of early complementary feeding in the development of oral tolerance: concerns and controversies. Pediatr Allergy Immunol. 2008;19(5):375–80.
74. Roduit C, Frei R, Depner M, Schaub B, Loss G, Genuneit J, Pfefferle P, Hyvärinen A, Karvonen AM, Riedler J, Dalphin JC. Increased food diversity in the first year of life is inversely associated with allergic diseases. J Allergy Clin Immunol. 2014;133(4):1056–64.
75. Agostoni C, Decsi T, Fewtrell M, Goulet O, Kolacek S, Koletzko B, Michaelsen KF, Moreno L, Puntis J, Rigo J, Shamir R. Complementary feeding: a commentary by the ESPGHAN Committee on Nutrition. J Pediatr Gastroenterol Nutr. 2008;46(1):99–110.
76. Praticò AD, Leonardi S. Immunotherapy for food allergies: a myth or a reality? Immunotherapy. 2015;7(2):147–61.
77. Wang J, Sicherer SH. Immunologic therapeutic approaches in the management of food allergy. Expert review of clinical immunology. 2009;5(3):301–10.

Chapter 9
Discipline Techniques

Overview

Discipline is a widely researched and controversial area in parenting studies [1]. This research area often employs a number of terms or euphemisms that impede understanding if they are not first carefully defined. As a starting point, many parenting programs or parenting literature are often not discussing parenting as a whole. The term "parenting" is used frequently as a stand-in for discipline. From this careful avoidance of the word discipline, we infer that discipline carries a negative connotation for some. In this chapter, we refer to **discipline** as the practice of attempting to increase children's appropriate behaviors and decrease their unacceptable ones. The goals of discipline aim to make children **prosocial**, that is, act in accordance with their larger social culture. Many behaviors children exhibit that discipline seeks to reduce are not inherently "wrong," or "bad"; they are simply unacceptable in the larger social context of adult functioning. For example, throwing a temper tantrum when the store is out of a needed product is not an acceptable behavior in adults. When children are young, discipline is used to guide them away from this behavioral response and toward a more acceptable and effective one.

This definition of discipline does not sound particularly ominous or frightening. What then, accounts for the avoidance of using the word? We pose that just as "parenting" stands in for "discipline," "discipline" stands in for "punishment." Here the negative connotation is not only more likely, it is apt. Punishment necessarily refers to introducing a negative element after an unacceptable behavior to reduce it over time [2].

Equating punishment with discipline is a gross oversimplification, and an erroneous one at that. More precisely, discipline almost always involves some forms of punishment. No child is born knowing the societal guidelines and legal statutes for aggression, fairness, appropriate language, and the like. Therefore, all children will at least occasionally display behaviors their parents wish to decrease. Parents have at their disposal a variety of options for punishment. Some forms are nonphysical and others are physical. Nonphysical punishments are any responses that introduce an element of negativity into a child's life following a behavioral infraction [2]. Examples include time-outs, removals of privilege, and brief reprimands. Physical punishments range in widely in definition and application. Some researchers define spanking as a type of corporal punishment, while others define corporal punishment as physical punishments more severe than spanking. When reviewing the literature, it is important for practitioners to note which definition the study authors are using. In this chapter, we use **spanking** to refer to a mild, open-handed strike to the child's buttocks or extremities [3]. We use **corporal punishment** to refer to the more severe forms of physical punishments that include hitting the child's face, hitting the child with an object, and shaking or shoving the child [4]. Actions harsher than corporal punishment (striking the child with a closed fist, burning, etc.) are considered **abuse**.

While discipline often involves some punishment for misbehavior, effective discipline techniques also include methods to teach children how to increase their rates of prosocial behaviors. Furthermore, we argue that the research shows the emphasis should be on these strategies, with punishment used on an as-needed basis. We discuss the current evidence-based approaches for using these positive parenting strategies. Moving forward, when we refer to **positive parenting**, we specifically refer to behavioral approaches other than punishment that increase appropriate behavior.

Overlapping terms cause confusion about the topic of discussion. While a pediatrician may want to assist parents with discipline, parents may interpret that their pediatrician wants them to physically punish their child. Parents may object to physical punishments only and not be aware of nonphysical punishments. Preferences come into play, but clarifying confusion is the first step toward understanding parents' preferences. If we take seriously the idea that there will never be only one correct way to parent, by extension, there will never be only one way to discipline. Parent and child factors will interact to determine the best possible discipline methods, and even these will not be employed "perfectly" by fallible parents.

The pediatrician's task is to provide parents with the information that will guide them to the best possible methods given their starting point. While very harsh and strict parents may need education about the effects of this mode of discipline, parents who are too lax and lack firmness in limit setting may require information about the consequences of raising children without teaching them through the use of discipline. Just as in other forms of medicine in which one size does not fit all, pediatricians will need to first assess where parents fall along this continuum before making recommendations.

A Note about Warmth

Before moving forward into discussing discipline, we will briefly address the wider scope of "parenting." The field responsible for studying discipline techniques, developmental psychology, largely utilizes a specific framework developed by Diana Baumrind for understanding parenting style [5]. Baumrind's typology examines parents' style along two dimensions—demandingness and responsiveness [6]. As a general rule, the recommended parenting style is the **authoritative** style. Authoritative parents exert control over their children's behavior in order to ensure desirable outcomes. However, they modify how these outcomes are achieved in response to their children's needs, maintaining a warm and supportive relationship with their children [6].

While this chapter focuses on discipline, note that discipline only addresses the control dimension of Baumrind's authoritative parenting. Ideally, good discipline occurs along with high levels of parental responsiveness, characterized by warmth, understanding, love, reciprocity, communication, and unconditional regard.

Common Parental Concerns

Best Approach to Discipline

As Chris Gottlieb, an attorney for parents accused of abuse, notes wryly, "parenting is something we are inclined to judge harshly at the same time that it is impossible to do in anything but an extremely flawed way.... We all know this... [y]et we couple this knowledge with extreme intolerance for the shortcomings of other parents" [7]. Her unique perspective, from working with parents at the outer fringes of acceptable parenting, informs about how even much more temperate parents are judged today. There is a current drive to impose perfectionistic standards on parenting. Gottlieb considers the "[l]egitimate efforts to protect children from serious abuse have morphed into second guessing decisions well within parental prerogative" [7].

Parents and researchers typically have two questions about discipline: Does it work? and Is it harmful? Statements in their physicians' offices reflect parents' concerns about the challenge of implementing discipline successfully. As we will explore, the evidence base shows that there are effective discipline techniques [8–10]. However, parents can find the strategies difficult to understand, stressful to implement, and impossible to use with 100% consistency every time. Many authors of popular, nonclinical parenting books try to mollify parents by proclaiming that the use of one simple approach (found in their book, of course) will result in effective discipline [11, 12]. Parents and researchers are also concerned about the possible effects of discipline. The evidence typically seeks to understand the direct and indirect effects of different forms of discipline [1]. Positive parenting and punishment techniques have undergone cycles of popularity and scorn as the evidence-based shifts according to new findings [1].

As is so often the case in deciding which approach, among many, to take, either extreme (either all-positive or all-punishment) is unlikely to provide the optimal balance. For example, any recommendations to avoid physical punishment should not be confused with an injunctive to avoid discipline altogether [13]. As we will examine, parents do not deliver discipline techniques in a vacuum. Their relationship with their child, their emotional state while delivering punishment, and their balance of using positive reinforcement in addition to punishment all affect the overall discipline experience.

When to Seek Help

Parents cannot know the ins and outs of what is developmentally normative when it comes to childhood behavior, and that includes defiance, tantrums, sharing, physical aggression, and other behaviors implicated in discipline. Parents' concerns vary according to their children's ages. Concerns about discipline have been shown to peak around a child's age of 3 years [14]. During the preschool years from ages 3–5, children in nonclinical samples show a gradual decrease in the kinds of behaviors that warrant discipline, such as tantrums, hyperactivity, attentional problems, and fighting with peers [15]. Difficulties with sharing, noncompliance with parental commands, and emotional dysregulation, while frustrating to parents, are par for the developmental course [15]. We provide a table outlining expected child behavior according to developmental level to help streamline understanding among parents (Table 9.1).

Discipline in toddlerhood is almost universally challenging, as children seek autonomy while learning to understand limit setting from authority figures [15]. The primary reason parents seek help from mental health professionals is for child noncompliance [16, 17]. **Noncompliance** is defined as one of two interactions. The first is when children fail to do as their parents ask, even when the request is age-appropriate [10]. The other is when children intentionally do the opposite or something other than their parent requested [10]. In some cases, noncompliance reflects a lack of understanding of the parents' limits [15]. When children do understand the limit but choose not to comply, this stems from either emerging self-assertion or from defiance [15]. Children who can state their preferences and dislike when authority figures' limits stand in the way of their preferences are said to engage in self-assertion [18]. Self-assertion is apparent when the child's choice of noncompliance is understandable. For example, a child who was told to clean up his toys but instead continues playing is not complying due to a specific preference for playing [18]. Defiance is more likely when the child's resistance to authority figures' directives result in a suboptimal outcome for the child [18].

Table 9.1 General guidelines for normal development [23]

	Negative emotional behaviors	Oppositionality	Aggression
Infancy	• cries in response to hunger, fatigue, frustration, no specific reason (particularly in the late afternoon, evening, and nighttime) (*frequently*)	• flails • pushes away • shakes head • gestures to indicate refusal • dawdles in response to frustration, need for control, stress separation from parents, intrusive interactions, etc.	• cries • refuses comfort • kicks • bites (*intermittently*)
Early childhood	• cries • whines in response to hunger, fatigue, frustration (*frequently*) • hits • bites in response to anger • tantrums in response to not getting a desired outcome	(same as Negative Emotional Behaviors, but in a more mature fashion, including:) • uses words in response to dissatisfaction • briefly argues • uses bad language • intentionally defies • dawdles in response to anger	• grabs toys • shows hostility toward siblings/peers • kicks • shows verbal hostility toward others (*intermittently*) typically responds to parental reprimand
Middle childhood	• tantrums • pounds fists • screams (*occasionally*)	[same as Negative Emotion Behaviors, but in a more mature fashion, including:] • shows defiance to commands for chores or daily living tasks to be completed • gives excuses • uses bad language • displays negative attitude • gestures to indicate refusal	[same Negative Emotion Behaviors but with more intention, such as:] • gets even in response to a perceived injustice • causes pain to others • uses profanity • bullies • hits peers in response to provocation (*intermittently*)
Adolescence	• hits objects • slams doors • curses • screams (*occasionally*)	• verbally argues • demands reasons from parents • gives excuses	• uses profanity • argues • speaks disrespectfully (*infrequently*) • physical aggression in response to provocation (*infrequently*)

After being told to clean up the toys, the defiant child does not continue playing but instead begins strewing the toys around the room [18]. This distinction marks the difference between normative child development that requires basic discipline techniques, and non-normative child development that increases the likelihood that the parent will need professional help for more challenging parent–child interactions [15].

Parents, particularly new parents, have always had questions about when their children's behavior is "normal" or when it requires help. In addition to their doctors, parents typically turn to their social circles to gauge how much of their children's behavior is in line with what other children exhibit. Now that many parents utilize social media for sharing about their children, this process has become complicated. Parents share to a much wider audience than they did before this mode of communication was available [19]. Consequently, parents see posts about children they barely know. Without a broader understanding of that child, the parent may not understand whether the sharing parent is highlighting an exceptionally positive or negative aspect of that child. Even when parents are presenting something positive about their child, they may use "humblebragging," a method for bragging about one's child that seems at first blush to be self-deprecating [19]. This behavior can be confusing to parents who are already worried about their children's misbehavior, as they see parents purportedly complaining about their children's positive behaviors.

Despite these challenges, social media and blogging are immensely popular among new parents [20]. While some studies show that parents with higher Internet use disconnect from in-person relationships [21], others show no negative impact on in-person connection and feelings of loneliness [22]. One study of 157 mothers of children 1.5 years or younger reported daily use of social media and feelings of social connection, social support, and wellbeing [20]. While this study was purely correlational (study authors cannot conclude that social media use caused these feelings), it is unlikely that parents will leave social media en masse any time soon. It is therefore all the more important that primary care physicians take the time to assess parents' primary behavioral concerns, as we outline below in the Conclusion.

Common Misconceptions

Spanking is universally cruel versus spanking is a necessary component of discipline

This misconception requires stating both extremes of opinion, as research has evidence refuting both statements. Over 30 countries have now established laws that prohibit the use of any corporal punishment for children, including spanking [24]. The United States is not among that group (nor is Canada) [24]. Accordingly, spanking in the United States is still fairly common according to repeated surveys. One survey found that 7 out of 10 American parents reported using some corporal punishment with their children [25]. The benefits and risks of spanking have been hotly contested in the child development literature for decades [1, 4, 13]. Parents will typically have their own impressions about spanking, often formed by their childhood experiences. The value of spanking is often in the eye of the beholder: parents with more positive attitudes toward spanking are more likely to spank their children [26].

It is not unusual to encounter parents who speak well of spanking. They may have been spanked as a child and did not experience any ill effects. They may also cite the fact that it works. While this statement would be based on parental observation, the data back up this assertion. In one of the most cited meta-analyses of spanking—which is notoriously anti-spanking—the author did concede that spanking is effective in gaining children's compliance in the short-term [27]. An original experimental design found that while other discipline methods could be just as effective as spanking, spanking was still more effective than doing nothing in response to children's behavior [28].

Other parents may be staunchly against spanking. They could have upsetting memories of their parents using this technique. Others could have observed children responding with tears when their parents spanked them in a public setting, such as a park. Or they may recognize that spanking does nothing to teach the child what behavior they should have exhibited instead of whichever one preceded the spanking. They would also be correct. Research shows that while spanking effectively changes children's behavior in the immediate term, it does not result in children internalizing a particular moral code in the longer term [27].

Despite this array of opinions, there is evidence that parental attitudes regarding spanking can be altered [29]. One study compared parents who interacted with a computer-based psychoeducational program about various discipline techniques [30]. Specifically with regard to spanking, parents who viewed the program responded differently about how they would manage their children's aggression compared to a control group of parents who did not receive the information [30].

Mirroring parents' strong opinions, the research in the area of spanking as a discipline technique remains hotly contested. A widely-cited meta-analysis of spanking and other forms of punishment concluded that spanking caused detrimental long-term outcomes in children who were spanked [27]. Measures of long-term outcomes tend to measure concepts such as aggression in children and academic performance. Critics of this work have noted that the statistical methods used to arrive at these conclusions were not appropriate for the data [4, 31]. Illustrating this point, researchers applied the same statistical methods to measure nonphysical forms of punishment, such as sending children to their rooms and removing privileges [32]. The statistical method told the same story—that these punishments had similar effects on long-term outcomes [32]. Similarly unadjusted correlational analyses show similar effects for time-out, another nonphysical punishment [33].

Instead, when researchers account for pre-existing differences between children who were spanked compared to children who were not, any long-term negative outcomes associated with disruptive behaviors disappear [4]. This is presumably because parents are more likely to spank children who are already misbehaving, rather than children who are not. Looking at children who were spanked according to how much they misbehave later in life may not represent an effect of spanking, as much as it shows that these children are continuing to have trouble controlling their behavior despite having been spanked [4, 31].

Analyses that use these unadjusted correlations to draw their conclusions do not consider other pre-existing characteristics of families where the spanking occurred, such as parent education, age, income, marital status, and depression [34–38]. Once these kinds of factors are incorporated into the analysis, the effect sizes become minuscule [4]. This means that while there may be a statistically significant difference between children who are spanked and not spanked on these long-term outcomes, the size of the difference between them is not only not causational, but the difference is very small. These small differences can disappear completely if other factors are considered, such as how frequently the children were spanked [39].

Analyses that group together children who are spanked only occasionally with children who are routinely spanked do not give an accurate impression for children whose parents may use spanking only in select circumstances [31]. Other analyses that many use as evidence against spanking also include harsher forms of physical punishment such as beatings with whips, belts, and sticks [40]. A recent meta-analysis shows that while there may be some remaining influences of spanking on long-term child outcomes, they are small and may be accounted for by other factors not yet identified [4].

What is clear is that spanking does not occur in a vacuum. Spanking and other forms of physical punishment are more or less problematic within a wider context that includes the parent/child relationship, cultural norms, child factors, frequency, and harshness.

- **Parent/child relationship**: There is some evidence that spanking that occurs within an overall loving and warm parent/child relationship is not viewed poorly by children. A Canadian study surveying 818 college students found that young adults had more favorable views regarding corporal punishment if they were spanked by parents they perceived as warm and supportive in general [41]. Alternatively, students who noted that their parents seemed to use corporal punishment impulsively had less favorable attitudes [41]. Otherwise supportive and loving parents seem to mitigate possible poor outcomes of these punishments [42]. Children are also more likely to accept the punishment if they feel it was objective, that is, formed by preplanned parental thought rather than in a heated parental emotional reaction [27].
- **Cultural norms**: Research among several nations indicates that harsh punishments cause different child outcomes, based on whether those punishments are normative in those countries [43]. A study of eleven countries examined the

relationship between corporal punishment and maternal warmth on children's aggression and anxiety [43]. Results indicated that the level of authoritarian makeup of the country (or cultural subgroup within a country) influenced reported child outcomes [43]. Countries or cultures with more authoritarian values showed fewer negative effects of corporal punishment [43].

- **Child factors**: While it appears that harsh punishments act differentially on children depending on their age, sex, and ethnic background, the research literature has not determined these effects in a way that are clinically useful [1]. Many studies contradict one another, creating a lack of clarity as to specific interactions between these child characteristics and outcomes [1]. For example, while one study shows that Hispanic preschoolers' cognitive development may be enhanced by the use of harsh physical and verbal punishment [42], another finds that Hispanic preschoolers' adjustment suffers more than other children's when subjected to these kinds of punishments [3]. The research comparing boys' and girls' responses to harsh punishments are similarly varied and inconclusive [27, 44].

In addition to demographic characteristics, one study sought to determine if children's knowledge of emotions moderated the effects of harsh punishment [1]. These researchers found that in their sample of 250 preschool children, those with better emotional knowledge were affected more detrimentally by their parents' harsh punishments. In comparison to their emotionally attuned peers, those with poorer emotion knowledge either benefitted or were neutrally affected by their parents' harsh punishments. Study authors interpreted their findings to mean that children who understand their parents are angry or upset when using harsh punishment are more likely to feel frightened or think that the punishment is unfair. However, this is only a hypothesis. Because the mechanism causing these results is unclear, it is possible other explanations may account for these observed differences.

- **Frequency**: Frequency of physical punishment has a rather obvious influence on child outcomes. Infants who experienced physical punishment frequently were shown to exhibit a high hormonal stress response [45]. Parents who rely primarily on spanking for directing their children's behavior must often increase the rate and intensity of spanking over time for it to maintain its desired effect [46]. This is suboptimal for children and parents. There is a concern that the escalation required to maintain spanking's efficacy can, over time, turn into abuse [46].
- **Harshness**: In one retrospective study of over 34,000 adults, those who reported harsh physical punishment prior to age 18 displayed higher odds of developing adult health conditions such as cardiovascular disease, arthritis, and obesity [13]. This effect held even among participants who did not report other forms of child abuse or maltreatment that commonly occur in situations where harsh physical punishments are used [13]. Regardless of stances on spanking, the evidence base categorically rejects discipline techniques that use harsh punishments [1]. Even those who criticize the research methods that provide arguments against spanking eschew harsh forms of corporal punishment [31].

Rather than deciding between advocating spanking or prohibiting it, a moderation approach is recommended. The very small (or in some cases trivial) effects of spanking should be communicated carefully to the public [4]. Some small amount of spanking is likely not harmful to children [31]. Without necessarily endorsing spanking, parents can be aware that spanking may not be as detrimental as they thought, but that there are still other, preferred methods for disciplining young children that are effective and "least negative" [4].

> **To Explain to a Patient**
>
> Research in spanking is a contentious issue because of the moral undertones. Parents who believe spanking is effective and safe consider parents who do not use this method to be too lax and likely to raise their children to be reckless. Those who believe spanking is primitive and harmful judge parents who use this method because they believe they are intentionally inflicting harm on defenseless children. Both options sound terrible, and both sides are already convinced they are correct. Researchers have biases and opinions just like everyone else. Research will likely never arrive at one straight answer that can either exonerate or fully support spanking. What the current research seems to show is that if you are not spanking your child now, you should not start. If you do spank your child, make sure that you do so very sparingly and not in anger.

As long as parents do not physically punish their children, their discipline is not harsh

Harsh verbal punishment falls short of emotional abuse. **Emotional abuse** is characterized by direct attacks on the child's sense of self, occurs without regard to children's behavior, and is not culturally normative (i.e., a reasonable parent would not engage in these attacks in a public location for fear of negative feedback from observers) [1]. In contrast, harsh verbal punishments may include yelling or cursing but do not directly attack the child's sense of self [1]. Because these verbal onslaughts occur in response to children's misbehavior, they are classified as punishments [1]. Yet they often occur in the context of parental frustration, thus typically serving an emotional function for the parent rather than a disciplinary function in the true sense of teaching the child [1].

Some level of harsh verbal punishment may be culturally normative. Anecdotally, many parents concede that they at times "lose it and blow up," or describe some other form of yelling in response to their children's misbehavior. Although it is not emotional abuse, harsh verbal punishment is still not a recommended strategy for discipline. Research has found an association between harsh verbal punishment and negative outcomes in child aggression, cognitive development, self-concept, and academic achievement [42, 47].

Parents should avoid punishment entirely

Positive parenting strategies can and should be used as part of a parent's disciplinary repertoire. Discipline should both teach the child what not to do and also provide guidance as to what the child should do instead [30]. Teaching children what is acceptable need not mean lectures for every infraction. Instead, positive parenting practices are excellent for accomplishing this goal. Positive parenting includes [30]:

- stating rules firmly without explanation (e.g., "We don't hit in this house.")
- providing children with alternative appropriate behavior options (e.g., "Please put your hands in your lap.")
- asking children to provide alternative options (e.g., "What can you do with your hands right now?")
- praising children when they behave appropriately at another time, using specific, labeled praise as to what the child is doing well (e.g., "I like how you're keeping safe hands when playing with your little sister.")

These strategies are not punishment and they guide children to display the desired behavior. But children will inevitably test what happens if they do not follow these injunctions. Children are not born with the knowledge of socially appropriate behavior or the motivation to engage in prosocial behaviors [48, 49]. It is consequently the parents' role to teach them [10]. Children test parents' limits to varying degrees, from the quite frequently (for example, as is seen in children diagnosed with Oppositional Defiant Disorder) to regularly (as occurs in the context of normative learning about consequences for actions) to rarely (as occurs in children who are more temperamentally compliant, easygoing, eager-to-please, or anxious). If parents respond to limit testing with no punishment (even a small one, such as saying "No" in a firm tone), the child cannot be expected to learn that their behavior was inappropriate. Without punishment, parents send their children the message that the behavior was acceptable.

It is unlikely that more than a very small number of children could be effectively disciplined without the occasional use of punishment. Where positive parenting guides children's behaviors in the desired direction, punishment serves to alert children that what they have done is not acceptable. Both the American Academy of Pediatrics and the Canadian Pediatric Society recommend that providers inform parents about nonphysical forms of punishment to discipline their children [46]. Developers of parenting programs that include punishment strive for the least amount of punishment possible while still achieving the desired outcome [31].

Time-outs don't work. Time-outs harm children

A common refrain from parents in attempting discipline practices with their children is that time-outs don't work. We will also explore a minority opinion that time-outs are psychologically harmful to children.

In one author's clinical experience, the primary reason time-outs fail to provide desired outcomes is because parents are not providing a true time-out. "Time-out" is shorthand for "time out from positive reinforcement" [50]. **Reinforcement** is any response to a child's behavior that increases that behavior [2]. Reinforcements are defined by their outcomes. As such, they vary widely. For one child, receiving stickers will increase their cooperation for going to the dentist. For another child, stickers do not have that effect. In this example, stickers are a reinforcer for the first child but not the second. Reinforcement also occurs from intangibles, such as praise [2].

One common mistake of parents who try to reduce problem behaviors is that of giving a great deal of negative parental attention to each infraction: they display an emotional response like frustration with sighs and stern looks, they proceed to lecture their children as to what they did wrong, and they may engage in a protracted conversation with their children about why what they did was wrong. What many parents do not realize is that most children find parental attention—all parental attention, whether good or bad—reinforcing [10]. Thus, the very behavior parents try to eliminate is strengthened by this response. This is particularly true for children who have difficulty getting positive parental attention for their appropriate behaviors [10]. Some children show appropriate behaviors very infrequently by nature, making it harder for parents to provide positive attention at the times when their child behaves well [10]. Other children may not receive much positive parental attention because their parents are busy, stressed, or depressed [51]. If not able to obtain positive parental attention, children learn to pull for negative parental attention via inappropriate behaviors, rather than receive no attention at all [2].

As such, a time-out is meant to remove any responses to children's misbehavior that may, even inadvertently, strengthen it. Subsequently, time-outs in conjunction with copious negative parental attention are not true time-outs. Parents who place their children in time-outs where siblings are present and engaging with the child are not providing true time-outs. Parents who respond to whines, comments, crying, or screams from children in time-out are also providing reinforcement with their responses, nullifying the time-out.

Another error is to have children sit in time-out sessions that do not immediately follow the misbehavior. For reinforcement to be effective, particularly when learning a new behavior, it should directly follow the behavior [2]. To reduce behaviors, removal of reinforcement should follow directly as well [2]. Having children serve time-outs "later" (e.g., once they get home from the park, after dinner, etc.), renders the time-out ineffective because the reinforcement is too far removed temporally from the misbehavior.

Finally, time-outs must be delivered consistently over time for children to sufficiently learn the connection between their misbehavior and the time-out. This is logistically challenging for parents. Also, children will often respond to limit setting with an increase in their misbehavior, called an **extinction burst**, hoping to achieve outcomes similar to those they used to receive [2]. Many parents understandably interpret the extinction burst as proof the time-out is not working. Due to this misconception, the extinction burst phenomenon should be explained to parents beforehand so that they understand it is their cue to continue with their efforts [2].

The research shows time-outs are effective for children ages 3–12 [2]. Use of time-out with younger or older children is not indicated [2]. Finally, children should be aware of the reason they are going to time-out, but with minimal parental involvement to make this clear [2]. For example, "You didn't do what I told you to do, so you have to sit on the time-out chair," is a brief and effective explanation, and if delivered in a calm tone of voice, does not provide enough parental attention to reinforce the misbehavior [52]. When time-outs are delivered following these principles, they are highly effective among both clinical and nonclinical populations of children [53, 54].

Despite clear evidence in favor of time-out as an effective and safe method for punishment in both the short and long term, a small but vocal minority of non-researcher clinicians present the impression that time-outs are hotly contested [53]. A nonclinical book warning of the psychological dangers of time-outs generated a flurry of attention in lay media [12, 55]. Parents who do not follow this field of research closely could easily be led to believe that these authors represent the best scientific knowledge at this time. In fact, a number of the authors' claims about time-outs were not based in scientific evidence [56]. After receiving pushback from a significant number of child development experts, the authors began to walk back their statements [31, 57]. Among their responses to the criticisms they received, they placed responsibility for the overstating of their claims and their equation of time-outs with physical punishment on the media outlet that printed a story about their book [57]. They also took the opportunity to hedge their statement about time-outs, stating they only meant to apply those statements to time-outs improperly used, namely, used in anger [57]. While this response may have mollified some, the authors did not go so far as to acknowledge that proper time-outs are a recommended part of parents' disciplinary toolkits. Instead, they suggested that because time-outs are sometimes delivered in an angry fashion, time-outs should not be encouraged at all [57]. Instead, they advocate that parents give copious amounts of attention, in the form of comfort and soothing, to children who have just disobeyed them [12]. While it is understandable that at times parent may give time-outs while angry, it is less clear how parents are expected to reduce their anger sufficiently to hug and cuddle their misbehaving children any more easily. Additionally, children learn the opposite lesson—that misbehavior is appropriate—when they receive warmth and comfort from their parent as a consequence. These authors fail to acknowledge that their recommended alternative is just as challenging for parents to implement in moments of frustration and it additionally reinforces misbehavior through parental attention. There are multiple opportunities throughout parents' interactions with their children to provide warmth and love such that a brief (approximately 3 minute) removal of parental attention during a time-out would not damage or hurt a child [56].

Some parents are not concerned that time-outs are ineffective or directly damage their children, but worry that highly compliant children are vulnerable. Clearly, compliance is only one aspect of social development [10]. Children who are only compliant could find themselves following directives of adults who do not have the children's best interest at heart. However, compliance itself is not inherently bad. Compliance should be combined with supportive parenting, and an attached relationship between parents and children [10]. Children who are supported by their parents develop a sense of self that they can trust. We discussed above the difference between child misbehavior that is due to an assertion of self or of the child's own preferences and misbehavior that due to defiance [18]. Parents concerned about using discipline techniques with their children because it will stifle their children's sense of self are only addressing one side of the equation. The ability to assert oneself in the real world is predicated on two things: knowing one's preferences and advocating for them. Even young children develop preferences early, a large part of why parents bemoan the "Terrible Twos." But children must comply when compliance is needed and assert themselves using words when the situation allows. Discipline techniques should be coupled with language development in parent–child interactions. In this way, parents address both sides of the equation: raising children who understand and respect authority, and who can appropriately advocate for themselves when warranted.

Children who believe themselves to be in a reciprocal relationship with their parents, in which their opinions are heard and considered in child-appropriate domains are actually *more* likely to comply with parental directives [58]. For example, parents who provide their child more autonomy and direction in times of play experience an increase in compliance from those children during a parent-directed clean up task [58]. Parents whose children use self-assertion in parent-appropriate domains should, rather than pull back on discipline in those instances, consider other areas in which they have been too tightly controlling of their children's behavior. In those domains, they can loosen the reins and let their children have more say.

Current Research

Authoritative parenting, which necessarily includes some boundary setting, assists positive child outcomes [59]. On either side of authoritative parenting are the harsh and lax parenting styles. Harsh parenting is classified as the kind that heavily emphasizes yelling, physical punishment, and coercive or severe means of control [60]. Lax parenting is typified by parents who are inconsistent and permissive in their parenting [60]. Not only do the harsh and lax parenting styles both predict child misbehavior [61], but children's misbehavior in turn promotes harsh and lax parenting responses [60]. This bidirectional interaction results in a coercive cycle that is hard to break [62]. Therefore, it is recommended that parents avoid either of these styles and focus on authoritative parenting.

It is typically easy to convince parents that harsh parenting is not a desired goal. Lax parenting presents a greater challenge. Permissive parenting is generally not too taxing on parents in the short term, as it allows parents to avoid difficult confrontations with their children following misbehavior. Yet evidence-based parenting programs for clinical populations include some component of punishment [31]. Anecdotally, in these authors' clinical experience, positive-only approaches fail to address common parental concerns about how to manage children's inappropriate or undesirable behaviors.

Many evidence-based parenting programs effectively leverage modes of developmentally appropriate discipline, both positive and punishment [8, 9]. Studies of treatments for children with clinical diagnoses (such as Oppositional Defiant Disorder or Attention Deficit/Hyperactivity Disorder) have found that parents can be taught to use a balance of positive and punitive parenting strategies to teach their children appropriate behavior. Parents in these programs are coached to use simple, direct commands when they would like their children to comply, a single warning if their children do not comply quickly, and a nonphysical punishment such as use of a time-out chair if their children still do not comply [63].

Parents referred to clinic training programs to discipline their children are often at their wits' end [9]. They are frustrated with their children and their relationship has begun to suffer [9]. While a time-out is uncomfortable for both parents and children as they occur, the benefit of reducing parent/child conflict, for most, outweighs this cost. These programs also include the use of positive parental attention to guide children's behavior. Positive attention is delivered as labeled praise ("I like how gently you're playing!"), unlabeled praise ("Good job!"), behavioral description ("You're using the crayons to draw on the paper."), and reflection (i.e., reflecting back what the child says to show the parent is listening) [52]. These positive strategies provide children with the information they need to behave correctly while simultaneously bolstering a warm parent–child relationship [63].

To Explain to a Patient

Research shows that both positive parenting techniques and punishment have their place in appropriate and effective discipline. Using only one or the other is like trying to control a thermostat with only one temperature control: warm or cool. If a room is too warm, of course turning the temperature down is a good response. But what if the room is too cold? All the turning the temperature down in the world will not address this situation. Sometimes children behave well, and they should learn from their parents that they are doing a good job. Things like verbal praise or physical signs of affection can be used so children associate their good behavior with a response they like. But as any parent knows, all children misbehave sometimes. Praise cannot be used here. In the case of minor behaviors (like whining) sometimes ignoring the behavior will make it go away. In cases that involve physical safety (like a child who runs into the street or strikes another child), ignoring is not appropriate. Parents need to be able to use some form of either redirection or punishment so their children can learn not to do this again. While it takes many repeated attempts to learn appropriate behavior (just as it does to learn anything!) without both positive and negative feedback in discipline, children cannot learn.

Conclusion

Young children with exceptionally challenging behavioral difficulties are more likely to develop significant problems later in life [8]. Research shows improved outcomes when these children are helped prior to 8 years old using an evidence-based parenting treatment [8]. These treatments follow similar formats, providing parents with strategies for handling children's challenging behaviors on a day by day basis, giving them more effective parenting techniques, and teaching them coping and communication skills [8]. Thus, identification and referral are crucial to positive long-term outcomes.

While pediatricians are often parents' first line of help, many do not systematically screen for clinical disorders such as Oppositional Defiant Disorder due to constraints on time, available resources in the community to provide referrals, and only brief training in identifying these disorders [64]. Even when physicians can recognize a behavioral disorder, reimbursement for screening and treatment presents another hurdle [8].

Doctors can take steps to reduce the challenge of connecting parents with appropriate strategies and treatments for their children. The first recommendation is for physicians to directly ask parents for their top one or two behavioral concerns at the moment [8]. By letting the parent set the agenda, the physician can be sure to address the parents' needs and reduce time spent giving advice that is either not needed or not a top priority for that particular child.

Second, physicians can familiarize themselves with some of the evidence-based parenting treatments, such as Helping the Non-Compliant Child, Parent–Child Interaction Therapy, and Incredible Years [8, 52, 65, 66]. By perusing some of these treatments, pediatricians can note the similarities in recommended strategies, many of which they can explain to parents within the context of an office visit [8].

Third, physicians should take a collaborative approach whenever possible, utilizing the system as a whole to address parents' concerns [8]. For example, scheduling visits at the end of the day when the physician feels less rushed and utilizing other practitioners when available (such as nurse practitioners, social workers, psychologists, and psychiatrists) reduce the burden on the pediatrician and provide the parent with a network of helpers [8].

Fourth, pediatricians can help parents—often in the trenches of exasperating behaviors—see the "bigger picture." Parents benefit from assurance from a professional that it is normal for their children's abilities to wax and wane throughout the day and over time [8].

Finally, pediatricians should offer parents an overall framework for their discipline strategies that emphasizes positive practices whenever possible (using positive parental attention for increasing prosocial behaviors and ignoring children when they engage in low-level inappropriate behaviors) with the supplementation of punishment for behaviors that are dangerous [8]. Pediatricians can be a powerful and effective bridge for families to reach positive discipline strategies with their children [8].

References

1. Berzenski SR, Yates TM. Preschoolers' emotion knowledge and the differential effects of harsh punishment. J Fam Psychol. 2013;27(3):463.
2. Armstrong KH, Ogg JA, Sundman-Wheat AN, Walsh AS. Behavioral terms and principles. In: Evidence-based interventions for children with challenging behavior. New York: Springer;2014. p. 111–3.
3. McLoyd VC, Smith J. Physical discipline and behavior problems in African American, European American, and hispanic children: emotional support as a moderator. J Marriage Family. 2002;64(1):40–53.
4. Ferguson CJ. Spanking, corporal punishment and negative long-term outcomes: a meta-analytic review of longitudinal studies. Clin Psychol Rev. 2013;33(1):196–208.
5. Baumrind D. Differentiating between confrontive and coercive kinds of parental power-assertive disciplinary practices. Hum Dev. 2012;55(2):35–51.
6. Maccoby EE, Martin JA. Socialization in the context of the family: parent-child interaction. In: Mussen PH editor. Handbook of child psychology: formerly Carmichael's Manual of child psychology 1983.
7. Belkin L. Parenting under scrutiny [Internet]. Motherlode Blog. 2016. http://parenting.blogs.nytimes.com/2010/08/26/parenting-under-scrutiny/. Accessed 2 March 2016.
8. Bauer NS, Webster-Stratton C. Prevention of behavioral disorders in primary care. Curr Opin Pediatr. 2006;18(6):654–60.
9. Kane GA, Wood VA, Barlow J. Parenting programmes: a systematic review and synthesis of qualitative research. Child Care Health Dev. 2007;33(6):784–93.
10. Owen DJ, Slep AM, Heyman RE. The effect of praise, positive nonverbal response, reprimand, and negative nonverbal response on child compliance: a systematic review. Clin Child Fam Psychol Rev. 2012;15(4):364–85.
11. Phelan T. 1-2-3 magic. Glen Ellyn, Ill.: ParentMagic, Inc.;2003.
12. Siegel D, Bryson T. No-drama discipline.
13. Afifi TO, Mota N, MacMillan HL, Sareen J. Harsh physical punishment in childhood and adult physical health. Pediatrics. 2013;132(2):e333–40.
14. Jenkins S, Bax M, Hart H. Behaviour problems in pre-school children. J Child Psychol Psychiatry. 1980;21(1):5–17.
15. Campbell SB. Behavior problems in preschool children: a review of recent research. J Child Psychol Psychiatry. 1995;36(1):113–49.
16. Chamberlain P, Smith DK. Antisocial behavior in children and adolescents: The Oregon Multidimensional Treatment Foster Care Model. 2003.
17. Schuhmann E, Durning P. Screening for conduct problem behavior in pediatric settings using the Eyberg child behavior inventory. Ambulatory Child Health. 1996;2(1):35–41.
18. Crockenberg S, Litman C. Autonomy as competence in 2-year-olds: maternal correlates of child defiance, compliance, and self-assertion. Dev Psychol. 1990;26(6):961.
19. Bartels JS. Parents' growing pains on social media: modeling authenticity. Character and.... 2016;1:51–70.
20. McDaniel BT, Coyne SM, Holmes EK. New mothers and media use: associations between blogging, social networking, and maternal well-being. Matern Child Health J. 2012;16(7):1509–17.
21. Nie NH, Hillygus DS, Erbring L. Internet use, interpersonal relations, and sociability. Internet Everyday Life. 2002;13:215–43.
22. DiMaggio P, Hargittai E, Neuman WR, Robinson JP. Social implications of the internet. Ann Rev Sociol. 2001;1:307–36.
23. The Broad Continuum of Conduct and Behavioral Problems [Internet]. UCLA School Mental Health Project. http://smhp.psych.ucla.edu/qf/behaviorprob_qt/continuum.pdf. Accessed 11 March 2016.

24. Durrant J, Ensom R. Physical punishment of children: lessons from 20 years of research. Can Med Assoc J. 2012;184(12):1373–7.

25. Simons DA, Wurtele SK. Relationships between parents' use of corporal punishment and their children's endorsement of spanking and hitting other children. Child Abuse Negl. 2010;34(9):639–46.

26. Vittrup B, Holden GW, Buck J. Attitudes predict the use of physical punishment: a prospective study of the emergence of disciplinary practices. Pediatrics. 2006;117(6):2055–64.

27. Gershoff ET. Corporal punishment by parents and associated child behaviors and experiences: a meta-analytic and theoretical review. Psychol Bull. 2002;128(4):539.

28. Day DE, Roberts MW. An analysis of the physical punishment component of a parent training program. J Abnorm Child Psychol. 1983;11(1):141–52.

29. Reich SM, Penner EK, Duncan GJ, Auger A. Using baby books to change new mothers' attitudes about corporal punishment. Child Abuse Negl. 2012;36(2):108–17.

30. Chavis A, Hudnut-Beumler J, Webb MW, Neely JA, Bickman L, Dietrich MS, Scholer SJ. A brief intervention affects parents' attitudes toward using less physical punishment. Child Abuse Negl. 2013;37(12):1192–201.

31. Larzelere RE, Gunnoe ML, Roberts MW, Ferguson CJ. Children and parents deserve better parental discipline research: critiquing the evidence for exclusively "Positive" parenting. Marriage Family Rev. 2016 (just-accepted).

32. Larzelere RE, Cox RB, Smith GL. Do nonphysical punishments reduce antisocial behavior more than spanking? a comparison using the strongest previous causal evidence against spanking. BMC Pediatrics. 2010;10(1):1.

33. Gershoff ET, Grogan-Kaylor A, Lansford JE, Chang L, Zelli A, Deater-Deckard K, Dodge KA. Parent discipline practices in an international sample: associations with child behaviors and moderation by perceived normativeness. Child Dev. 2010;81(2):487–502.

34. Day RD, Peterson GW, McCracken C. Predicting spanking of younger and older children by mothers and fathers. J Marriage Family. 1998;1:79–94.

35. Pinderhughes EE, Dodge KA, Bates JE, Pettit GS, Zelli A. Discipline responses: influences of parents' socioeconomic status, ethnicity, beliefs about parenting, stress, and cognitive-emotional processes. J Fam Psychol. 2000;14(3):380.

36. Smith JR, Brooks-Gunn J. Correlates and consequences of harsh discipline for young children. Arch Pediatr Adolesc Med. 1997;151(8):777–86.

37. Straus MA, Stewart JH. Corporal punishment by American parents: national data on prevalence, chronicity, severity, and duration, in relation to child and family characteristics. Clin Child Fam Psychol Rev. 1999;2(2):55–70.

38. Wissow LS. Ethnicity, income, and parenting contexts of physical punishment in a national sample of families with young children. Child Maltreatment. 2001;6(2):118–29.

39. Lansford JE, Wager LB, Bates JE, Pettit GS, Dodge KA. Forms of spanking and children's externalizing behaviors. Fam Relat. 2012;61(2):224–36.

40. Larzelere RE, Baumrind D, Cowan P. Ordinary physical punishment: is it harmful. Psychol Bull. 2002;128(4):580–90.

41. Bell T, Romano E. Opinions about child corporal punishment and influencing factors. J Interpersonal Violence. 2012;18:0886260511432154.

42. Berlin LJ, Ispa JM, Fine MA, Malone PS, Brooks-Gunn J, Brady-Smith C, Ayoub C, Bai Y. Correlates and consequences of spanking and verbal punishment for low-income white, African American, and Mexican American Toddlers. Child Dev. 2009;80(5):1403–20.

43. Lansford JE, Sharma C, Malone PS, Woodlief D, Dodge KA, Oburu P, Pastorelli C, Skinner AT, Sorbring E, Tapanya S, Tirado LM. Corporal punishment, maternal warmth, and child adjustment: a longitudinal study in eight countries. J Clinical Child Adolesc Psychol. 2014;43(4):670–85.

44. Chang L, Schwartz D, Dodge KA, McBride-Chang C. Harsh parenting in relation to child emotion regulation and aggression. J Fam Psychol. 2003;17(4):598.

45. Bugental DB, Martorell GA, Barraza V. The hormonal costs of subtle forms of infant maltreatment. Horm Behav. 2003;43(1):237–44.

46. [AAP] American Academy of Pediatrics, American Academy of Pediatrics. Guidance for effective discipline. Pediatrics. 1998;101(4):723–8.
47. Solomon CR, Serres F. Effects of parental verbal aggression on children's self-esteem and school marks. Child Abuse Negl. 1999;23(4):339–51.
48. Kochanska G, Murray K, Coy KC. Inhibitory control as a contributor to conscience in child-hood: from toddler to early school age. Child Dev. 1997;68(2):263–77.
49. Strand PS. Coordination of maternal directives with preschoolers' behavior: influence of maternal coordination training on dyadic activity and child compliance. J Clin Child Adolesc Psychol. 2002;31(1):6–15.
50. Kazdin AE. Behavior modification in applied settings. Waveland Press;2012.
51. Elgar FJ, McGrath PJ, Waschbusch DA, Stewart SH, Curtis LJ. Mutual influences on mater-nal depression and child adjustment problems. Clin Psychol Rev. 2004;24(4):441–59.
52. Eyberg S, Funderburk B. PCIT. [Gainesville, FL]: PCIT International, Inc.; 2011.
53. Quetsch LB, Wallace NM, Herschell AD, McNeil CB. Weighing in on the time-out contro-versy: an empirical perspective. Clin Psychol. 2015;68(2):4–19.
54. Everett GE, Hupp SD, Olmi DJ. Time-out with parents: a descriptive analysis of 30 years of research. Educ Treat Child. 2010;33(2):235–59.
55. Siegel D, Bryson T. 'Time-Outs' are hurting your child [Internet]. TIME.com. 2014. http://time.com/3404701/discipline-time-out-is-not-good/. Accessed 11 March 2016.
56. Atkins M, Albano A, Fristad M, Pelham B, Piacentini J, Abidin D et al. Outrageous claims regarding the appropriateness of time outs have no basis in science [Internet]. Society of Clinical Child & Adolescent Psychology. 2014. http://effectivechildtherapy.org/sites/default/files/files/Time%20In-Out%20Press%20Release.pdf. Accessed 11 March 2016.
57. How Many Parents Use Time-Outs Inappropriately [Internet]. The Huffington Post. 2016. http://www.huffingtonpost.com/daniel-j-siegel-md/time-outs-overused_b_6006332.html. Accessed 11 March 2016.
58. Parpal M, Maccoby EE. Maternal responsiveness and subsequent child compliance. Child Dev. 1985;1:1326–34.
59. Steinberg L, Lamborn SD, Dornbusch SM, Darling N. Impact of parenting practices on ado-lescent achievement: authoritative parenting, school involvement, and encouragement to suc-ceed. Child Dev. 1992;63(5):1266–81.
60. Del Vecchio T, O'Leary SG. Predicting maternal discipline responses to early child aggres-sion: the role of cognitions and affect. Parenting: Sci Pract. 2008;8(3):240–56.
61. Smith AM, O'Leary SG. Attributions and arousal as predictors of maternal discipline. Cogn Therapy Res. 1995;19(4):459–71.
62. Granic I, Patterson GR. Toward a comprehensive model of antisocial development: a dynamic systems approach. Psychol Rev. 2006;113(1):101.
63. Eyberg SM, Nelson MM, Boggs SR. Evidence-based psychosocial treatments for children and adolescents with disruptive behavior. J Clin Child Adolesc Psychol. 2008;37(1):215–37.
64. Perrin E, Stancin T. A continuing dilemma: whether and how to screen for concerns about children's behavior. Pediatr Rev/Amer Acad Pediatr. 2002;23(8):264.
65. Forehand RL, McMahon RJ. Helping the noncompliant child: a clinician's guide to parent training. New York: Guilford press; 1981.
66. Webster-Stratton C. The Incredible Years® Series. Family-Based Prevention Programs for Children and Adolescents: Theory, Research, and Large-Scale Dissemination. 2015. p. 42.

Chapter 10
Medications

Overview

When medications are taken as recommended—that is, when instructions are adhered to—they play a crucial role in modern medicine. The World Health Organization defines **adherence** as "the extent to which a person's behavior—taking medication, following a diet, and/or executing lifestyle changes, corresponds with agreed recommendations from a health care provider" [1]. Medications lose their ability to prevent negative health outcomes and unnecessary health service usage when they are not taken as agreed upon by patient and doctor [2]. If physicians are not aware that their patients have been non-adherent, poor medication response may prompt physicians to increase the dosage or request more tests to achieve desired outcomes [2].

Physicians in pediatric practices encounter additional struggles with adherence [2]. Multiple accounts from parents and children create ambiguity when assessing for adherence [2]. Parental education during office visits is crucial, yet there is evidence that parents do not understand and recall all that is presented to them. One study found that within a 15 minute physician visit, parents remember approximately half of the information their doctors presented [3]. In particular, parents are most likely to recall the information presented in the first third of the visit, which typically focuses on diagnosis rather than treatment [3]. Not only must parents understand and agree to medication regimens, pediatricians must also, in many cases, obtain minimal levels of cooperation from juvenile patients [2]. Without children's cooperation, parents frequently experience children spitting out medications, making adherence an even greater challenge [4]. Similar to other adult patients, parents may forget to deliver the medication or misunderstand the instructions [5]. Yet for pediatric patients, multiple caretakers may assume responsibility for medication administration, adding another level of complexity to an already fraught process [2]. The largest hurdles to medication adherence among pediatric

© Springer International Publishing AG 2017

C.A. Di Bartolo and M.K. Braun, *Pediatrician's Guide to Discussing Research with Patients*, DOI 10.1007/978-3-319-49547-7_10

populations are daily living stressors and family conflict [6]. One study found that the risk of medication non-adherence was 1.53 times higher in families with high levels of reported conflict than in families with low levels [7].

Among chronically ill patients, multiple factors undermine adherence: the extended nature of the illness, bouts of periodic symptom remission, and the common practice of prescribing more than one medication simultaneously. Estimates place adherence among chronically ill patients anywhere between 30% and 70% [8–10]. Pediatric rates of adherence in chronic conditions are even more variable, with studies reporting rates between 11% and 93% [2]. Adherence in chronically ill children therefore presents a double-barreled challenge [11]. Over the past 2 decades, child and adolescent diagnoses of chronic illness has steadily increased [12]. One study determined that approximately 68% of children diagnosed with a chronic illness subsequently receive a prescription for treatment [13].

Particularly among children who are chronically ill, parents may not give their children medications if they require more information to comprehend the diagnosis, worry that the medication will not produce the desired outcome, or fear medication side effects [14]. These uncertainties may cause the parent to discontinue treatment. For example, a child with asthma may experience a brief period of symptom remission, which is common in chronic illness. A parent with side effect concerns may use this opportunity to temporarily discontinue medication in order to mitigate what they perceive to be the risks of side effects [14]. Parents may also weigh the cost versus benefit of giving their children medication if they perceive any side effects or fail to observe improvements after initiating treatment [5].

This chapter reviews parental medication concerns in three areas: antibiotics, asthma, and Attention-Deficit/Hyperactivity Disorder (ADHD).

Antibiotics

Antibiotics are one of the most commonly prescribed medications in pediatrics for acute illness. Effective use of antibiotics have extended life expectancy, assisted cancer treatments, and made possible extensive surgeries and organ transplants [15]. Since the inception of modern medicine, bacteria have evolved to resist antibiotics. Even as penicillin underwent clinical trials, 50% of the Staphylococcus aureus bacteria developed resistance in just 10 years [15]. A persistent problem, antibiotic-resistant bacteria had been kept at bay in part by continuous development of new antibiotics [15]. In the past 2 decades, the number of pharmaceutical companies investing in antibiotic development has dwindled from 18 to 4 [15]. As bacteria develop resistance to antibiotics, strains emerge for which the scientific and medical community has no treatment, creating a significant public health threat [16].

While there are likely many causes for the increase in antibiotic-resistant bacteria, one proposed factor is the overuse of antibiotics [17, 18]. It is estimated that between 80% and 90% of antibiotics are prescribed within primary care settings

[19]. Prescriptions for antibiotics in outpatient doctors' offices are written more frequently for children than for any other age group [17]. As such, promoting careful use and avoiding overuse of antibiotics in pediatric practice has the potential to help stem the tide of antibiotic-resistant bacteria [20]. Extensive research has examined parents' difficulties understanding the indicators for antibacterial treatment and the pressure physicians experience to prescribe antibiotics even when they are not indicated [21]. At the same time, press covering the overuse and dangers of antibiotics has created a subculture of parents who are wary of any antibiotic use for their children [22]. We review the current literature to familiarize practicing clinicians with the current landscape of parental concerns and the reality of the interactional nature of the consultation between patient and physician.

Asthma

We will also examine parental concerns regarding medication treatment for the most common chronic pediatric medical condition: asthma [23]. Asthma affects approximately 8.3% of American children [24]. There is evidence that uncontrolled asthma not only produces symptoms such as wheezing and difficulty breathing in the short-term but, over time, can also cause a restructuring of the airway, making normal breathing difficult to sustain in the long-term [25]. As asthma is caused by chronic inflammation of the airway, treatments focus on reducing this inflammation and preventing further deterioration of the airway [26, 27]. The most commonly used asthma control medications are inhaled corticosteroids, which are anti-inflammatory agents [28]. Research shows that when used as prescribed, inhaled corticosteroids are effective in reducing asthma symptoms and preventing future hospitalizations [27]. As such, physicians globally recommend them for asthma treatment [28].

Despite medical benefits, estimates suggest that only half of all asthmatic children adhere to their treatment plan [29]. Asthma control medications are subject to the three major components that negatively affect adherence to treatment: regular use, inconvenient delivery, and no immediately observable benefits [30]. In some cases, parents' concerns about negative side effects contribute to lower medication adherence. Improving care to asthmatic children depends in part on sufficiently addressing parental beliefs and concerns regarding asthma control medicine [27]. We will review two common concerns in the research base regarding inhaled steroids for use with children.

Attention-Deficit/Hyperactivity Disorder (ADHD)

Attention-Deficit/Hyperactivity Disorder (ADHD) is a chronic psychiatric condition affecting children's ability to control their attention, motor movements, and impulses [31]. While estimates vary, prevalence studies estimate that approximately 5% of American children are affected by ADHD, with higher rates observed in males [31]. Symptoms of ADHD typically reduce gradually with age, but individuals diagnosed with ADHD in childhood continue to show greater impairments than their unaffected peers throughout adolescence and often into adulthood [31]. Children diagnosed with ADHD show higher rates of other impairing behaviors such as opposition, aggression, temper tantrums, and unco-operativeness [31]. In adolescents with ADHD, higher rates of negative outcomes are observed than in peers without ADHD, such as discontinuing education, inter-action with law enforcement, early onset substance use, conduct disorders, dan-gerous driving, gambling, and early parenthood [31–34]. Children and adolescents with ADHD also experience higher rates of learning disorders and emotional dif-ficulties, such as anxiety, mood disorders, and low self-esteem [31].

Substantial debate among the public and some within the scientific commu-nity seeks to understand the nature of ADHD, both as a disorder and in terms of whether it requires medical treatment [35]. Because many symptoms of ADHD outwardly reflect normative child behavior (albeit to an extreme degree), some have argued against its classification as a psychiatric illness [36, 37]. The debate about ADHD as a diagnosis is closely linked to medical treatment of the disor-der [35]. In addition to behavioral approaches, one of the primary recommended interventions for ADHD is stimulant medication [38]. Stimulants are the class of drug used to treat ADHD that most polarize and concern parents [39]. Despite its overall efficacy in treating the core symptoms of ADHD, most parents exhibit hes-itancy and uncertainty regarding the decision to initiate medication treatment for their children with ADHD [40]. We will review the founded and unfounded con-cerns about side effects of this medication.

Common Parental Concerns

Better Safe Than Sorry Versus Antibiotics Are Overused

A commonly cited reason for parents' misunderstanding about the correct usage of antibiotics is their lack of knowledge about differentiating between viral and bac-terial infections. A survey of 400 parents inquiring into their past experiences with antibiotics provides evidence in favor of this argument [22]. In this sample, 32% of parents reported that they thought antibiotics were useful for treating colds, 58% thought antibiotics should be used to treat coughs, and 58% said antibiotics are appropriate for treating fevers [22].

Another study of over 1,000 parents showed that one-third believed antibiot-ics could help treat viral illness [41]. This study found lower knowledge about antibiotics was associated with parents with lower educational attainment, fewer children, and less exposure to information about antibiotic resistance [41]. Indeed, nonspecific symptoms such as fever and respiratory difficulties can proceed to more dangerous illnesses, a fact many parents are aware of [42]. Particularly for parents who cannot afford to take time off work to take care of a sick child, antibiotics are seen as a form of preventative treatment to ensure their child's illness will not progress [42].

A subset of parents takes an opposing stance, that antibiotics are harmful or overused. In the sample of 400 parents surveyed in the study above, nearly one-third (29%) of parents reported concern that their children receive too many antibiotics [22]. 85% thought that too many antibiotics could cause problems [22]. Among the problems caused by over-prescription of antibiotics, 55% cited resistance, and 15% thought efficacy would be affected [22].

Even parents who are rationally aware that antibiotics are not currently indicated for their sick children still consider treatment options within a context of distress [42]. When concerned about risks, people tend to show a preference for choices that will mitigate risks, even when those risks are low in likelihood [42]. Parents can cognitively comprehend that antibiotics are not currently indicated, but their emotional state prompts a different line of thinking. This emotional component explains the failure of education-alone interventions to improve judicious antibiotic use.

Asthma Control Medication Slows Growth

Despite the proven efficacy of inhaled steroids for the treatment of pediatric asthma, parents remain concerned about potential side effects [43]. In particular, the effect of steroid use on growth has been extensively examined [43]. There is evidence that high doses of inhaled steroids temporarily slow growth trajectories in children [44, 45]. One meta-analysis reviewed pre-pubescent children with mild to moderate asthma who were in research trials that also tracked their growth [46]. Among these children, those who received higher doses of inhaled steroids experienced slower growth trajectories when compared to children on lower dosages [43]. The highest impact on growth occurs in the first year of steroid treatment [43]. Growth also appears to be more affected by older forms of steroid treatment than new ones, although the research in this area is less robust [47].

Pediatric care strives to effectively treat illness without affecting normal development [43]. Before the extensive research of the past 2 decades, researchers estimated that steroid use could slow growth by as much as 1.5 cm per year [43]. After many well-controlled and longitudinal studies, researchers conclude that steroid use does slow growth in children, but not by as much as was originally hypothesized [43]. Only one study was conducted that examined an older formulation of steroids and tracked growth longitudinally [43]. This "worst-case" condition resulted in an average 1.2 cm total loss in adult height [48]. While most conclude the benefits of controlling asthma outweigh these risks, parents are correct in weighing a legitimate risk of slowed growth trajectory against their children's ability to breathe when considering treatment initiation.

Ambivalence Regarding Initiation of Stimulant Treatment

On a wide scale, the proliferation of stimulant prescriptions, such as Adderall (amphetamine and dextroamphetamine) and Ritalin (methylphenidate), for children with diagnoses of ADHD has troubled health professionals and parents alike [35]. In fact, the decision to start medication does not at all appear to be an easy one [49]. Parents decide to give their children stimulant medication because of the difficulties in raising a child with impairing symptoms [35]. Anecdotally, clinicians do not find that most parents quickly decide to initiate stimulant treatment. Backing up this clinical impression, a review of a Medicaid database revealed that approximately half of children diagnosed with ADHD do not begin stimulant treatment, and half of those who do discontinue within 1 year [50].

Initially, parents must decide how they feel about the ADHD diagnosis. The concept of behavioral challenges as stemming from a neurological disorder is not universally accepted [35]. Parental attitudes about ADHD medication are influenced by their general conceptions of psychiatric illness in children and the specific behavioral challenges of ADHD [51]. Among families, fathers generally show less willingness to accept the ADHD diagnosis than mothers [52–54].

Parents are commonly reluctant to try stimulant medication until other interventions have been attempted [55]. Some interventions parents try before initiating stimulants are evidence-based (e.g., behavioral modification) while others are not (e.g., dietary changes or homeopathic strategies) [55]. In cases where children are not at imminent risk of harm or school expulsion due to their ADHD symptoms, attempting other evidence-based interventions first is sensible [55]. However, exploring numerous unproven treatments before considering an efficacious stimulant treatment is conceptually similar to delaying treatment altogether [55].

Parents' worries about stimulant side effects shed light on the individual struggles that underlie each prescription [35]. In one small study, a majority of parents cited academic goals as the primary driver for stimulant medication initiation [35]. Similarly, parents in another study who initiated stimulant treatment were most likely to do so when a clear functional impairment, such as academic difficulties, was present [56]. Fear for their child's physical safety when not medicated also generally overrides parents' fears about stimulant medication side effects [55]. Other parents who recognize that withholding medication in the short-term will likely create more significant problems later in the child's life also tend to show higher adherence to medication [55]. Parents weigh the benefits of symptom improvement and subsequent functional strides against their concerns regarding side effects [35]. Each parent is willing to accept different types and severity levels of side effects to achieve desired outcomes for his or her child [35].

Even parents who choose to begin treatment for their children are typically concerned about the implications of their decision, both medically (as in the case of side effects) and philosophically. In addition to side effects, parents report concerns about using medication to improve behavioral outcomes [56].

Conceptualizing ADHD within a biomedical model facilitated medication acceptance in some parents [55, 56]. While some parents consider medication a temporary fix until their children age, others think of medication as a long-term mainstay in their children's lives [35]. In some cases parents terminate treatment due to side effects or at their children's request [35]. Many of these parents find themselves second-guessing treatment termination [35]. In other cases, parents exhibit continued ambivalence about continuing medication even after observing the clear positive effects of the medication on their child's functioning [56].

Rather than think of stimulant medication initiation as a one-time decision, physicians should understand that over the course of many years, most parents revisit their decision to begin, delay, stop, or restart medication [56]. One study found that parents who thought of the medication decision as a process involving trial and error to find the right medication had more realistic expectations and a more positive experience with stimulant medications overall [55]. While current American Academy of Pediatrics guidelines do not explicitly recommend starting and stopping stimulant treatment, physicians will likely find themselves treating families who seek to understand the correct medication dosage and amount on this trial basis [56, 57].

Common Misconceptions

Parents routinely pressure physicians for antibiotics and will be disappointed if they do not receive a prescription

Among physicians, the concern that parents ask for antibiotics remains a persistent challenge. Physicians report pressure from parents (54%), lack of time (19%), and fear of litigation (12%) as contributing to their decision to prescribe antibiotics against clinical indicators [58]. One study queried 61 physicians as to their impressions about the state of affairs in antibiotics [22]. Among these physicians, 71% reported parents asked them for antibiotic prescriptions when not indicated at least 4 times in the previous month [22]. Of this set, 35% acknowledged they wrote the prescription against their better clinical judgment [22]. Those who study this phenomenon commonly point out that physicians in busy practices struggle to find the time to carefully review the indicators for antibiotic use with parents [22]. These researchers consider the issue a matter of cost–benefit analysis: physicians find it easier to write the prescription than trying to explain why they will not prescribe antibiotics [22]. Legal considerations are also hypothesized to affect clinicians' decisions, particularly in cases where nonspecific fever could progress into an illness requiring antibiotic treatment [22]. The risk assessment for one child (which typically favors the "better safe than sorry" approach) stands in contradistinction to population risks, wherein a meaningful negative outcome arises from unnecessary antibiotic use [42].

However, this interpretation of the position in which physicians find themselves presupposes that the patient–physician relationship will be deleteriously affected by failing to provide an antibiotic prescription when requested. Studies have generally not found a link between patient satisfaction and whether or not they received an antibiotic prescription [59, 60]. In light of persistent physician concerns regarding parental pressure to prescribe, researchers have undertaken the process of examining how these conversations unfold.

One study reviewed 60 videotaped interactions between parents and physicians [61]. Researchers found that the interactions were more complex than a pressuring parent and resistant physician. Parents brought in their children to see the pediatrician for one of two reasons—either to obtain reassurance that their child is not critically ill or to receive validation of the severity of their child's illness [61]. Whether or not parents were expecting an antibiotic was tied to their perception of the severity of their children's illness [61]. Parents upset about their children's symptoms did not appear to be seeking antibiotics per se, but rather, clinical concern and appreciation for the severity of their child's suffering [61].

Regrettably, researchers found that when physicians explained the difference between viral and bacterial infections, they inadvertently projected subtle cues that viral infections are less severe in nature [61]. Researchers hypothesized that parents who are worried about the severity of their children's illness are more upset by receiving the message that their child is not significantly ill more than they may be about not receiving an antibiotic prescription. These parents want guidance as to how their child will be treated. Rather than directly compare viral infections to bacterial ones, physicians who find a viral infection in children can focus on the treatments and symptom management they would recommend for those children [61]. By focusing on what the child has (a viral infection) rather than what the child does not (a bacterial infection) physicians focus their time on the interventions that are likely to be successful, thus sending the message that they care about delivering good care [61]. If a parent were to subsequently make a direct inquiry about antibiotics, the clinician could explain that viral infections are caused by a mechanism that antibiotics have no influence over, without comparing symptoms or severity between viral and bacterial infections.

Children will build a tolerance to their asthma medication, requiring increasingly higher doses over the years

Inhaled corticosteroids, the mainstay treatment for pediatric asthma, unfortunately touch on two considerable fears among parents. Parents may have trouble separating the dangers of inhalants as a form of drug abuse (i.e., "huffing" toxic substances to obtain a high) from medications with an inhaled delivery [62]. Second, parents are likely aware of the dangers of anabolic steroid use, given their prevalence in the world of professional sports [62]. As a result, it is supposed that parents project these fears onto inhaled corticosteroid use for their children [62]. Stories of steroid abuse and general addiction cause concern among parents that giving their children an inhaled steroid daily will drive addiction [62]. Education alone does not appear to be sufficient—among one sample of parents with addiction fears, two-thirds reported that they felt they had received sufficient education about their child's treatment [62]. This finding supports the growing body of evidence that education alone is not capable of allaying parental concerns and, by extension, increasing adherence.

Even parents who agree to initiate treatment for their children show ongoing fears, some of which may prompt them to reduce adherence [27]. Just over 20% of a sample of parents who agreed to medication initiation still believed that their children could become addicted to the steroids in their medication [63]. Another study found that while 75% of parents felt asthma control medications were necessary for their children's health, 34% still voiced strong concerns about those medications [27]. When weighing the necessity of medication against perceived risks, it would appear the concerns about medication regularly overtake necessity: only approximately 20% of this sample reported complete adherence [27]. One-third of parents in another study wanted to stop their children's steroid treatment as soon as they possibly could [63].

Parents of children with more severe symptoms are more concerned about medication risks than parents of children with mild symptoms [27]. Parents' concerns about the medication were associated with medication adherence—the more concern they had, the less adherent they were [27]. Taken together, these results imply that less adherent parents are not less concerned about their children's health—in fact, these parents witness more severe symptoms than more adherent parents. However, their concerns about medication outstrip their worries about the illness itself. As children with more severe symptoms receive higher doses of medication, it appears that parents' concerns about medications are in proportion to the prescribed dosage.

A study examining parents' concerns regarding asthma medication in a Malaysian sample supports this conclusion. Among 170 parents of children with asthma, 112 expressed concerns regarding medication [62]. Among these parents, the 2 most commonly cited fears were side effects (94%) and that their children would become dependent on the medication and require higher dosages over time to maintain proper lung functioning (86%) [62]. Again, parents with concerns showed increased likelihood of missing dosages of their children's medications [62]. Their children also visited medical offices more frequently than children of parents without these concerns [62]. Overall, parents with concerns about medication had children who were prescribed higher doses of medication [62]. This supplements the above finding that more concerned/less adherent parents have children with more severe symptoms [62].

Counter to many parents' impressions, guidelines recommend beginning children on the optimal dosage according to symptoms and then gradually decreasing the dosage over time in accordance with response to treatment [64]. Parents who stop their children's treatment outside of this protocol will see a re-emergence of symptoms. One controlled study measured outcomes of children who are first optimally treated on an inhaled steroid and then cease to take it [65]. Children who stopped (compared to others who continued) experienced an increase in asthmatic symptoms, increased need for emergency bronchodilator use, and increased airway responsiveness [65]. Halting children's medications from fear of side effects unintentionally creates an acute condition from symptom re-emergence [64]. Increased medications, exactly what parents are attempting to avoid, become necessary to stabilize the child's condition [64]. Daily control medication with dosage reduced in a stepwise fashion better controls asthma than relying on fast-acting treatment for emergent symptoms [64]. Following the recommended downward stepwise approach helps avoid the rapid cycling between managed and acute asthma symptoms [64].

Parents concerned about their children's ability to breathe in the long-term without medication should be aware that uncontrolled asthma appears to have negative long-term effects on breathing owing to airway restructuring caused by the disease [25]. In a double-blind randomized controlled trial, patients with mild to moderate asthma who used inhaled steroids as prescribed experienced greater improvements in airway restructuring than those who did not use the medication [66]. Although some children will require inhaled corticosteroid treatment into adulthood, there is no evidence that they require increasing dosages due to tolerance; and they are less likely to require extensive treatments in future.

Stimulant medication for ADHD comes with widespread side effects in both the long- and short-term

While parents may have the impression that stimulant treatment is still relatively new and untested, the history of treating disruptive behaviors in children with stimulants dates as far back as 1937 [67]. Since the 1960s, hundreds of randomized controlled trials have shown that stimulants provide significant and robust improvements in ADHD symptoms [67]. These improvements are observed in individuals as young as preschool-age through adulthood [68]. Contrary to persistent concerns, numerous longitudinal studies have yielded limited long-term negative side effects of stimulant medications [67]. The long-term side effect with the most evidence is growth rate, with literature reviews suggesting possible decreases in growth rates in the first 1–3 years of stimulant treatment [69, 70]. In the short-term, the most common side effects of stimulant medication are difficulty sleeping, decreased appetite, and headache [67]. Difficulty sleeping, decreased appetite, stomachaches, social withdrawal, and lethargy are more commonly reported in children receiving higher doses than lower doses [71].

In addition to these established side effects, parents continue to voice concerns about side effects that have no basis in evidence [56]. More alarming possible side effects, such as sudden cardiac arrest, mania, or psychosis have been reported in the media despite being unfounded in any studies [67]. Sudden death has not been found to occur in higher rates among stimulant-treated children than in the general population [72].

Concerns that stimulant medication promotes substance use disorders later in life is also a persistent fear that has dogged stimulant treatment despite the lack of evidence supporting this theory [73]. Parents concerned about substance use disorders may not be aware that rates of substance use in adults are higher in those who were diagnosed with ADHD than those who were not, irrespective of medication [74]. While the exact mechanism is still not understood, the irregular transmission of dopamine implicated in ADHD is possibly related to the dopaminergic response of substances such as nicotine [73]. Also proposed is that children with ADHD experience more challenges academically and socially due to their symptoms, which may in turn moderate their use of substances later in life [73]. A review of studies examining this hypothesis found that prescribed stimulant use may actually be associated with a decrease in the risk for developing a substance use disorder [75]. Subsequent studies continue to show no evidence for increased risk of substance use disorders in a stimulant-treated sample, and in some cases, decreased risk is observed [76, 77].

Current Research

Antibiotics

Current research shows a shift in parents' concerns regarding antibiotics that mirrors the recent decline in pediatric antibiotic usage [78]. Focus groups conducted with parents find a general understanding that not all infections require antibiotic treatment [78]. Essentially all parents reported attempting home remedies to provide symptom relief before bringing their children into the doctor [78]. This reflects what many physicians suspect: namely, by the time they see a child, the parent has surpassed their personal threshold for concern. Research shows that physicians' perceptions that parents are requesting antibiotics are not truly reflective of the parents' desires, but rather, are related to parents' expectations that their children will be treated if the parent perceives them to be significantly ill [60, 79].

Far from requesting antibiotics across the board, more parents are showing concerns regarding overuse of antibiotics [78]. In light of this new knowledge, new misconceptions have emerged, in particular with regard to who is the antibiotic-resistant subject: the patient or the bacteria. Parents report fears that their children will become resistant to antibiotics [78]. These parents think of antibiotics as a substance that their children can develop a tolerance to, eventually rendering the medication ineffective [78]. In this current landscape, physicians should take care to clarify that antibiotic resistance refers to the bacteria becoming resistant to the antibiotic, and not the child becoming resistant to antibiotics' effects.

Asthma

Asthma management involves dynamic interactions between parents and children. Thus, adherence to regular medication usage can be viewed through the lenses of both child adherence and parental adherence [30]. Parental versus child adherence is a particularly important distinction as children age and parents begin to shift more of the responsibility for taking medication to their children [30]. Many parents shift responsibility for medication administration to their children based on age rather than maturity level or the child's comprehension [30].

Research shows that both parents and children have wide variability in their knowledge of asthma and how medications treat it [80]. Until recently, clinicians were unaware as to how lack of knowledge affected medication adherence [30]. Children's knowledge alone is likely not sufficient to explain adherence (or lack thereof), so researchers examined the interaction effects of child knowledge and children's responsibility [30].

In a study of 106 asthmatic children, results showed that age was significantly related to knowledge—older children knew more about asthma and treatment [30]. Older children also exhibited higher ability to reason through the causes and effects of asthma [30]. Yet older children were less likely to be adherent to asthma medication [30]. Taken together, these results indicate that older children can understand asthma, its causes and consequences, and still remain less adherent than younger children whose parents remain primarily responsible for their treatment [30].

While the study did not assess why older children—with more knowledge—adhere less to treatment, the researchers suggested possible explanations that practicing physicians can consider [30]. Even if older children understand more, they may lack the memory capacity or daily living strategies to follow through with medication administration [30]. They may also use their time of increased responsibility and decreased supervision to test out not using medication, particularly if they were not brought on board with the treatment when it was initially managed by their parents [30]. There is also the possibility that the social stigma associated with taking asthma medication increases as children age [30].

These factors may seem trivial, but they have direct bearing on medication adherence. One study of adults found that when adult concern for medication outweighs their perception of the benefits, adherence is low [81]. Study authors of the sample of asthmatic children pose that the same issues may influence older children [30]. As such, it is recommended that clinicians remain mindful of explaining asthma, its causes, effects, and need for treatment, but also to assess the health beliefs of the pediatric patient [30]. Physicians should anticipate a likely dip in adherence as children reach adolescence and proactively address adolescents' concerns at that time [30].

Attention-Deficit/Hyperactivity Disorder

Despite ongoing debate among the lay public, stimulant medications provide meaningful symptom relief in children with ADHD and are typically taken for months to years at a time without significant side effects [82]. Some differences between primary care prescribers and psychiatrists emerge in the treatment of ADHD [82]. Compared to primary physicians, psychiatrists are more likely to begin treatment at lower doses, titrate up to higher maximal doses, and see the patient 3 times in the first 90 days (an indicator of increased monitoring) [83]. Primary care physicians are helpful in the broad identification and education of ADHD; pediatricians without the time to see a patient multiple times to monitor stimulant medication and parents' concerns should consider referring parents directly to a psychiatrist.

Any physician who prescribes stimulant medications should take careful note of parents' beliefs and attitudes about the diagnosis and medication before prescribing [84]. These factors play a large role in whether or not the parent initiates and sustains treatment [84]. One study of 50 parents found that their understanding of the scientific literature—which theoretically should allay concerns about stimulant side effects—did not, in fact, dispel such fears [39]. This may be partially due to the fact that 40% of parents in the sample consulted, in addition to their physicians, non-medical sources regarding their questions about stimulant medications [39]. Even among parents whose children have taken stimulants long-term (on average, approximately 2 years), only 80% were convinced of the medication's safety [39]. Parents do not view all side effects equally. Many symptoms, such as mild appetite suppression or sleep initiation difficulty, are tolerated for years [85]. When psychological side effects, such as increased moodiness or irritability or a change in personality, occur, they frequently prompt discontinuation [86].

Patients benefit when physicians anticipate the commonly occurring side effects and provide relief. If any of the below common side effects cannot be managed, non-stimulant alternatives can be tried. For appetitive suppression, parents can give their children medication with or after meals [73]. Additional snacking may also be included throughout the day to ensure children are receiving adequate nutrition [73]. Evidence is mixed regarding the practice **medication holidays**, when parents suspend their children's medication when they are not in school (either over weekends or longer breaks) [73]. Therefore physicians should not directly recommend drug holidays, but can support parents who choose to try this method. Evidence shows wide variability between patients in the effects of stimulant medication on sleep disturbance [73]. Because sleep initiation is influenced by a number of factors, physicians should ascertain the child's sleep patterns before initiating treatment and keep records for a baseline [73]. Physicians should note the following factors: bedtime resistance, difficulty initiating sleep, awakening during the night, trouble waking in the morning, any breathing-related sleep dis-orders, and daytime sleepiness [73]. In some cases of stimulant treatment, the dif-ficulty sleeping is due to a rebound effect, wherein the hyperactive symptoms of ADHD that have been suppressed throughout the day emerge as the medication wears off [73]. The hyperactive ADHD symptoms themselves can inhibit sleep [73]. In other cases, the stimulant itself appears to impede sleep [73]. Physicians should assess which is occurring before providing recommendations, as the solu-tions may differ. Changing stimulant schedules to provide smaller, more frequent doses throughout the day can reduce rebound effects on sleep [73]. If the stimulant is causing difficulty sleeping, physicians should prescribe the lowest effective dose to be given as early in the day as possible [73].

Adherence

Given the current research of medication adherence, practicing physicians should maintain a high level of acknowledgement for and understanding of low adher-ence in their patients [2]. Given the high variability of adherence displayed in the pediatric population, physicians should consider adherence as among the top most likely contributors when children are unresponsive to treatment [2]. Parents can experience negative feelings associated with non-adherence, such as guilt or shame, which may reduce the likelihood of their willingness to share their true adherence rates [2]. Rather than assume perfect adherence, physicians can ask par-ents how treatment administration is proceeding in an open, non-confrontational manner that presupposes some level of non-adherence at the outset [2]. Physicians should take care to emphasize that all but a very limited number of individuals are fully adherent to medication regimens [2].

When parents acknowledge lapses in medication administration, physicians can recommend techniques to improve adherence [2]. No techniques can guaran-tee perfect adherence; however, a combination of strategies has been found to be most effective [2, 87, 88]. Reviews of interventions to assist families in increasing medication adherence often include injunctions to consider developmental needs of the children and families [87]. However, there is no available research that sys-tematizes how this can be achieved [87]. For example, it is still unclear from the research base whether interventions should focus primarily on interventions for the parent, child, or both [87].

Education is almost always provided within researched adherence strategies [87]. In written or verbal format education typically includes information about the illness, treatment rationale, and positive outcomes of adhering to such a treatment [87]. This technique of providing information is nearly universally recommended for use in clinical practice [89]. However, reviews of the literature have found that education alone produces negligible effects on adherence [88]. Education contin-ues to be recommended because although it is unlikely to improve adherence inde-pendently, lack of education certainly works against adherence rates [90].

Provided parents understand the diagnosis, treatment-effect potential, and side effects, physicians can shift to providing concrete strategies. Techniques should minimize the cognitive load on parents, such as, for example, setting alarms rather than asking them to remember a medication schedule [2]. Doctors should also provide instruction in written format whenever possible, further reducing the need for parents to retain and recall information during the stresses of daily life [2]. Behavioral approaches are suggested, such as goal setting, monitoring, providing positive reinforcement to the child for medication adherence (such as small rewards), and linking medication administration to other daily living tasks, such as brushing teeth [87].

Given the above discussion on parents' fears of medication side effects, tactics that frighten parents regarding adverse outcomes of medication non-adherence should be avoided [2]. While it may seem appropriate to emphasize the need of medications by focusing on negative outcomes of low adherence, this strategy has the unfortunate effect of pitting fear against fear. Focusing instead on the anticipated desired health outcomes that will occur with medication adherence amplifies the reasons for medication prescription as well as provides reassurance that side effects, if they do arise, are not being tolerated unnecessarily.

Conclusion

Interventions to increase adherence gradually decrease in efficacy over time, suggesting the importance of sustained reassessment and follow up [88]. Physicians must balance the need for optimal treatment with the need to maintain a positive, collaborative, long-term relationship with patients. Pediatric practice regularly involves ongoing relationships for both acute and chronic illness. Rather than aim for complete adherence, physicians should strive to help their patients achieve clinically meaningful adherence [2].

References

1. Sabaté, E. Adherence to long-term therapies: evidence for action. World Health Organization. 2003.
2. Matsui D. Current issues in pediatric medication adherence. Pediatric Drugs. 2007;9(5):283–8.
3. Beers MH, Berkow R. The Merck manual of diagnosis and therapy. Merck and Co. Inc, 1999.
4. Mattar ME, Markello J, Yaffe SJ. Pharmaceutic factors affecting pediatric compliance. Pediatrics. 1975;55(1):101–8.
5. Shope JT. Medication compliance. Pediatr Clin North Am. 1981;28(1):5.
6. Penkower L, Dew MA, Ellis D, Sereika SM, Kitutu JM, Shapiro R. Psychological distress and adherence to the medical regimen among adolescent renal transplant recipients. Am J Transplant. 2003;3(11):1418–25.

7. DiMatteo MR. Social support and patient adherence to medical treatment: a meta-analysis. Health Psychol. 2004;23(2):207.

8. Lask B. Motivating children and adolescents to improve adherence. J pediatrics. 2003;143(4):430–3.

9. Nevins TE. Non-compliance and its management in teenagers. Pediatr Transplant. 2002;6(6):475–9.

10. Haynes RB, McDonald H, Garg AX, Montague P. Interventions for helping patients to follow prescriptions for medications. The Cochrane Library. 2002.

11. Winnick S, Lucas DO, Hartman AL, Toll D. How do you improve compliance? Pediatrics. 2005;115(6):e718–24.

12. Van Cleave J, Gortmaker SL, Perrin JM. Dynamics of obesity and chronic health conditions among children and youth. JAMA. 2010;303(7):623–30.

13. Newacheck PW, Taylor WR. Childhood chronic illness: prevalence, severity, and impact. Am J Public Health. 1992;82(3):364–71.

14. Gardiner P, Dvorkin L. Promoting medication adherence in children. Am Fam Physician. 2006;74(5):793–8.

15. Shallcross LJ, Davies DS. Antibiotic overuse: a key driver of antimicrobial resistance. Br J Gen Pract. 2014;64(629):604–5.

16. Spellberg B, Bartlett JG, Gilbert DN. The future of antibiotics and resistance. N Engl J Med. 2013;368(4):299–302.

17. McCaig LF, Hughes JM. Trends in antimicrobial drug prescribing among office-based physicians in the United States. JAMA. 1995;273(3):214–9.

18. Neu HC. The crisis in antibiotic resistance. Science. 1992;257(5073):1064–73.

19. Goossens H, Ferech M, Vander Stichele R, Elseviers M. ESAC project group. outpatient antibiotic use in Europe and association with resistance: a cross-national database study. The Lancet. 2005;365(9459):579–87.

20. Hersh AL, Jackson MA, Hicks LA, Brady MT, Byington CL, Davies HD, Edwards KM, Maldonado YA, Murray DL, Orenstein WA, Rathore M. Principles of judicious antibiotic prescribing for upper respiratory tract infections in pediatrics. Pediatrics. 2013;132(6):1146–54.

21. Vaz LE, Kleinman KP, Lakoma MD, Dutta-Linn MM, Nahill C, Hellinger J, Finkelstein JA. Prevalence of parental misconceptions about antibiotic use. Pediatrics. 2015:peds-2015.

22. Palmer DA, Bauchner H. Parents' and physicians' views on antibiotics. Pediatrics. 1997; 99(6):e6-.

23. American Lung Association. Trends in asthma morbidity and mortality. epidemiology and statistics unit, Research and Scientific Affairs.

24. Akinbami LJ, Simon AE, Rossen LM. Changing trends in asthma prevalence among children. Pediatrics. 2016;137(1):1–7.

25. Bousquet J, Jeffery PK, Busse WW, Johnson M, Vignola AM. Asthma: from bronchoconstriction to airways inflammation and remodeling. Am J Respir Crit Care Med. 2000;161(5):1720–45.

26. National Heart Lung and Blood Institute. National asthma education and prevention program. Expert panel report. 2007;3.

27. Conn KM, Halterman JS, Fisher SG, Yoos HL, Chin NP, Szilagyi PG. Parental beliefs about medications and medication adherence among urban children with asthma. Ambul Pediatr. 2005;5(5):306–10.

28. Azizi HO, Lee EL, Mohan J. Guidelines for the management of childhood asthma. Med J Malaysia. 1997;52:416–27.

29. Bender B, Milgrom H, Rand C. Nonadherence in asthmatic patients: is there a solution to the problem? Ann Allergy Asthma Immunol. 1997;79(3):177–87.

30. McQuaid EL, Kopel SJ, Klein RB, Fritz GK. Medication adherence in pediatric asthma: reasoning, responsibility, and behavior. J Pediatr Psychol. 2003;28(5):323–33.

31. Charach A, Dashti B, Carson P, Booker L, Lim CG, Lillie E, Yeung E, Ma J, Raina P, Schachar R. Attention deficit hyperactivity disorder: effectiveness of treatment in at-risk preschoolers; long-term effectiveness in all ages; and variability in prevalence, diagnosis, and treatment. Comparative effectiveness reviews. 2011;44.

32. Barkley RA, Fischer M, Smallish L, Fletcher K. Young adult outcome of hyperactive children: adaptive functioning in major life activities. J Am Acad Child Adolesc Psychiatry. 2006;45(2):192–202.

33. Reimer B, Mehler B, D'Ambrosio LA, Fried R. The impact of distractions on young adult drivers with attention deficit hyperactivity disorder (ADHD). Accid Anal Prev. 2010;42(3):842–51.

34. Faregh N, Derevensky J. Gambling behavior among adolescents with attention deficit/hyperactivity disorder. J Gambl Stud. 2011;27(2):243–56.

35. Hansen DL, Hansen EH. Caught in a balancing act: parents' dilemmas regarding their ADHD child's treatment with stimulant medication. Qual Health Res. 2006;16(9):1267–85.

36. Breggin P. Talking back to Ritalin: What doctors aren't telling you about stimulants and ADHD. Da Capo Press; 2007.

37. Diller LH. Running on Ritalin: A physician reflects on children. Society, and Performance in a. 1999.

38. Zuvekas SH, Vitiello B, Norquist GS. Recent trends in stimulant medication use among US children. Am J Psychiatry. 2006.

39. Berger I, Dor T, Nevo Y, Goldzweig G. Attitudes toward attention-deficit hyperactivity disorder (ADHD) treatment: parents' and children's perspectives. J Child Neurol. 2008;23(9):1036–42.

40. Bussing R, Gary FA, Mills TL, Garvan CW. Parental explanatory models of ADHD. Soc Psychiatry Psychiatr Epidemiol. 2003;38(10):563–75.

41. Kuzujanakis M, Kleinman K, Rifas-Shiman S, Finkelstein JA. Correlates of parental antibiotic knowledge, demand, and reported use. Ambul Pediatr. 2003;3(4):203–10.

42. Meropol SB, Votruba ME. Decision-making and the barriers to judicious antibiotic use. Pediatrics. 2015;136(2):387–8.

43. Kuzik BA. Inhaled corticosteroids in children with persistent asthma: Effects on growth. Paediatrics Child Health. 2015;20(5):248.

44. Todd G, Dunlop K, McNaboe J, Ryan MF, Carson D, Shields MD. Growth and adrenal suppression in asthmatic children treated with high-dose fluticasone propionate. The Lancet. 1996;348(9019):27–9.

45. Wolthers OD, Pedersen S. Controlled study of linear growth in asthmatic children during treatment with inhaled glucocorticosteroids. Pediatrics. 1992;89(5):839–42.

46. Pruteanu AI, Chauhan BF, Zhang L, Prietsch SO, Ducharme FM. Inhaled corticosteroids in children with persistent asthma: dose-response effects on growth. Evid Based Child Health: A Cochrane Rev J. 2014;9(4):931–1046.

47. Zhang L, Prietsch SO, Ducharme FM. Inhaled corticosteroids in children with persistent asthma: effects on growth. Evid Based Child Health: A Cochrane Rev J. 2014;9(4):829–930.

48. Kelly HW, Sternberg AL, Lescher R, Fuhlbrigge AL, Williams P, Zeiger RS, Raissy HH, Van Natta ML, Tonascia J, Strunk RC. Effect of inhaled glucocorticoids in childhood on adult height. N Engl J Med. 2012;367(10):904–12.

49. Froehlich TE, Lanphear BP, Epstein JN, Barbaresi WJ, Katusic SK, Kahn RS. Prevalence, recognition, and treatment of attention-deficit/hyperactivity disorder in a national sample of US children. Arch Pediatr Adolesc Med. 2007;161(9):857–64.

50. Winterstein AG, Gerhard T, Shuster J, Zito J, Johnson M, Liu H, Saidi A. Utilization of pharmacologic treatment in youths with attention deficit/hyperactivity disorder in Medicaid database. Ann Pharmacother. 2008;42(1):24–31.

51. Pescosolido BA, Jensen PS, Martin JK, Perry BL, Olafsdottir S, Fettes D. Public knowledge and assessment of child mental health problems: findings from the National Stigma Study-Children. J Am Acad Child Adolesc Psychiatry. 2008;47(3):339–49.

52. Bussing R, Gary FA. Practice guidelines and parental ADHD treatment evaluations: friends or foes? Harvard Review of Psychiatry. 2001;9(5):223–33.
53. Singh I. Boys will be boys: fathers' perspectives on ADHD symptoms, diagnosis, and drug treatment. Harv Rev Psychiatry. 2003;11(6):308–16.
54. Mychailyszyn MP, Myers M, Riley AW. Coming to terms with ADHD: how urban African-American families come to seek care for their children. Psychiatr Serv. 2007.
55. Coletti DJ, Pappadopulos E, Katsiotas NJ, Berest A, Jensen PS, Kafantaris V. Parent perspectives on the decision to initiate medication treatment of attention-deficit/hyperactivity disorder. J Child Adolesc Psychopharmacol. 2012;22(3):226–37.
56. Brinkman WB, Sherman SN, Zmitrovich AR, Visscher MO, Crosby LE, Phelan KJ, Donovan EF. Parental angst making and revisiting decisions about treatment of attention-deficit/hyperactivity disorder. Pediatrics. 2009;124(2):580–9.
57. Brown RT, Amler RW, Freeman WS, Perrin JM, Stein MT, Feldman HM, Pierce K, Wolraich ML. American academy of Pediatrics subcommittee on attention-deficit/hyperactivity disorder. Treatment of attention-deficit/hyperactivity disorder: overview of the evidence. Pediatrics. 2005;115(6):e749–57.
58. Bauchner H, Pelton SI, Klein JO. Parents, physicians, and antibiotic use. Pediatrics. 1999;103(2):395–401.
59. Hamm RM, Hicks RJ, Bemben DA. Antibiotics and respiratory infections: are patients more satisfied when expectations are met? J Fam Pract. 1996;43(1):56–63.
60. Mangione-Smith R, McGlynn EA, Elliott MN, Krogstad P, Brook RH. The relationship between perceived parental expectations and pediatrician antimicrobial prescribing behavior. Pediatrics. 1999;103(4):711–8.
61. Cabral C, Ingram J, Lucas PJ, Redmond NM, Kai J, Hay AD, Horwood J. Influence of clinical communication on parents' antibiotic expectations for children with respiratory tract infections. Annals Fam Med. 2016;14(2):141–7.
62. Chan PW, DeBruyne JA. Parental concern towards the use of inhaled therapy in children with chronic asthma. Pediatr Int. 2000;42(5):547–51.
63. Yoos HL, Kitzman H, McMullen A. Barriers to anti-inflammatory medication use in childhood asthma. Ambul Pediatr. 2003;3(4):181–90.
64. Eid NS. Update on national asthma education and prevention program pediatric asthma treatment recommendations. Clin Pediatr. 2004;43(9):793–802.
65. Waalkens HJ, Van Essen-Zandvliet EE, Hughes MD, Gerritsen J, Duiverman EJ, Knol K, Kerrebijn KF. Cessation of long-term treatment with inhaled corticosteroid (budesonide) in children with asthma results in deterioration. Am Rev Respi Dis. 1993;148(5):1252–7.
66. Ward C, Pais M, Bish R, Reid D, Feltis B, Johns D, Walters EH. Airway inflammation, basement membrane thickening and bronchial hyperresponsiveness in asthma. Thorax. 2002;57(4):309–16.
67. Pliszka SR. Pharmacologic treatment of attention-deficit/hyperactivity disorder: efficacy, safety and mechanisms of action. Neuropsychol Rev. 2007;17(1):61–72.
68. Spencer T, Biederman J, Wilens T, Harding M. O'DONNELL DE, Griffin S. Pharmacotherapy of attention-deficit hyperactivity disorder across the life cycle. J Am Acad Child Adolesc Psychiatry. 1996;35(4):409–32.
69. Poulton A. Growth on stimulant medication; clarifying the confusion: a review. Arch Dis Child. 2005;90(8):801–6.
70. Faraone SV, Biederman J, Morley CP, Spencer TJ. The effect of stimulants on height and weight: a review of the literature (manuscript in preparation).
71. Greenhill L, Kollins S, Abikoff H, McCracken J, Riddle M, Swanson J, McGough J, Wigal S, Wigal T, Vitiello B, Skrobala A. Efficacy and safety of immediate-release methylphenidate treatment for preschoolers with ADHD. J Am Acad Child Adolesc Psychiatry. 2006;45(11):1284–93.

72. Villalaba L. Follow up review of AERS search identifying cases of sudden death occurring with drugs used for the treatment of attention deficit hyperactivity disorder ADHD. Available at http://www.fda.gov/ohrms/dockets/ac/06/briefing/2006-4210b_07_01_safetyreview.pdf.

73. Cortese S, Holtmann M, Banaschewski T, Buitelaar J, Coghill D, Danckaerts M, Dittmann RW, Graham J, Taylor E, Sergeant J. Practitioner review: current best practice in the management of adverse events during treatment with ADHD medications in children and adolescents. J Child Psychol Psychiatry. 2013;54(3):227–46.

74. Charach A, Yeung E, Climans T, Lillie E. Childhood attention-deficit/hyperactivity disorder and future substance use disorders: comparative meta-analyses. J Am Acad Child Adolesc Psychiatry. 2011;50(1):9–21.

75. Wilens TE, Faraone SV, Biederman J, Gunawardene S. Does stimulant therapy of attention-deficit/hyperactivity disorder beget later substance abuse? a meta-analytic review of the literature. Pediatrics. 2003;111(1):179–85.

76. Biederman J, Monuteaux MC, Spencer T, Wilens TE, MacPherson HA, Faraone SV. Stimulant therapy and risk for subsequent substance use disorders in male adults with ADHD: a naturalistic controlled 10 year follow-up study. Am J Psychiatry. 2008.

77. Mannuzza S, Klein RG, Truong NL, Moulton III JL, Roizen ER, Howell KH, Castellanos FX. Age of methylphenidate treatment initiation in children with ADHD and later substance abuse: prospective follow-up into adulthood. Am J Psychiatry. 2008.

78. Finkelstein JA, Dutta-Linn M, Meyer R, Goldman R. Childhood infections, antibiotics, and resistance what are parents saying now? Clin Pediatr. 2014;53(2):145–50.

79. Stivers T, Mangione-Smith R, Elliott MN, McDonald L, Heritage J. Why do physicians think parents expect antibiotics? What parents report vs what physicians believe. J Fam Pract. 2003;52(2):140–7.

80. McQuaid EL, Howard K, Kopel SJ, Rosenblum K, Bibace R. Developmental concepts of asthma: reasoning about illness and strategies for prevention. J Appl Dev Psychol. 2002;23(2):179–94.

81. Horne R, Weinman J. Patients' beliefs about prescribed medicines and their role in adherence to treatment in chronic physical illness. J Psychosom Res. 1999;47(6):555–67.

82. Charach A, Fernandez R. Enhancing ADHD medication adherence: challenges and opportunities. Curr Psychiatry Rep. 2013;15(7):1–8.

83. Chen CY, Gerhard T, Winterstein AG. Determinants of initial pharmacological treatment for youths with attention-deficit/hyperactivity disorder. J Child Adolesc Psychopharmacol. 2009;19(2):187–95.

84. Dosreis S, Myers MA. Parental attitudes and involvement in psychopharmacological treatment for ADHD: a conceptual model. Int Rev Psychiatry. 2008;20(2):135–41.

85. Charach A, Ickowicz A, Schachar R. Stimulant treatment over five years: adherence, effectiveness, and adverse effects. J Am Acad Child Adolesc Psychiatry. 2004;43(5):559–67.

86. Toomey SL, Sox CM, Rusinak D, Finkelstein JA. Why do children with ADHD discontinue their medication? Clin Pediatr. 2012;51(8):763–9.

87. Dean AJ, Walters J, Hall A. A systematic review of interventions to enhance medication adherence in children and adolescents with chronic illness. Arch Dis Child. 2010;95(9):717–23.

88. Kahana S, Drotar D, Frazier T. Meta-analysis of psychological interventions to promote adherence to treatment in pediatric chronic health conditions. J Pediatr Psychol. 2008;33(6):590–611.

89. Staples B, Bravender T. Drug compliance in adolescents. Pediatric Drugs. 2002;4(8):503–13.

90. Nevins TE. Why do they do that? Pediatric Nephrol. 2005;20(7):845–8.

Chapter 11
Sleep

Overview

The occurrence of childhood sleep problems is one of the most common challenges parents present to their physicians [1]. Parents report sleep difficulties throughout childhood at rates between 20 and 30% [2–6]. Problems span from typical but frustrating challenges to clinical sleep disorders. Among the numerous types of sleeping difficulties, some are psychological, others behavioral, and still others physical [7]. Prevalent sleep problems that do not typically warrant diagnosis but suggest that intervention is appropriate include disruptive bedtime routines, difficulty falling asleep, nighttime awakenings, and subsequent interactions in which children attempt to get out of bed after it is expected that they stay in bed [1, 8]. **Disruptive bedtime routines** refer to situations in which children actively resist their parents' attempts to get them to bed and then to sleep [9]. Diagnosable sleep problems cover a range of medical and biological abnormalities: insomnia, hypersomnolence, narcolepsy, breathing sleep disorders (including sleep apneas), circadian rhythm disorders, and parasomnias (including nightmare disorders and Restless Leg Syndrome) [10].

Sleep problems present a special challenge for pediatricians. Physicians must first recognize which behaviors are normal amidst the wide variability of healthy sleep. They also encounter parents who perceive a normal problem as pathologic. Finally, they must assess the numerous factors affecting children's sleep patterns: biological, psychological, cultural, social, and familial [6]. For example, a child may show bedtime resistance, which appears behavioral in nature. However, the child may suffer from a medical condition such as sleep apnea or nighttime enuresis (bedwetting) that makes sleep an unpleasant experience. The medical challenge leads the child to reject the bedtime routine because it signals the uncomfortable situation about to occur. A physician must identify the complex interplay of factors before deciding on appropriate referrals or initiation for treatment.

© Springer International Publishing AG 2017
C.A. Di Bartolo and M.K. Braun, *Pediatrician's Guide to Discussing Research with Patients*, DOI 10.1007/978-3-319-49547-7_11

On average, children with intellectual or developmental disabilities (IDD) experience a higher prevalence of sleep disorders and poor sleep habits than the general population [9]. Impaired sleep occurs widely in children with Down syndrome, Autism Spectrum Disorder, Angelman's syndrome, and Prader–Willi syndrome, who encounter higher than average rates of sleep problems [9]. Children with IDD display disruptive bedtime routines, vocally and/or physically resisting caretaker attempts to guide the children through their bedtime routine, into bed, and finally to sleep [9]. These children may also experience **delayed sleep onset**, a difficulty falling asleep according to typical circadian rhythms [9]. Children who exhibit disruptive bedtime routines frequently experience delayed sleep onset as a consequence of the difficult interactions preparing for bed [9]. A **sleep–wake cycle disturbance** is characterized by short episodes of sleep that occur in the evening or early morning hours as a result of premature awakening [9]. Disruptive bedtime routines, delayed sleep onset, and sleep–wake cycle disturbance contribute to difficulties in attaining sufficient and regular sleep in children with IDD [9].

Cultural and social influences of sleep are by no means new. However, of recent interest among Western parents and physicians alike is the practice of co-sleeping. Fairly common in Asian countries, **co-sleeping** is the practice of children sleeping in the same bed as their parents [6]. Infants and young childhood in Asian countries frequently co-sleep with their parents, but prevalence decreases as children age [6]. Social factors such as acceptability influence the prevalence of this practice [11]. For example, a survey of Korean mothers found a nearly 75% approval rate for co-sleeping with young children (ages 3–6 years) [11]. Co-sleeping is not the norm in Western countries, and is particularly rare among non-Hispanic parents [6]. Western parents are more likely to use **solo sleeping**, in which children sleep in their own bassinet, crib, and/or room. Researchers presume Western acceptability for co-sleeping is lower due to cultural taboos, drives to foster independence even in young children, and medical recommendations as to the safety hazards of co-sleeping [6].

This socially influenced practice affects sleep problems, as co-sleeping is related to changes in children's sleep patterns, disturbances, and sleepiness the following day [12, 13]. One study of Chinese children and American children compared a number of sleep variables to determine if co-sleeping in Chinese children (where it occurs more as the cultural norm) prompted later bed times, earlier wake times, higher report of sleep problems, and increased daytime sleepiness with lower total sleep times [6]. Researchers found that Chinese children went to bed an average of 30 minutes later and woke 30 minutes earlier than their American counterparts [6]. This resulted in a loss of 1 hour of sleep per night [6]. Daytime sleepiness in Chinese children was associated with shorter sleep times, whereas American children were more likely to show daytime sleepiness if their parents reported restless sleep and snoring [6]. While these results provide further evidence as to the detrimental effects of co-sleeping, study authors noted other cultural factors that may have influenced differences [6]. Chinese children have more homework than American children and take a 2 hour nap in the middle of the day [6]. Both of these factors could affect sleep quantity and quality, just as co-sleeping might.

Until a randomized controlled trial is conducted, wherein some parents are randomly assigned to co-sleeping and others assigned to solo sleeping, causality between co-sleeping and these detrimental effects cannot be established. The lack of evidence has prompted some Western parents to question advice to avoid co-sleeping with their young children. Specialists in sleep disorders do not specifically reject co-sleeping [14]. If parents choose to co-sleep with their children, physicians concern themselves with how parents can do so without risking their children's physical safety [14].

Despite the significant concerns regarding children's sleep and sleep problems, few pediatricians receive sufficient training in this area [1, 7]. This training deficit is at least partially due to the emerging nature of sleep research and sleep medicine [15]. Complicating matters, sleep disorders manifest differently in children than in adults [7]. A fair conclusion to this deficiency in training is that general practitioners likely struggle with appropriate assessment, diagnosis, treatment, and specialist referral for improving children's sleep [7]. One study of pediatricians found they commonly informed parents that children outgrow sleeping problems, and consequently did not recommend treatment [16]. In fact, there is little evidence to suggest that sleep problems remit without treatment [17]. When treatments *are* recommended, physicians frequently prescribe medication (prescription or nonprescription) despite both inadequate evidence such medications for sleep problems in children and a plethora of research promoting the efficacy of behavioral interventions [1, 14, 18]. When sleep problems are not properly assessed, they can be treated ineffectively or inappropriately [7].

Figures bear out these concerns. Despite sleep as a common parental concern, one study reviewed 50,000 patient-physician contacts and found sleep mentioned in less than 200 [19]. Without proactive screening from physicians, parents bear the responsibility of identifying whether their children may have sleep problems and bringing up their concerns for clinical consultation [20]. Parents identify sleep problems according to a number of factors: parental expectations for childhood sleep (realistic or not), parental knowledge of developmentally appropriate sleep, and cultural norms influencing parental perception of normative versus problematic sleep [20]. For example, regular awakenings during the night are an unremarkable aspect of healthy sleep patterns, yet parents may think these awakenings indicate a sleep problem [21]. In turn, parental cognitions and perceptions about children's sleep are influenced by culture, parental childhood experience of sleep, and experiences with their children's sleep [20]. Parents require assistance from a trained medical professional to help them assess their children's sleep and obtain evidence-based help when needed.

Common Parental Concerns

Physically and Emotionally Draining Nighttime Battles

Children's sleep problems are inherently intertwined with their parents' sleep [22]. Anecdotal reports from clinicians highlight an emerging pattern of stressed and tired parents of children with sleep difficulties [22]. In one author's experience, children who display bedtime resistance and nighttime awakenings prevent their parents from attaining maximum sleep. When children display disruptive bedtime routines, parents spend more time getting their children into bed than they would otherwise. This causes parents to do their other tasks later in the evening. This shift creates later bedtimes for already tired parents. Parents also find their opportunities to relax and unwind are diminished because of the extra time putting their children to sleep.

Once children are asleep, those who wake during the night cause specific challenges for their parents. Children may cry, call out, or climb into their parents' beds. These actions disrupt parents' sleep at various points in their sleep cycle, affecting their ability to achieve restful sleep. Additionally, abrupt awakenings can cause parents to be emotionally dysregulated or behaviorally uninhibited. This causes challenges in the parent–child interaction when "half-awake," possibly short-tempered parents must guide their children back to bed. Rather than engaging in the process of getting children back to bed, some parents elect to let their child sleep for the remainder of the night in their own bed. While some parents choose to co-sleep with their children, there is anecdotal evidence that parents who find themselves in a "reactive co-sleeping situation" experience stress, marital tension, and frustration [23]. Parents who take this path of less resistance may still end up tired and stressed.

Using these common anecdotes as an entry point, one research team studied whether children's sleep problems disrupt their parents' sleep and cause deleterious effects [22]. Researchers examined 47 parents, some of whom had children with sleep problems and others did not [22]. Tellingly, the researchers found no significant difference between children with and without sleep problems with regard to bedtimes, wake times, and total sleep time of the children [22]. What did differ was that parents of children with sleep problems got out of bed to respond to their children's awakenings more than the other parents [22]. These results indicate that the more parents get up in the middle of the night, the worse their perception of their children's sleep. More child sleep disruptions significantly predicted maternal sleep quality [22]. In turn, poor maternal sleep quality significantly predicted maternal depression, parental distress, fatigue, and sleepiness [22]. Confirming the common sense hypothesis that a tired parent is not an optimal parent, sleep disruptions of children significantly predicted parental functioning [22]. Mothers of children with sleep difficulties reported higher feelings of stress and overload, due in a meaningful part to their own poor sleep quality [22].

Study authors concluded that children's sleep is important for the functioning of the whole family [22]. In a sense, parents have to "put on their own oxygen first" to best care for their children. Parents who manage their children's awakenings in the night fight an uphill battle to be the best parents they can be in the daytime. Taking an example from the child abuse literature, preliminary evidence shows that one risk factor for child abuse is a parent with insufficient sleep [24]. On the other hand, when children's bedtime resistance and nighttime awakenings improve, so do rates of maternal depression, parenting ability, parental stress, and marital satisfaction [3, 25–27].

Children Need a Certain Number of Hours of Sleep Per Night

Assessing adequacy of sleep by number of hours is extremely challenging, given that children's needs vary according to age and other individual factors [7]. The ability to provide evidence-based sleep requirements would require very large controlled studies conducted cross-culturally, which are nearly impossible to undertake for practical reasons [28]. Most sleep duration recommendations come in the form of charts that display recommended number of hours of sleep for various age brackets. The recommendations tend to be based on studies of Western populations [29, 30]. This is despite clear cultural differences in the perceived need for sleep among children [30]. These cultural differences emerge in other considerations for sleep sufficiency, such as napping practices [30]. Numerous factors affect an individual's need for sleep, and while not all are currently known, growth rates, stress, and illness are all likely implicated [31]. As a result, there is no optimal level of sleep based on age that parents should aim for [31].

Parents concerned with whether their children are getting sufficient sleep are served by examining their children's daytime functioning rather than timing their sleep [31]. In children, insufficient sleep can manifest as, for example, becoming frustrated more easily than that child normally would for their temperament, or an increase in impulsiveness relative to that child's baseline level of impulsivity [32]. Children who remain sleepy after waking in the morning are likely not attaining sufficient sleep [31]. Tired children also tend to have trouble focusing and may fall asleep quickly when given the opportunity (such as during a car ride) [31].

Common Misconceptions

The only effect of lack of sleep is feeling tired the next day

When children beg to stay up "just ten more minutes," or point out that they are not finished with their homework, parent may be tempted to relent. Extensive research from a variety of methods shows that deficits in sleep quality and quantity cause numerous negative outcomes, with strong potential for adverse long-term outcomes [33]. The research-established outcomes of disrupted sleep indicate wide-ranging negative effects on mood, affect, energy, weight, behavior, learning, memory, and executive functioning (an aspect of cognitive functioning associated with higher order thinking) [7, 22, 33–35]. Based on psychometric tasks, disturbances in sleep have variable effects on functioning based on the task's demands and duration, as well as children's level of motivation, personality, and personal sleep requirements [36]. In some children, it seems possible that activity levels may actually increase in response to sleep deprivation, rather than display the sluggishness more typically associated with fatigue [7]. This paradoxical response has led some to hypothesize that a subset of children diagnosed with Attention-Deficit/Hyperactivity Disorder may actually be suffering from impaired sleep [32].

One study experimentally reduced children's sleep to capture subsequent teacher ratings [34]. Verifying common impressions, even children with no sleep disorders experienced a decline in academic performance as rated by their teachers when they received less sleep [34]. Interestingly, the teachers in this study were aware that their students were participating in a study where their sleep would be restricted, but teachers were blind as to when the students were sleep deprived versus when they slept as usual [34]. This allows for a more objective rating than reports of parents who are fully aware of when their children receive more or less sleep. Most parents are aware that sleep is a biological imperative. That it commonly takes a lower priority than schoolwork is counterproductive, the given loss of sleep's effect on behavioral, emotional, and cognitive functioning is needed for school success.

Giving children antihistamines or other medications is a good way to get them to sleep

Only a limited number of studies provide any evidence of efficacy for using medications to help children sleep [37, 38]. A very small number of studies specifically examined medications to assist sleep onset in children [8]. These studies either found no effect, effects when used in conjunction with behavioral interventions, or have not examined sleep aides in children younger than 3 years [39–41]. As such, the Food and Drug Administration does not recommend the use of any sleep medications for children [8].

Despite the lack of evidence, pharmacologic treatments are commonly used both in clinical practice and in homes without physician recommendation [8]. For example, about half of the respondents in one survey of 670 pediatricians reported that they recommended a nonprescription antihistamine to be used off-label for the purposes of promoting sleep in children younger than 2 years [42]. Until further evidence in favor of medications presents itself, physicians should not prescribe medications or suggest over-the-counter interventions to parents [8]. Parents should be specifically advised not to give their children over-the-counter medications for the reduction of sleep problems [8]. Physicians who recommend medication should do so only in conjunction with a behavioral intervention, for the purposes of mirroring how medications in research were examined [8].

Using behavioral interventions to improve children's sleep cause attachment problems and possibly trauma

Behavioral Interventions Overview

Given parents' struggles with sleep, clinicians developed and tested behavioral interventions to fill this need. Many parents turn to these established behavioral interventions to address their concerns [8]. These interventions vary in application, but different versions have been shown to be effective in helping parents assist their young children to sleep [43]. Some parents use these interventions with a clinician's help and support, and others read books or articles to implement the intervention independently [43].

Behavioral sleep interventions utilize basic behavioral approaches to increase desired sleep-related behaviors (e.g., staying in bed, self-soothing). Behaviorists work from a theory that examines the antecedents and consequences that occur before and after (respectively) a behavior occurs [44]. By adjusting antecedents before the behavior occurs and the consequences after a behavior occurs, the learning of new behaviors can be achieved [44].

A Note About Implicit Learning

Behaviorists speak in terms of "learning." Most people are familiar with explicit learning, whereby children learn how to tie their shoes or recite times tables. The kind of learning behaviorists refer to is implicit learning. **Implicit learning** is what allows children to realize gradually over time that certain actions are connected with certain outcomes. This process is often unconscious. When behaviorists explain concepts such as children learning that their cries will gain them parental attention, they do not propose that infants are consciously thinking, "If I keep crying, I'll keep getting cuddles from Mom." Instead, they are referring to the learning that occurs beneath conscious awareness, over time, with regard to repeating patterns of interactions.

Whenever possible, behaviorists prefer providing reinforcement after a desired behavior has occurred, whether it be providing something positive (e.g., praise, pat on the back) or removing something negative (e.g., nagging stops once child has displayed the desired behavior). Either of these reinforcement mechanisms increase the likelihood that the child will display the desired behavior again.

Some behaviors, however, are undesired and should not be reinforced. Many parents believe that if they yell, frown, lecture, or scold such behaviors, that they will occur less frequently. In many cases, this is a misguided principle. Children are highly influenced by interactions with their parents, whether those exchanges are positive or negative in nature. In the case of sleep, infants who cry when they should be sleeping often receive cuddles and rocking, teaching the child that to receive such attention, they should continue to cry. Older children who get out of bed and/or negotiate with their parents for more time awake often receive extensive responses from parents (in the form of answering questions, reading books, getting water, etc.). If parental attention reinforces crying or out-of-bed behavior, removing parental attention should result in a diminishment of these behaviors. Any time behaviors do not receive reinforcement over a prolonged period of time, the behavior is very likely to decrease and then stop completely. Behaviorists refer to this as "extinction," because the behavior stops [8].

Regardless of the differences among behavioral interventions for sleep, they all rest on two key principles: parental attention maintains a behavior; children older than 3 months old can soothe themselves to sleep if given the chance [8]. Applying a behavioral approach to sleep is fairly straightforward in theory, though challenging to implement in practice. When infants cry prior to falling asleep, many parents seek to comfort and soothe them. To maintain that parental attention, infants may continue to fuss. Crying is not consistent with sleeping. Older children may get out of bed or negotiate or argue with parents around bedtime. Parents who engage in these discussions inadvertently help their children in accomplishing their goal—staying awake. Talking is not consistent with sleep. When parents withdraw their attention, infants, and children will (eventually) naturally fall asleep on their own.

A Vocal Minority

There is extensive research showing that behavioral approaches improve children's sleep [43]. Despite the clear evidence in favor of using behavioral interventions for children (at least 3 months of age) with sleep problems, debate continues in the academic and public sphere as to the advisability of using this approach [8]. In part, some of the behavioral terms sound jarring, such as "extinction" [8]. The colloquial terms often sound just as negative, such as "cry-it-out" [8]. A vocal minority of researchers and, in many cases, non-researchers argue that behavioral approaches should not be used with children [45]. Instead, these critics of behavioral sleep interventions believe parents should be unilaterally responsive to their children's every need [45]. These critics uphold the theory that children should control every parent–child interaction. They refer to this theory in various ways. Some misapply attachment psychology literature [46]. Others lift terms from sociocultural fields, such as anthropology [45]. Critics of behavioral interventions recommend extensive interactions between parent and child, such as **proximal care**, which employs extensive holding, frequent breastfeeding, near-immediate responses to children's crying or fussing, and co-sleeping [45]. Others use terms such as "external womb," in which mothers are expected to provide the same level of support, holding, and responsiveness as supposedly occurs in the womb [47].

These critics are strongly and often emotionally against the concept that a child might cry without receiving immediate attention from a caregiver. They consider the matter one of morality and ethics rather than science [46]. After sleep researchers and clinicians challenged their stance, some have subsequently sought to find empirical evidence to promote their opinion. To explain why their approach is misguided, it is first necessary to understand in detail their objections to behavioral interventions.

The critics posit that young children who cry during the night are always signaling for parental attention to have a need to be met [46, 47]. They argue that evolutionarily, a crying child was a dangerous child, because the cries would signal to predators that humans were in the vicinity. As such, crying must always be stopped immediately, and it must be stopped by parental attention [47]. That someone may cry for reasons other than to gain attention from another are not addressed.

Critics of behavioral sleep interventions acknowledge that children's sleep disruptions wake their parents [46]. They do not address how lack of parental sleep affects the children they are trying to protect [14]. In rare cases, parents who become frustrated by children's crying have been known to become abusive, with actions such as smothering, shaking, or hitting their infants to make the crying cease [48, 49]. Critics of behavioral approaches assume that all parents can respond to their children's needs with infinite patience, which is unlikely to be true in practice. Instead, these critics focus on behavioral sleep interventions as a way to force modern sociological context (wherein many parents must work to support their families and need to be rested to do so) onto a natural biological function of children [46]. While some parents may be in a financial position to quit their jobs or take on more flexible hours to allow for the lack of sleep their children cause, this is likely not the norm. Critics of behavioral sleep interventions do not provide parents with the practical assistance they would need to implement their recommended approach. In some cases, they argue that a midline approach can be taken, but do not address how responding to a child's every need can be modified to be less extreme [46]. The unilateral responsiveness approach also disproportionately affects women and single parents.

Their argument appears to rest on the idea that humans should avoid any behaviors or actions that deviate from pure biological urges. These theoretical arguments that behavioral sleep training is not biologically advisable hinge on whether a child's emotional and physiological needs can still be met if they ever experience bouts of short-term crying without gaining immediate attention [50]. Without supporting evidence, these critics state that parents must make themselves available to their children when they cry, no matter the circumstances, and after no delay between onset of crying and parental response, otherwise children may experience significant long-term consequences [47]. Again, without evidence, these critics widely write about how behavioral interventions may cause such effects as: neuronal abnormalities, an abnormal stress reactivity that has lifelong consequences, weakened ability to self-regulate, meaningfully undermined trust in caregivers (and other attachment figures later in life), a decrease in caregiver sensitivity and responsiveness [47]. They draw on wide-ranging fields such as attachment theory and neuroscience to attempt to bolster their claims [47]. In some cases, critics equate the practice of not responding to children's crying at all times as tantamount to neglect [47]. Yet these critics have found no evidence that long-term health effects they fear will occur in children who learn to self-soothe [14]. Studies that directly examined their concerns regarding long-term outcomes are discussed below.

These critics would not have remained vocal for long without an audience. They are correct that research shows some parents express worry over intense crying from their children [51]. In some cases, parents themselves may feel as through they are insensitive or even abusive if they do not respond when their children cry [50]. One study assessed parent's impressions of whether or not a child who cried was signaling distress [50]. Parents who, prior to their child's birth, held cognitions that a crying child is a distressed child subsequently spent more time soothing their children at night and had children with more disrupted sleep [50]. Parents form the concept that crying must mean distress before their children are born, and it appears parents interact with their children based on this belief more than specific child needs. Critics often do not acknowledge that most behavioral approaches include some form of parents responding to their children crying, and consequently, parents may also be unaware of this fact [14].

Sleep Training Limitations

Sleep researchers acknowledge limitations and gaps in the current knowledge of behavioral sleep interventions. For one, the current research does not have evidence as to the precise age that is most effective to begin sleep training [8]. The age to start sleep training rests on a few developmental considerations: when infant sleep consolidates to allow sleep for stretches at a time, when infants no longer require feeding at night, and when infants can soothe themselves. One review of the infant sleep consolidation literature found limited change in consolidation amounts between 3 and 12 months old [52]. Similarly, infants younger than 3 months may still require multiple feedings during the night; therefore their cries should not be ignored [8]. Clinical experience shows that children can effectively learn to soothe themselves to sleep by approximately 3–4 months of age [8]. Meanwhile, there is no evidence that children younger than 3 months can soothe themselves [8]. This information leads sleep researchers to conclude that sleep training prior to 3 months of age is not advisable [8]. However, the precise age beyond that when an individual child may respond best to a behavioral intervention is still unanswered in the literature [8]. No trial has been conducted comparing different age start times, so there are no studies showing that a specific age is more effective or that another may result in negative consequences [8]. Overall, several studies show the efficacy of behavioral interventions with toddlers, pre-school-aged children, and school-aged children [8].

Another limitation of behavioral interventions is the knowledge required to implement them as they are intended, called **fidelity**. If behavioral interventions are not conducted with fidelity, parents may encounter suboptimal or even counterproductive outcomes to their efforts. One feature of extinguishing a behavior is that the removal of attention to the behavior often causes a phenomenon called an "extinction burst" [8]. An **extinction burst** is when children, recognizing that they are no longer receiving the reinforcement they used to receive for a behavior, increase the intensity of the behavior in an attempt to reestablish the response they were expecting [44]. Parents who have not been coached in advance about extinction bursts may easily misunderstand the increase in crying as proof that their children cannot soothe independently. The extinction burst phenomenon should be explained to parents beforehand so that they understand it is their cue to continue with their efforts [44, 53]. If this is not explained, parents who try to withstand crying for a time but then give in once the crying increases inadvertently teach their children that they can gain parental attention by crying louder than they were previously [8, 53, 54].

Parents' fears about crying children should also be addressed prior to beginning a behavioral intervention. Parents concerned that crying causes their children permanent harm are observed to have reduced ability to successfully implement evidence-based behavioral interventions to improve their children's sleep [51]. Parents also need information about what normal sleep looks like in childhood and that even children who have successfully learned to sleep can experience re-emergence of problems from time to time. Without this knowledge, parents may also behave in ways that inadvertently promote worse sleep [51]. Researchers in the field recommend providing concrete guidelines to parents, follow-up phone calls, and problem-solving from clinicians so parents can feel more confident in trying behavioral interventions [51].

Behavioral Interventions Safety

Despite these limitations and critic objections, sleep training arose out of a clinical need [14]. Researchers did not develop and test behavioral interventions to improve children's sleep so that adults could "impose" on children's needs, as critics suggest [14]. Physicians want parents to use whatever strategies work for their babies, whether it be co-sleeping or solo sleeping, using a behavioral intervention, or not [14]. As long as the child and parent are sufficiently rested, behavioral interventions are not clinically indicated. Sleep specialists continue to encounter parents who suffer from a lack of sleep, which has negative consequences for both themselves and their children [14].

One claim of behavioral intervention critics is that children must experience negative long-term outcomes as a result of being taught to "give up" on gaining parental attention through crying [46]. Researchers of a study that randomly assigned over three hundred 8–10 month-olds to receive either behavioral interventions or no treatment (what these critics recommend) examined this very question [55]. Their longitudinal study of these children at 6 years old is the longest study to date testing this hypothesis [55]. Their results found no such negative outcomes among the 225 families they were able to reconnect with after the main portion of the study ended [55]. Researchers assessed the children and parents on numerous factors for differences depending on which group they were assigned to [55]. Child factors consisted of emotional and behavioral outcomes, sleep problems and habits, psychosocial functioning and chronic stress [55]. Parents were assessed for depression, anxiety, stress, and authoritative parenting style (the recommended parenting style) [55]. The study authors found no difference on any of these measures [55]. They conclude that, as there is still no evidence that behavioral interventions cause long-term detriment to children, physicians can confidently recommend this approach to parents struggling with their children's sleep problems [55].

Critics frequently assert that sleep training must have a negative effect on the parent–child attachment relationship [46]. They argue that behavioral sleep training puts parental wants over child needs, leaving children with lifelong feelings of insecurity [46]. The research shows no such negative impact on the parent–child relationship [8]. Clinical trials have found the opposite to be true [8]. In one study, mothers reported feeling better about their relationship with their children after implementing a behavioral intervention for sleep [56]. Studies examining infant security and attachment after sleep training find that infants felt more secure after just 3 days of sleep training, with security increasing again by week 6 [17, 57]. In the long-term follow-up study of 225 children discussed above, the children randomly assigned to sleep training displayed no difference on measures of child–parent closeness, conflict, attachment, or overall relationship with their parents than children who were not sleep trained [55]. Extensive research has concluded that there is still no evidence supporting fears that sleep training negatively affects the parent–child attachment or child security [8].

When It Comes to Behavioral Sleep Training, One Size Fits All

Many parents encounter non-clinical versions of behavioral sleep training without speaking with a doctor [58]. Parenting books often include some information about sleep training, and many non-clinical books are available for public consumption [36, 59]. When reading a step-by-step approach, parents may conclude that there is only one way to sleep train their children. Research shows the opposite: behavioral plans are most effective when they are tailored to the child's specific sleep challenges [9]. More simplistic explanations of sleep training may also give the impression that standard extinction is required. Standard extinction procedures typically advise parents to ignore all child cries when putting the child to bed. In contrast, **graduated extinction** is a behavioral sleep training process by which parents gradually remove parental attention for crying [60]. For example, parents may decide to check on their children after 1 minute of crying the first time in the evening, 5 minutes the third time, and 10 minutes every time thereafter. The research base shows that using a graduated extinction procedure helps both typically developing children and children with disabilities to overcome sleep difficulties [60]. It appears that both graduated extinction and standard extinction are effective, and both are more effective than doing nothing [54]. This conclusion stems from a small study of parents who were randomly assigned to standard extinction, graduated extinction, or waitlist (no treatment) [54]. Children in both treatment groups experienced improvement in sleep, maintained those gains 2 months after the intervention concluded, and did not experience negative side effects [54]. None of these outcomes were found for children whose parents were assigned to continue checking on their children as they had been prior to study enrollment [54].

Parents not only concern themselves with what treatments work. They also want a treatment that is relatively easy to implement. Researchers measure parent acceptance by examining drop-out rates (a **drop-out** is a participant who leaves the study before its conclusion) and treatment satisfaction ratings. Parents in the standard extinction condition were not more likely to drop-out of treatment [54], indicating minimal acceptance even for the treatment that is harder to implement. Treatment satisfaction ratings indicate that those who completed the treatment found the graduated extinction version easier to use [54]. Notably, children in the graduated extinction group experienced benefits on the same timeline as children in the standard extinction group [54]. This finding addresses concerns that graduated extinction, which may be perceived as "watered down," still works as rapidly as the more intensive version. No studies have been done to date to compare different checking schedules within graduated exposure [8]. Therefore, parents can set the graduated schedule that works for their schedule and personal beliefs about how long a child should cry unattended.

Some parents may find extinction of any kind too challenging to implement [54]. A survey of approximately 200 parents sought to understand how parents implement behavioral interventions without support from clinicians [58]. Among the sample, about half of parents tried graduated extinction with their children [58]. Tellingly, the majority tried it for less than a week, and only 12.7% tried for over a month [58]. On average, parents reported feeling stressed by using the intervention, though they overall felt "fairly" supported by those close to them as they attempted it [58]. This study highlights an unresolved research question: whether parents comprehend the difference between attempting a "cry-it-out" method in an evidence-based way (with high fidelity) and in a community setting [58]. The results of this survey suggest that parents who use behavioral sleep training in the community use it with less fidelity and with less success than in clinical or research settings [58].

Child age is a relevant factor when deciding what kind of behavioral intervention to use. For older children, the use of graduated extinction with a bedtime pass has been shown to be effective and received high satisfaction ratings from parents [61]. In this version of sleep training, parents use common extinction procedures and add the use of a bedtime pass [61]. Parents in the study told their children (ages 3 through 6 years old) that after being tucked into bed for the night, they could use their bedtime pass for one time out of bed past that point [61]. The pass could only be turned in for select reasons, such as asking for a glass of water or a hug [61]. Requests antithetical to sleep, such as asking to stay up later, do not count for pass usage [61]. After the children use the pass for the evening, parents ignore all further requests for the night (the extinction portion of the procedure) [61]. Variations of the bedtime pass can be used, such as providing incentives if the child does not use the pass (e.g., special breakfast the next morning) [61]. While the study examined the use of the pass in children ages 3 through 6 years old, the treatment may be effective for children up to 10 years of age [61].

Guidance that is relevant to all children of parents who strive for solo sleep is to start early by putting infants to bed drowsy but still awake [8, 53]. Behavioral approaches used later in the child's life rest on children's ability to soothe themselves to allow for independent sleep [8]. By putting infants to bed drowsy but awake, they begin practicing at an early age to fall asleep on their own [3]. Later in the night when they awake naturally, they can also fall back asleep on their own [3]. In contrast, children who fall asleep only while being nursed or rocked begin to associate those conditions with falling asleep. This sets up the child to continually need help to fall back to sleep when they wake throughout the night.

Current Research

While many behavioral treatments have proven effective in research trials, wide-scale studies observing their success in homes are lacking [1]. Because sleep interventions necessarily occur in children's homes, parents become the primary interventionist [1]. Even parents who are invested in implementing a sleep training program with fidelity encounter difficulties in their environment, such as when their children sleep at another caretaker's house, on vacation, and during special occasions [62]. Research trials have had to rely on parents to provide the intervention and accurate reports as to the resulting effects [1]. Subsequently, trials are not blinded (that is, parents who provide data are aware of what the intervention is, because they are delivering it) [1].

The field of sleep research is still evolving, as are the behavioral interventions that researchers are developing and testing [9]. For example, many researchers have tested multi-component programs, and while they have been effective, the interventions may be similarly effective without all the components [9]. As such, there are a number of options for physicians to choose from and difficulties with implementation that have not yet been addressed. Behavioral approaches are the first-line recommended treatment for sleep problems [53]. Within this broad category, options consist of standard extinction, graduated extinction, extinction with the bedtime pass, and extinction with parental presence (in which parents stay in their children's room when they cry but do not pick their children up or talk to them) [53]. At minimum, physicians can always provide sleep hygiene information for parents to set consistent bed *and* wake times, which are fundamental components to improving sleep quality [9].

Like most behavioral interventions, sleep interventions are time-consuming, challenging to implement with precision, and provoke undesirable reactions from children who are not happy about the change [9]. Where behavioral sleep interventions are uniquely challenging is that they must be implemented when parents are tired and usually pressed for time [9]. The Selecting Sleep Interventions Questionnaire is one method clinicians can use for selecting treatment recommendations based on the concerns and needs of specific patients [63]. Rather than asking parents to implement procedures that they are not equipped to handle, assessing first how much parents can take on increases their chances of success and reduces the likelihood they make the situation worse using behavioral approaches only inconsistently.

Conclusion

A rule of thumb when physicians make recommendations is that it appears parents prefer simple advice with few components [62]. Particularly because parents show a preference for simpler interventions, taking recommendations from research can be challenging when the evidence-based treatments are still complicated [62]. Before implementing a behavioral intervention, parents benefit from being informed about the extinction burst and that about the reality that sleep problems that had improved may appear again after a child comes back from a vacation, has a change in bedtime routine, spends time with a different caretaker, etc. [53]. At a minimum, parents can be coached to initiate basic sleep hygiene, which includes setting consistent bedtimes and wake times, engaging their children in relaxing activities for at least 30 minutes prior to bedtime, and avoiding giving their children caffeinated foods and beverages [9]. When making recommendations as to how parents can improve their children's sleep through their own actions, physicians must walk a fine line between explaining how parents can assume responsibility for improving the problem without parents feeling blamed [53]. Clinicians should ask parents questions to assess their concerns and find out what they would like to happen differently with regard to their children's sleep [1]. Because no method for graduated extinction has been found superior to others, it is currently acceptable to allow parents to follow whichever schedule works best for them [8]. Overall customization is recommended so that the intervention chosen can be suited to the child's sleep environment and the parents' tolerance [8]. This approach is not only patient-centered, but strongly recommended for implementing an evidence-based intervention in a successful manner [1].

References

1. Jin CS, Hanley GP, Beaulieu L. An individualized and comprehensive approach to treating sleep problems in young children. J Appl Behav Anal. 2013;46(1):161–80.
2. Anders TF, Eiben LA. Pediatric sleep disorders: a review of the past 10 years. J Am Acad Child Adolesc Psychiatry. 1997;36(1):9–20.
3. Mindell JA, Durand VM. Treatment of childhood sleep disorders: generalization across disorders and effects on family members. J Pediatr Psychol. 1993;18(6):731–50.
4. Owens JA, Maxim R, Nobile C, McGuinn M, Msall M. Parental and self-report of sleep in children with attention-deficit/hyperactivity disorder. Arch Pediatr Adolesc Med. 2000;154(6):549–55.
5. Sadeh A, Raviv A, Gruber R. Sleep patterns and sleep disruptions in school-age children. Dev Psychol. 2000;36(3):291.
6. Liu X, Liu L, Owens JA, Kaplan DL. Sleep patterns and sleep problems among schoolchildren in the United States and China. Pediatrics. 2005;115(1):241–9.
7. Stores G. Children's sleep disorders: modern approaches, developmental effects, and children at special risk. Dev Med Child Neurol. 1999;41(8):568–73.
8. Thomas JH, Moore M, Mindell JA. Controversies in behavioral treatment of sleep problems in young children. Sleep Medicine Clinics. 2014;9(2):251–9.
9. Luiselli JK. Sleep and sleep-related problems. In: Behavioral health promotion and intervention in intellectual and developmental disabilities. Springer International Publishing; 2016. pp. 163–176.
10. DSM-5 American psychiatric association. diagnostic and statistical manual of mental disorders. Arlington: American Psychiatric Publishing. 2013.
11. Yang CK, Hahn HM. Cosleeping in young Korean children. J Dev Behav Pediatr. 2002;23(3):151–7.
12. Liu X, Liu L, Wang R. Bed sharing, sleep habits, and sleep problems among Chinese school-aged children. Sleep-N Y Then Westchester. 2003;26(7):839–44.
13. Blader JC, Koplewicz HS, Abikoff H, Foley C. Sleep problems of elementary school children: a community survey. Arch Pediatr Adolesc Med. 1997;151(5):473–80.
14. Sadeh A, Mindell JA, Owens J. Why care about sleep of infants and their parents? Sleep Med Rev. 2011;15(5):335–7.
15. Pagel JF, Pegram GV. Sleep medicine: Evidence-based clinical practice. In: Primary care sleep medicine. New York: Springer; 2014. pp. 11–20.
16. Mindell JA, Moline ML, Zendell SM, Brown LW, Fry JM. Pediatricians and sleep disorders: training and practice. Pediatrics. 1994;94(2):194–200.
17. France KG, Hudson SM. Behavior management of infant sleep disturbance. J Appl Behav Anal. 1990;23(1):91–8.
18. Rosen CL, Owens JA, Scher MS, Glaze DG. Pharmacotherapy for pediatric sleep disturbances: current patterns of use and target populations for controlled clinical trials. Curr Ther Res. 2002;31(63):B53–66.
19. Chervin RD, Archbold KH, Panahi P, Pituch KJ. Sleep problems seldom addressed at two general pediatric clinics. Pediatrics. 2001;107(6):1375–80.
20. Sadeh A, Mindell J, Rivera L. "My child has a sleep problem": a cross-cultural comparison of parental definitions. Sleep Med. 2011;12(5):478–82.
21. Sadeh A. Assessment of intervention for infant night waking: parental reports and activity-based home monitoring. J Consult Clin Psychol. 1994;62(1):63.
22. Meltzer LJ, Mindell JA. Relationship between child sleep disturbances and maternal sleep, mood, and parenting stress: a pilot study. J Fam Psychol. 2007;21(1):67.
23. Gulli C. Co-sleeping and a battle for the bed—Macleans.ca [Internet]. Macleans.ca. 2013 [cited 8 April 2016]. http://www.macleans.ca/society/life/battle-of-the-bed/. Accessed.
24. Owens JA. Epidemiology of sleep disorders during childhood. Principles and practices of pediatric sleep medicine. Philadelphia: Elsevier; 2005. p. 27–33.

25. Hiscock H, Wake M. Randomised controlled trial of behavioural infant sleep intervention to improve infant sleep and maternal mood. BMJ. 2002;324(7345):1062.
26. Wolfson A, Lacks P, Futterman A. Effects of parent training on infant sleeping patterns, parents' stress, and perceived parental competence. J Consult Clin Psychol. 1992;60(1):41.
27. Eckerberg B. Treatment of sleep problems in families with young children: effects of treatment on family well-being. Studies 2004;11:12.
28. Hunt CE. National sleep disorders research plan. Bethesda: National Center on Sleep Disorders Research; 2003.
29. Blair PS, Humphreys JS, Gringras P, Taheri S, Scott N, Emond A, Fleming PJ. Childhood sleep duration and associated demographic characteristics in an English cohort. Sleep. 2012;35(3):353–60.
30. Jenni OG, O'Connor BB. Children's sleep: an interplay between culture and biology. Pediatrics. 2005;115(1):204–16.
31. Dement WC, Vaughan C. The Promise of Sleep. 1999.
32. Dahl RE. The impact of inadequate sleep on children's daytime cognitive function. In: Seminars in pediatric neurology. WB Saunders; 1996. 3(1):44–50.
33. Beebe DW. Cognitive, behavioral, and functional consequences of inadequate sleep in children and adolescents. Pediatr Clin North Am. 2011;58(3):649–65.
34. Fallone G, Acebo C, Seifer R, Carskadon MA. Experimental restriction of sleep opportunity in children: effects on teacher ratings. Sleep-N Y Then Westchester. 2005;28(12):1561.
35. Hart CN, Cairns A, Jelalian E. Sleep and obesity in children and adolescents. Pediatr Clin North Am. 2011;58(3):715–33.
36. Ferber R. Solve your child's sleep problems. 2nd ed. New York: Fireside Books; 2006.
37. Owens JA, Babcock D, Blumer J, Chervin R, Ferber R, Goetting M, Glaze D, Ivanenko A, Mindell J, Rappley M, Rosen C. The use of pharmacotherapy in the treatment of pediatric insomnia in primary care: rational approaches. A consensus meeting summary. J Clin Sleep Med. 2005;1(1):49–59.
38. Mindell JA, Emslie G, Blumer J, Genel M, Glaze D, Ivanenko A, Johnson K, Rosen C, Steinberg F, Roth T, Banas B. Pharmacologic management of insomnia in children and adolescents: consensus statement. Pediatrics. 2006;117(6):e1223–32.
39. Merenstein D, Diener-West M, Halbower AC, Krist A, Rubin HR. The trial of infant response to diphenhydramine: the tired study—a randomized, controlled, patient-oriented trial. Arch Pediatr Adolesc Med. 2006;160(7):707–12.
40. France KG, Blampied NM, Wilkinson P. Treatment of infant sleep disturbance by trimeprazine in combination with extinction. J Dev Behav Pediatr. 1991;12(5):308–14.
41. Rossignol DA, Frye RE. Melatonin in autism spectrum disorders: a systematic review and meta-analysis. Dev Med Child Neurol. 2011;53(9):783–92.
42. Owens JA, Rosen CL, Mindell JA. Medication use in the treatment of pediatric insomnia: results of a survey of community-based pediatricians. Pediatrics. 2003;111(5):e628–35.
43. Sleep P. Behavioral treatment of bedtime problems and night wakings in infants and young children. Sleep. 2006;29(10):1263.
44. Armstrong KH, Ogg JA, Sundman-Wheat AN, Walsh AS. Behavioral terms and principles. In: Evidence-based interventions for children with challenging behavior. New York: Springer; 2014. 111–123.
45. St James-Roberts I, Alvarez M, Csipke E, Abramsky T, Goodwin J, Sorgenfrei E. Infant crying and sleeping in London, Copenhagen and when parents adopt a "proximal" form of care. Pediatrics. 2006;117(6):e1146–55.
46. Blunden SL, Thompson KR, Dawson D. Behavioural sleep treatments and night time crying in infants: challenging the status quo. Sleep Med Rev. 2011;15(5):327–34.
47. Narvaez D. Dangers of "crying it out": damaging children and their relationships for the long-term. Psychol Today. http://www.psychologytoday.com/blog/moral-landscapes/201112/dangers-crying-it-out2011. Accessed Dec 2011.

48. Barr RG. "Colic" is something infants do, rather than a condition they "have": a developmental approach to crying phenomena, patterns, pacification, and (patho) genesis. New evidence on unexplained early crying: its origins, nature, and management. Cincinnati; 2001:87–104.
49. Reijneveld SA, Brugman E, Hirasing RA. Excessive infant crying: definitions determine risk groups. Arch Dis Child. 2002;87(1):43–4.
50. Tikotzky L, Sadeh A. Maternal sleep-related cognitions and infant sleep: a longitudinal study from pregnancy through the 1st year. Child Dev. 2009;80(3):860–74.
51. Tse L, Hall W. A qualitative study of parents' perceptions of a behavioural sleep intervention. Child: care, health and development 2008;34(2):162–72.
52. Henderson JM, France KG, Blampied NM. The consolidation of infants' nocturnal sleep across the first year of life. Sleep Med Rev. 2011;15(4):211–20.
53. Kuhn BR. Practical strategies for managing behavioral sleep problems in young children. Sleep Med Clin. 2014;9(2):181–97.
54. Reid MJ, Walter AL, O'Leary SG. Treatment of young children's bedtime refusal and nighttime wakings: a comparison of "standard" and graduated ignoring procedures. J Abnorm Child Psychol. 1999;27(1):5–16.
55. Price AM, Wake M, Ukoumunne OC, Hiscock H. Five-year follow-up of harms and benefits of behavioral infant sleep intervention: randomized trial. Pediatrics. 2012;130(4):643–51.
56. Hiscock H, Bayer JK, Hampton A, Ukoumunne OC, Wake M. Long-term mother and child mental health effects of a population-based infant sleep intervention: cluster-randomized, controlled trial. Pediatrics. 2008;122(3):e621–7.
57. France KG. Behavior characteristics and security in sleep-disturbed infants treated with extinction. J Pediatr Psychol. 1992;17(4):467–75.
58. Loutzenhiser L, Hoffman J, Beatch J. Parental perceptions of the effectiveness of graduated extinction in reducing infant night-wakings. J Reprod Infant Psychol. 2014;32(3):282–91.
59. Giordano Twelve hours' sleep by twelve weeks old. A step-by-step plan for baby sleep success. New York: Dutton; 2006.
60. Meltzer LJ, Mindell JA. Nonpharmacologic treatments for pediatric sleeplessness. Pediatr Clin North Am. 2004;51(1):135–51.
61. Moore BA, Friman PC, Fruzzetti AE, MacAleese K. Brief report: evaluating the bedtime pass program for child resistance to bedtime—a randomized, controlled trial. J Pediatr Psychol. 2007;32(3):283–7.
62. Knight RM, Johnson CM. Using a behavioral treatment package for sleep problems in children with autism spectrum disorders. Child Fam Behav Ther. 2014;36(3):204–21.
63. Durand VM. Sleep problems. In: Luiselli JK, editor. Children and youth with autism spectrum disorder (ASD): recent advances and innovations in assessment, education, and intervention. 1st ed. New York: Oxford University Press; 2014. p. 174–92.

Chapter 12
Screen Time

Overview

Usage studies reveal that children of all ages currently consume more screen content than at any other time [1]. On average, American children spend about half of their waking time (approximately 7.5 hours) watching screens [2]. Original research on child development and electronics was limited to television. The profusion of electronic games has complicated the situation, including stationary and handheld devices dedicated to gaming [3]. Video games must be included in research endeavors, as over 90% of American children and adolescents play video games [4, 5]. As soon as personal computers became ubiquitous in homes, game developers rushed to provide content that would appeal to children. The subsequent proliferation of various handheld devices—essentially small computers—such as laptops, tablets, and smartphones has made the opportunities for children to engage in screen time essentially limitless [6]. In response, parents, pediatricians, psychologists, nutritionists, education professionals, ophthalmologists, game developers, and policy makers have striven to understand the possible benefits and drawbacks to these modes of playing, communicating, and relaxing. The use of these devices in combination is colloquially referred to as **screen time**. The resulting dialogue and research tend to focus on two extreme views—that screen time is either all good or all bad [7]. The truth likely lies between these two extremes. Research into screens shows benefits in some areas and drawbacks in others [8].

Original research into screens could focus only on television. Even within this narrow field, the research agenda was comprised of two main areas of inquiry: concern about violent or sexual content, and the developmental implications of passive viewing [9, 10]. Most agreed that children should be shielded from inappropriate content, while some debated whether screens could foster child development (as educational programs such as *Sesame Street* aimed to do) [10]. While a limited number of programs are proven to convey cognitive benefits, early

© Springer International Publishing AG 2017
C.A. Di Bartolo and M.K. Braun, *Pediatrician's Guide to Discussing Research with Patients*, DOI 10.1007/978-3-319-49547-7_12

childhood television viewing presents the brain with only passive experiences. The early childhood period requires interactive engagement with people in the environment for the brain to develop attention and behavioral regulation [11]. Once interactive games entered the market, the issues gained an additional layer of complexity. Parents and healthcare professionals alike became concerned about the potentially "addictive" nature of games, especially as these games provide reinforcement for continued play in the form of winning points or advancing to higher levels [7].

As screen time has become an undeniable part of children's lives, current research commonly emphasizes how it fits into the child's life as a whole. Excessive screen time is associated with numerous negative health outcomes, the promotion of other unhealthy behaviors (e.g., extended sedentary time, eating meals in front of a screen), and the displacement of other, more positive, activities [12]. Any time spent in front of a screen is necessarily not spent in another activity. Those concerned with child development commonly want to know whether the displaced activity would have benefitted the child more than the screen time. Except for those who ascribe to an extreme form of enrichment parenting, most also believe that children's time does not need to be optimized at every moment. Children can enjoy periods of fun and relaxation that have no developmental aim. Yet parents and professionals question whether children are capable of using screen time judiciously for this purpose.

In this chapter, we will explore research findings regarding the extent to which screen time displaces sleep, physical activity, and psychosocial development. As for content, we will review the contentiousness around violence in games, particularly whether they cause aggression in children. We will address whether programs or games billed as educational deliver the outcomes they claim. We will also review the literature about screens for the very young, particularly as it pertains to their psychosocial development. Finally, we cover barriers to parents implementing recommendations to limit screen time in children.

Common Parental Concerns

Screen Time Displacement

1. Sleep

Years of mounting research has led to an unambiguous conclusion that televisions in children's bedrooms are detrimental to healthy sleep [13–15]. Light-emitting diodes (LEDs) are found in most screens children encounter [16]. The light emitted by LEDs contains more blue wavelength light than typical incandescent light bulbs [16]. Blue wavelength light is found naturally in the morning hours and is important for regulating the circadian system [17]. This type of light cues the suprachiasmatic nucleus to suppress melatonin production, the hormone that promotes sleep [17]. As such, blue wavelength light in the evening hours is detrimental to sleep. Accordingly, research has found that prolonged exposure to screens prior to bedtime is associated with poorer sleep patterns [18]. Practically, children who play electronic games in their rooms past their bedtimes sleep less than their peers [19]. Of the sleep they do get, these children experience poorer quality and feel more tired after awakening than peers who attain sufficient sleep [20]. Children who play electronic games or who use the computer for nonacademic purposes for more than 2 hours have higher odds of attaining insufficient sleep [21].

With regard to gaming in particular, various models have been proposed to explain how gaming may displace sleep. One model argues for a displacement effect, whereby the more time children spend on games, the less they tend to sleep [17]. Another theorizes that the excitement of game play arouses children physiologically, making subsequent sleep difficult to initiate [17], although evidence that physiological arousal detracts from sleep onset has not been found [22]. Prolonged gaming, however, does reduce total sleep time. One study assigned one group of adolescents to play fast-paced, violent video games for 50 minutes. A second group played for 150 minutes [22]. While the adolescents who played for the longer time period lost, on average, close to half an hour of sleep, measures of physiological arousal did not detect differences between them and the more moderate players [22]. All participants still fell asleep within 30 minutes, a clinically acceptable sleep latency [22]. While slow wave sleep was significantly affected in the longer gaming group, the difference was small [22]. No other changes in sleep architecture, the structure and pattern of sleep along a number of variables, were observed [22]. After stopping, researchers also asked participants if they would like to continue playing, and if so, for how long [22]. On average, adolescents who played for the longer time period still wanted to play for another quarter hour [22]. Among both groups, participants who wanted to play for longer took longer to fall asleep than those who wanted less additional time [22]. Study authors hypothesize that continued cognitive involvement in the game may create a desire to continue playing, thereby inhibiting sleep onset [22].

2. Physical Activity

Common sense would suggest that the more time children spend on screens, the less they spend in physical activity. Interestingly, recent evidence shows only a small negative relationship between video game use and children's physical activity [3]. One large meta-analysis of previous studies could not find sufficient evidence in support of the theory that video game usage displaces physical activity [23]. Out of all these studies, only one used a randomized design where games were removed from the home and any resulting changes in physical activity were monitored [3]. This study found a statistically significant but clinically negligible increase in daily amount of physical activity once all games were removed from the home [24]. The physical activity of children who had games removed increased by only 3.8 minutes per day [24]. No increase in weekly physical activity was found [24]. The lack of displacement can be understood in conjunction with related findings. Children who spend a great deal of time on video games can also spend sufficient time in physical activity, and children who do not play video games can also refrain from physical activity if their activity preferences are sedentary (e.g., reading, music, art) [25, 26].

The emergence of active-input electronic games—games requiring players to move their bodies to continue and influence game play—has added a new element to the research on electronic games and physical activity. Active-input games have been shown to increase light-to-moderate-intensity physical activity in the short term (i.e., the activity observed in the laboratory while the children are playing) [3]. However, research so far indicates that active-input games are not effective for maintaining an increase in physical activity over time [3]. The few studies that measured physical activity during active-input game play over longer periods of time found that children gradually became less and less interested in playing these games over time [3]. As such, active-input games may be best recommended only insofar as they can engage currently inactive children in some physical activity. Once children are sufficiently engaged, other forms of physical activity should be encouraged. Continuing active-input games as the sole method for activity is unlikely to be helpful [3].

There is a distinction between sedentary behavior and not engaging in activity vigorous enough to meet the criteria for moderate-to-vigorous physical activity [3]. When a child engages in activities in which he remains relatively still—such as when playing traditional video games, watching television, and reading—he is said to be sedentary. A child who is engaged in moderate-to-vigorous physical activity might be playing soccer or swimming. Between these two extremes, a child might be engaged in light activities that are neither sedentary nor vigorous enough to count as "physical activity," such as walking to school, cleaning her room, or playing a board game. This distinction explains how children who play video games can engage in physical activity while *also* having higher rates of sedentary behavior than their nongaming peers [3]. Playing traditional (i.e., not active-input) video games is an example of sedentary behavior [3]. Prolonged epochs of sedentary behavior are associated with a host of negative health outcomes [3]. Because children who play games can also be physically active, the conclusion cannot be drawn that all video games present excessive sedentary behavior [3]. However, children who play for long stretches at a time should be encouraged to take breaks to reduce the negative influence of sedentary behaviors [3].

Because obesity is related to physical activity and sedentary behaviors, it has been studied with regard to video games [3]. Overall, research in this area is mixed. Some studies find effects on cardiometabolic health based on game play, and others find no such association [3]. While causality has not been established, the amount of time children spend on video games is associated with increased risk of obesity [27]. One study randomly assigned some 4–7-year olds to have their TV and computer time cut in half, while others continued to play as they had been [28]. After 3 years, the group with halved screen time showed a significant reduction in their body mass index (a weight-to-height ratio commonly used as an indicator of healthy weight) [28]. Children who were not assigned to receive a reduction in screen time displayed no such BMI reduction [28]. Taken with the findings that excessive sedentary behavior negatively affects health, results continue to suggest the positive outcomes of limiting video game usage without necessarily advocating for complete elimination [3].

3. Psychosocial Development

Psychosocial development refers to the development of personality, and it encompasses the psychological and social attitudes and skills children acquire as they age and mature. Parent–child interactions are typically among the first rich opportunities for infants and young children to begin learning about normal face-to-face interactions. Screen time takes away from the time that children would otherwise interact with parents [29]. Before addressing children's screen time among a number of psychosocial aspects, we briefly mention parents' screen time. Parents' use of screens also detracts from parent–child interactions [30]. In particular, being occupied with their own screens inhibits parents from monitoring and interacting with their children [30].

Part of normative social interactions is tolerating brief periods of non-stimulation, as may occur while waiting for the server at a restaurant, riding in a car, or accompanying parents on errands [29]. Parents are commonly observed to use screens to keep young children occupied during these times. The electronic device industry has termed this usage of their product as a "shut-up toy" [29]. Physicians and researchers are becoming concerned that this practice seriously impedes children from learning the internal mechanisms needed to occupy themselves for initially short and then gradually longer periods of time [30]. Anecdotally, parents' defense of using screens in this fashion typically includes some comment that their child "cannot" be quiet without it. Rather than argue with the truth of this statement, we acknowledge that children cannot do most psychosocial tasks until they learn to do so. Learning comes out of a necessity. If children never need to occupy themselves because the screen supplants the need, they are not expected to learn this skill in the long term [29]. Precisely because children "cannot" occupy themselves without screens justifies that screens should *not* be used in this manner.

Use of screens to access social media is extremely common among adolescents, who use the Internet for social interaction more than any other age group [31]. Before the proliferation of social media sites and applications used for connecting with people already in the adolescent's social circle, researchers and parents alike were concerned that Internet usage would cause adolescents to become withdrawn, socially isolated, and forge superficial connections with strangers [31]. Longitudinal studies bore out these concerns, with evidence that Internet usage was associated with social withdrawal among adolescents after less than one year [32].

This is in contrast to current usage studies, which show that adolescents now use the Internet primarily to maintain preexisting friendships [31]. Research to date suggests that forging social connections on the Internet may have differential effects on adolescents depending on a few factors: type of technology, gender, and social anxiety [31]. The Internet can facilitate social interactions when adolescents talk with preexisting friends or use instant messaging [33, 34].

Gender moderates outcomes as well. While the personal self-disclosure needed to form strong friendships is challenging for many early- and middle-adolescents, boys struggle more than girls to disclose in face-to-face communication [35]. Computer-mediated communication (CMC) eliminates almost all visual inputs and outputs [36]. CMC also provides time to prepare comments in advance and manage the timing of responses [36]. As hypothesized, CMC is effective at encouraging a higher rate of self-disclosures and more intimate self-disclosures [37]. Consequently, boys generally benefit from CMC more than girls [36].

Social anxiety influences how adolescents use the Internet and are affected by its usage. Researchers debate two approaches to this notion: the rich-get-richer hypothesis and the social compensation hypothesis [31]. **Rich-get-richer** presumes that adolescents who are already socially savvy simply translate those skills online and become socially competent on the Internet as well. By contrast, the **social compensation** theory proposes that adolescents who are socially unskilled are drawn to the Internet because of the lower stakes of online interaction [31]. Most research results provide support for the rich-get-richer theory [31]. However, adolescents who are socially anxious do prefer online disclosure over in-person disclosure [36]. As such, it is theorized that socially anxious adolescents can benefit from online communication with their preexisting friends to the extent that it allows them to deepen their relationships [31]. At this stage, it appears that Internet use likely does not teach social skills. It may, however, provide another outlet for already socially deft adolescents to engage socially and a more comfortable outlet for socially anxious or male adolescents to deepen preexisting friendships.

Excessive screen time also raises concerns about mood and anxiety. Video game play has been associated with higher levels of anxiety and depression [38]. Children who play for more than 30 min per day are more likely to feel negatively when they wake the next day [39]. There may be gender differences on games' impact on mood. One study found that girls reported increased stress in response to violent game play, whereas boys did not [40]. Researchers, clinicians, and parents voice concerns that some adolescents feel more negatively about themselves when they compare their social lives to those of their peers on social media [41]. Despite these concerns, there does not seem to be sufficient evidence to warrant recommending avoidance of social media to prevent or mitigate depression [41]. Issues regarding mood are challenging to study given their multiple influences and multiple screen modalities. Current research continues to recommend considering children and adolescents' mood and screen usage on an individual basis.

Violent Content and Aggression

Of all the video game research of the past 10 years, the most conclusive results were found in the area of violent video games and aggression [7]. Over one hundred research articles examining the relationship between violent video games and aggression were culled into a meta-analysis [42]. This analysis found that violent video games had a significant effect on the 6 aggression-related outcomes studied: aggressive behavior, aggressive cognition, aggressive affect, physiological arousal, empathy, and prosocial behavior [42]. Other meta-analyses have found an association between violent video game playing and aggressive behaviors [43, 44].

A challenge to assessing aggression as a result of violent video game play is that these studies often measure observable behaviors occurring just after game play in the laboratory. Yet very few parents have such a narrow concern—when people speak of aggression and violent video games, they refer to long-term outcomes or changes in children's brains as a result of playing. Consequently, researchers have begun using brain imaging technology to investigate underlying neuronal differences between players of violent games and nonviolent games. Specifically, researchers have hypothesized that extended exposure to violent game play causes a suppression of activity in the emotion-processing centers of players' brains [45]. One study compared violent game players to nonviolent ones and found no difference in suppression of emotion-processing centers of the brain [46]. Another fMRI study scanned the brains of 13 adolescents who were high consumers of either violent or nonviolent video games to examine how the emotion-processing centers of their brains responded to playing violent games. During violent video game play, researchers found increased activity in emotion-processing centers among players who did not regularly play violent games and reduced activity in players whose game of choice was typically violent in nature [45]. While the transference of neuroimaging studies to observable changes in behavior or mood is still tenuous, the authors hypothesize that these findings suggest a possible "desensitization" among regular players of violent video games [45]. Due to logistical challenges and financial constraints, most brain imaging studies in this area have enrolled only a small number of participants, so conclusions are limited.

The most vocal critic of violent video game research discovered many fewer connections between aggression and violent video game play in his own studies than are found in the field at large [47]. This researcher contends that the studies that found an association between aggression and violent video games report only negligible effect sizes [48]. In response, some researchers acknowledge a small effect size, but point out that children and adolescents play these games a great deal [7]. They argue that the effect sizes compound over time as game play continues, so that the association accumulates into a more meaningful difference over time [7]. Others do not agree that the reported effect size of the association between aggression and violent video game play is small—they point out that they are similar to the effects of secondhand smoke on lung cancer [7, 49].

The same critic referred to has also posited researcher bias as contributing to the evidence that violent games are associated with aggression [7, 48]. This claim was investigated using statistical tools to look for bias due to the following: a prominent scholar who influences others, a group of researchers who have formed a consensus, or a systemic bias that excludes findings that do not support the hypothesis that video games are associated with aggression [50]. This study found no evidence to support the presence of any of the three biases [50]. Even the most vocal critic of violent game research has found some results that violent games are connected with increased aggressive thoughts, increased physiological arousal, and decreased prosocial behavior [48, 50]. Despite ongoing debate within the research community about bias, study design, statistical methodology, and effect sizes, the literature increasingly supports the conclusion that violent video games cause more aggression in players than nonviolent ones [50].

Common Misconceptions

Screen time is beneficial if the content is educational

A limited number of television shows, such as *Sesame Street* and *Blue's Clues*, have been studied extensively and found to promote academic skills in preschool children [29]. In contrast, television shows with fast pacing and quick editing cuts have a deleterious effect on attention among child viewers [51]. Even taking into account shows with educational content and slow pacing, children younger than 30 months require real-life interactions for learning [52]. Therefore, even passive content that bills itself as "educational" cannot confer a benefit to very young children. With the proliferation of smart phones and downloadable applications ("apps"), many parents have come to believe that interactive games can help their very young children learn. Complicating matters, thousands of phone apps are marketed as "educational" without any research to support this claim [29]. So far, only one study has shown that children can learn some language skills from an interactive game at 2 years of age [53]. Outside of this study, there is no other research to support the use of interactive games with toddlers [29]. Some parents argue that their children must learn to use the devices at a young age so that they are not disadvantaged when they are older [54]. These parents can be reassured that even apes, such as Rhesus monkeys and Orangutans, can easily learn to use screen-based devices [55, 56]. Electronic books have been found to engage children with some dynamic characteristics such as narration, text highlighting, animation, sound effects, and games [53]. However, the very features that engaged the children simultaneously impaired their comprehension of the story [53]. This evidence suggests that while electronic books may not be harmful, they are not as beneficial as noninteractive, i.e., traditional, books.

Some parents observe their children watching television or playing video games for hours at a time and attribute this behavior to an increase in their capacity to pay attention. Research findings do not bolster this interpretation. In television shows, editing and pace influence underlying neural processes [54]. **Executive functioning** refers to the constellation of skills emerging from the prefrontal cortex that are implicated in goal-directed behaviors: attention, working memory, inhibitory control, problem-solving, self-regulation, and delay of gratification. One researcher found that 4-year olds who viewed just 9 minutes of a popular children's television program that consisted of fantastical characters inter- acting through fast-paced dialogue and images experienced immediate decreases in executive functioning [51]. A longitudinal study of 2,623 children found that duration of television viewing between the ages of 1 and 3 years of age was directly related to the likelihood that children would be diagnosed with attentional problems by the age of 7 [57].

The evidence about video games is similar to that of television. A longitudi- nal study of over 3,000 adolescents found that video game playing was associated with more attention problems later in life [58]. The most vocal critic of the current video game research again did not find such an association [47]. The discrepancy in findings may be explained by content: in one study, violent video games were associated with increased attention difficulties, while educational games were associated with attention improvements [59]. Neurological research has not found that video game play improves attention, but has discovered that fast-paced games can improve visual/spatial skills [60–62]. Regrettably, the evidence that these vis- ual/spatial skills transfer to non-video game settings is limited [63]. The visual/ spatial benefit within video game play is, on its own, not sufficient for physicians to begin recommending video game play [63].

Many parents intuit that video game play is negatively associated with aca- demic performance. Similarly, researchers' displacement theory argues that the time children spend on video games displaces the time they could otherwise spend on homework, reading, or other enriching activities [64]. A study that sampled a nationally representative group of children and adolescents between the ages of 10 and 19 found that those who played video games spent 34% less time doing home- work and 30% less time reading than the nongamers [65]. Research finds that the amount of video game play children engage in is associated with poorer academic performance [66].

As for research on video games marketed as educational, there remains insuf- ficient evidence in the field to conclude that these games result in academic improvement [3]. Some educational games have been shown to assist teaching children in a variety of topics [67]. Games have advantages in aiding teaching [7]. Well-designed games can grab students' attention, set clear learning objectives, give regular feedback and reinforcement, involve the learner actively, and can be set to the appropriate difficulty level for the learners' needs [68]. However, well- designed games are few and far between.

Electronic devices teach very young children to sit still and be quiet

In spite of the known and wide-ranging adverse health effects associated with passive screen viewing, watching television has become an integral part of the childhood experience [69]. The average preschool child watches between 3.2 and

5.6 hours of television per day [69], which is well above the 2 hour daily limit the American Academy of Pediatrics (AAP) recommends [70]. If parents are aware of this guideline, they presumably have some reason for permitting their young children to watch as much television as they do. Parents may view watching television favorably if it achieves desired outcomes like calming their children down or preparing them for sleep [71]. That screens babysit children is a common reason for their use—in one study, half of parental respondents acknowledged they benefit from using screens to babysit their children [72].

One study sought to understand parents' use of television to babysit their children by collecting data on over 800 parents of children ages 6 months through 6 years [70]. The study found that using television as a babysitter and strong, positive parental attitudes toward television predicted higher amounts of television viewing [70]. The best predictor of child television viewing amount, however, was the amount of parental television viewing [70]. Essentially, the more television parents watched, the more their children watched [70]. The study authors also found that while highly educated parents did not hold particularly favorable views of television or watch a great deal themselves, they still used it as a babysitter for their children [70]. Parents with less education were more likely to view more television themselves, which was associated with higher amount of viewing among their children [70].

Ultimately, while parents may use screens to occupy their children in the immediate-term, screens do not convey any skills for children to learn to regulate their attention in the long term. Research has already established that the more screen time children engage in when young, the more likely they are to have attention problems later in life [57]. When comparing screen time amounts among young children to academic qualities in fourth grade (as reported by teachers), researchers found that more time spent on screens predicted less task-oriented, persistent, and autonomous behaviors in the classroom, all of which are strategies related to learning [73].

Current Research

Despite many unknowns in screen time research, two guidelines with good evidence have been established: (1) children younger than 2 years of age should not be exposed to screens; and (2) older children should not spend more than 2 hours per day on screens [74]. Parents show poor awareness and knowledge of these guidelines [75]. We discuss the factors that hinder parents from following these guidelines. The first barrier to reducing screen time is that many parents are not even aware that such recommendations exist [73]. Other parents may be aware of the existence of the recommendations, but do not know what the guidelines suggest [73]. We also provide recommendations for physicians to increase adherence to these guidelines.

The next hurdle emerges in parents' and children's perceptions that a 2 hour maximum is unrealistic and impractical [12]. Some parents report that screen time reduction is challenging because video games are so integrated into children's lives [12]. Other parents feel even more strongly, reporting that video games are "addictive" [12]. Due to anecdotal reports of "addiction," researchers have begun examining pathological gaming, or "video game addiction" [7]. Similar to true addictions, video games can sometimes cross the line from relaxing activity to a practice causing deleterious effects on life functioning [76]. Despite initial research showing that video game play may be pathological in up to 8.5% of American children, pathological gaming is still not classified as an addiction [76, 77]. Even without an explicit diagnostic category, many parents find that they need help curbing their children's game play.

Parents' own media use also influences efforts to limit screen time for their children. Amount of television viewing is highly related in parents and their children [54]. Parents who view more than 4 hours per day are 3 times more likely to have girls watch over this amount, and 10.5 times more likely to have a boy watch this amount [78]. Interestingly, one meta-analysis found that when mentally tallying the amount of screen time their children engage in, parents do not include the hours spent "co-viewing" with their children [12]. Parents tend to conceptualize co-viewing as a family activity distinct from youth-only screen time [12].

Of course, children's resistance makes limit-setting challenging. While some youth feel the time they spend on screens is excessive and would like to cut back, others think they spend a reasonable amount of time on screens [12]. Many youth perceive high amounts of screen time as the norm, making change more difficult for parents to achieve [12]. Interventions to reduce screen time ultimately involve both parties: the child as the end user and the parent as the influencer [12]. Children and adolescents may acknowledge other activities they could participate in if not watching screens [12]. Parents tend to narrowly focus on reducing screen time, rather than more broadly seeking to reduce time on sedentary activities and increase time on beneficial activities [12].

Knowing how popular screens are with children and adolescents, pediatricians can assume they impact children's development in some manner. To assess the extent to which intervention may be needed, physicians should inquire about screen time at well-child visits [7]. To understand the rationale for the 2 hour maximum recommendation, parents may first need to hear about the implications of excessive screen time. Physicians should also inform parents that current guidelines do not yet address the ubiquity of screens on phones in addition to stationary screen time [29].

Some parents and teachers are already concerned about the physiological, cognitive, and psychosocial deficits that arise from excessive screen time [12]. Parents who are aware of the negative potential health outcomes are more likely to engage in efforts to reduce screen time [12]. On the other hand, parents struggle to limit screen time when they misperceive screens as providing benefits such as sleep facilitation and as a method for relaxation [12]. As discussed above, parents should be informed that screen time is not an appropriate method for readying children for sleep because it negatively impacts resulting sleep quality. While video games and television are popular options for relaxation among both children and adults, children can decompress with activities that do not involve screens. Parents with high levels of education may need information about avoiding reliance on television as a babysitter, while less educated parents may need counseling to reduce their personal time spent watching television [70].

Parents should be informed that setting limits plays a key role in how much screen time their children consume [7]. Screen limits can be conceptualized as limits on content, duration, and location. For content, parents are advised not to rely solely on industry ratings [7]. Instead, clinicians can recommend that parents observe previews of shows and video or computer games to determine if they find the content appropriate [7]. For duration, parents will need to consider multiple forms of screens and how these activities accumulate over the course of the week. Location of devices assists overall limit-setting because controlling content or duration of screen time is challenging when children are alone with their devices [7]. Therefore, game devices and other screens should be kept in areas of the home where others are present [7]. Televisions or other screens should not be in children's bedrooms [12, 54]. This includes adolescents giving their cell phones to their parents when they go to bed at night. Other environmental factors may be harder for parents to implement, but nonetheless facilitate a reduction in screen time: engagement in extracurricular activities, owning a dog, and access to either a sizable backyard or a community that promotes outdoor activities [12].

Parental limits on screen time have been shown to be effective in reducing excessive television-watching among adolescents [79, 80]. Limits are more effective when implemented during the school week—either immediately before school or directly following [12]. Children who live in multiple homes with different caregivers prefer when the same limits are applied consistently between houses [12]. In general, limits must be consistently applied and understood by children in order to be effective [4]. Children who agreed with researchers that their parents set limits on their screen time (television and video games) were less likely to exceed the recommended limit of 2 hours per day than those who disagreed that their parents had rules [81]. In some cases, discussing limits with children before implementing may help increase compliance later [12]. Others have found that these discussions with adolescents can turn into arguments between the teens and their parents [82]. When arguments arise, parents were better served by sticking with their original limits rather than giving into resistance [82]. Adolescents viewed parents who capitulated as ineffectual [82]. Physicians should continue to ask about screen time, as parents will need to periodically reassess the limits they have set as their children age and as new technology becomes available [7].

Conclusion

Research into the new types of electronic media lags behind the pace at which producers introduce these devices into the market. Interactive screen time that is readily accessible via phone and tablet has emerged so quickly that research in this area is struggling to catch up [29]. As physicians are without evidence-based guidelines to provide guidance, parents adopt new technologies for their children without hard data. When researchers try to conduct the multiyear studies needed to show effects over time, the rapid emergence of new games complicates the process. For example, one study terminated early because they could not enroll additional children once the game used in the study was supplanted with a new, more popular option [24]. Due to these challenges, the effects of regular involvement with smart phones and tablets on learning, behavior, and family dynamics are currently unknown [29]. Ultimately, physicians can focus their efforts on helping parents limit screen time in accordance with current evidence-based guidelines and urge caution when introducing new technology to their children.

References

1. Licencing TV. TeleScope: A focus on the nation's viewing habits from TV Licensing. 2011.
2. Rideout VJ, Foehr UG, Roberts DF. Generation M 2: media in the lives of 8–18 year-olds. Kaiser Family Foundation; 2010.
3. Straker L, Abbott R, Collins R, Campbell A. Evidence-based guidelines for wise use of electronic games by children. Ergonomics. 2014;57(4):471–89.
4. Gentile DA, Walsh DA. A normative study of family media habits. J Appl Dev Psychol. 2002;23(2):157–78.
5. Gentile D. Pathological video-game use among youth ages 8 to 18 a national study. Psychol Sci. 2009;20(5):594–602.
6. Colley RC, Garriguet D, Janssen I, Craig CL, Clarke J, Tremblay MS. Physical activity of Canadian children and youth: accelerometer results from the 2007 to 2009 canadian health measures survey. Health Rep. 2011;22(1):15.
7. Prot S, McDonald KA, Anderson CA, Gentile DA. Video games: good, bad, or other? Pediatr Clin North Am. 2012;59(3):647–58.
8. Anderson CA, Gentile DA, Dill KE. Prosocial, antisocial, and other effects of recreational video games.
9. Kennedy C. Examining television as an influence on children's health behaviors. J Pediatr Nurs. 2000;15(5):272–81.
10. Anderson DR. Educational television is not an oxymoron. Ann Am Acad Polit Soc Sci. 1998;557(1):24–38.
11. Duncan GJ, Dowsett CJ, Claessens A, Magnuson K, Huston AC, Klebanov P, Pagani LS, Feinstein L, Engel M, Brooks-Gunn J, Sexton H. School readiness and later achievement. Dev Psychol. 2007;43(6):1428.
12. Minges KE, Owen N, Salmon J, Chao A, Dunstan DW, Whittemore R. Reducing youth screen time: qualitative metasynthesis of findings on barriers and facilitators. Health Psychol. 2015;34(4):381.
13. Mistry KB, Minkovitz CS, Strobino DM, Borzekowski DL. Children's television exposure and behavioral and social outcomes at 5.5 years: does timing of exposure matter? Pediatrics. 2007;120(4):762–9.
14. Mindell JA, Meltzer LJ, Carskadon MA, Chervin RD. Developmental aspects of sleep hygiene: findings from the 2004 national sleep foundation sleep in America poll. Sleep Med. 2009;10(7):771–9.
15. Owens J, Maxim R, McGuinn M, Nobile C, Msall M, Alario A. Television-viewing habits and sleep disturbance in school children. Pediatrics. 1999;104(3):e27.
16. Czeisler CA. Perspective: casting light on sleep deficiency. Nature. 2013;497(7450):S13.

17. Cain N, Gradisar M. Electronic media use and sleep in school-aged children and adolescents: a review. Sleep Med. 2010;11(8):735–42.
18. Wood B, Rea MS, Plitnick B, Figueiro MG. Light level and duration of exposure determine the impact of self-luminous tablets on melatonin suppression. Appl ergonomics. 2013;44(2):237–40.
19. Chahal H, Fung C, Kuhle S, Veugelers PJ. Availability and night-time use of electronic entertainment and communication devices are associated with short sleep duration and obesity among Canadian children. Pediatr obes. 2013;8(1):42–51.
20. Van den Bulck J. Television viewing, computer game playing, and Internet use and self-reported time to bed and time out of bed in secondary-school children. Sleep-N Y Then westchester. 2004;27(1):101–4.
21. Foti KE, Eaton DK, Lowry R, McKnight-Ely LR. Sufficient sleep, physical activity, and sedentary behaviors. Am J Prev Med. 2011;41(6):596–602.
22. King DL, Gradisar M, Drummond A, Lovato N, Wessel J, Micic G, Douglas P, Delfabbro P. The impact of prolonged violent video-gaming on adolescent sleep: an experimental study. J Sleep Res. 2013;22(2):137–43.
23. Marshall SJ, Biddle SJ, Gorely T, Cameron N, Murdey I. Relationships between media use, body fatness and physical activity in children and youth: a meta-analysis. Int J Obes. 2004;28(10):1238–46.
24. Straker LM, Abbott RA, Smith AJ. To remove or to replace traditional electronic games? a crossover randomised controlled trial on the impact of removing or replacing home access to electronic games on physical activity and sedentary behaviour in children aged 10–12 years. BMJ open. 2013;3(6):e002629.
25. Jago R, Fox KR, Page AS, Brockman R, Thompson JL. Physical activity and sedentary behaviour typologies of 10–11 year olds-response to saunders and colleagues. Int J Behav Nutr Phys Act. 2011;8(49.10):1186.
26. Liu J, Kim J, Colabianchi N, Ortaglia A, Pate RR. Co-varying patterns of physical activity and sedentary behaviors and their long-term maintenance among adolescents. J Phys Act Health. 2010;7(4):465.
27. Berkey CS, Rockett HR, Field AE, Gillman MW, Frazier AL, Camargo CA, Colditz GA. Activity, dietary intake, and weight changes in a longitudinal study of preadolescent and adolescent boys and girls. Pediatrics. 2000;105(4):e56.
28. Epstein LH, Roemmich JN, Robinson JL, Paluch RA, Winiewicz DD, Fuerch JH, Robinson TN. A randomized trial of the effects of reducing television viewing and computer use on body mass index in young children. Arch Pediatr Adolesc Med. 2008;162(3):239–45.
29. Radesky JS, Schumacher J, Zuckerman B. Mobile and interactive media use by young children: the good, the bad, and the unknown. Pediatrics. 2015;135(1):1–3.
30. Radesky JS, Kistin CJ, Zuckerman B, Nitzberg K, Gross J, Kaplan-Sanoff M, Augustyn M, Silverstein M. Patterns of mobile device use by caregivers and children during meals in fast food restaurants. Pediatrics. 2014; peds-2013.
31. Valkenburg PM, Peter J. Social consequences of the Internet for adolescents a decade of research. Curr Dir Psychol Sci. 2009;18(1):1–5.
32. Kraut R, Kiesler S, Boneva B, Cummings J, Helgeson V, Crawford A. Internet paradox revisited. J Soc Issues. 2002;58(1):49–74.
33. Bessiere K, Kiesler S, Kraut R, Boneva BS. Effects of Internet use and social resources on changes in depression. Inf Community Soc. 2008;11(1):47–70.
34. Valkenburg PM, Peter J. Online communication and adolescent well-being: testing the stimulation versus the displacement hypothesis. J Comput Mediated Commun. 2007;12(4):1169–82.
35. McNelles LR, Connolly JA. Intimacy between adolescent friends: age and gender differences in intimate affect and intimate behaviors. J Res Adolesc. 1999;9(2):143–59.

36. Schouten AP, Valkenburg PM, Peter J. Precursors and underlying processes of adolescents' online self-disclosure: developing and testing an "internet-attribute-perception" model. Media Psychol. 2007;10(2):292–315.
37. Tidwell LC, Walther JB. Computer-mediated communication effects on disclosure, impressions, and interpersonal evaluations: getting to know one another a bit at a time. Hum Commun Res. 2002;28(3):317–48.
38. Mathers M, Canterford L, Olds T, Hesketh K, Ridley K, Wake M. Electronic media use and adolescent health and well-being: cross-sectional community study. Acad Pediatr. 2009;9(5):307–14.
39. Kondo Y, Tanabe T, Kobayashi-Miura M, Amano H, Yamaguchi N, Kamura M, Fujita Y. Association between feeling upon awakening and use of information technology devices in Japanese children. J Epidemiol. 2012;22(1):12.
40. Ferguson CJ, Trigani B, Pilato S, Miller S, Foley K, Barr H. Violent video games don't increase hostility in teens, but they do stress girls out. Psychiatr Q. 2015;21:1–8.
41. Jelenchick LA, Eickhoff JC, Moreno MA. "Facebook depression?" social networking site use and depression in older adolescents. J Adolesc Health. 2013;52(1):128–30.
42. Anderson CA, Shibuya A, Ihori N, Swing EL, Bushman BJ, Sakamoto A, Rothstein HR, Saleem M. Violent video game effects on aggression, empathy, and prosocial behavior in eastern and western countries: a meta-analytic review. Psychol Bull. 2010;136(2):151.
43. Janssen I, Boyce WF, Pickett W. Screen time and physical violence in 10 to 16 year-old Canadian youth. Int J Public Health. 2012;57(2):325–31.
44. Anderson CA. An update on the effects of playing violent video games. J Adolesc. 2004;27(1):113–22.
45. Gentile DA, Swing EL, Anderson CA, Rinker D, Thomas KM. Differential neural recruitment during violent video game play in violent-and nonviolent-game players. Psychol Popular Media Cult. 2016;5(1):39.
46. Szycik GR, Mohammadi B, Hake M, Kneer J, Samii A, Münte TF, te Wildt BT. Excessive users of violent video games do not show emotional desensitization: an fMRI study. Brain Imaging Behav. 2016;16:1–8.
47. Ferguson CJ. The influence of television and video game use on attention and school problems: a multivariate analysis with other risk factors controlled. J Psychiatr Res. 2011;45(6):808–13.
48. Ferguson CJ. Evidence for publication bias in video game violence effects literature: a meta-analytic review. Aggression Violent Behav. 2007;12(4):470–82.
49. Bushman BJ, Huesmann LR. Effects of televised violence on aggression. Handb Child Media. 2001;223–54.
50. Lishner DA, Groves CL, Chrobak QM. Are violent video game-aggression researchers biased? Aggression Violent Behav. 2015;31(25):75–8.
51. Lillard AS, Peterson J. The immediate impact of different types of television on young children's executive function. Pediatrics. 2011;128(4):644–9.
52. Anderson DR, Hanson KG. What researchers have learned about toddlers and television. Zero Three. 2013;33(4):4–10.
53. Roseberry S, Hirsh-Pasek K, Golinkoff RM. Skype me! socially contingent interactions help toddlers learn language. Child Dev. 2014;85(3):956–70.
54. Sigman A. Time for a view on screen time. Archives of disease in childhood. 2012 Oct 8; archdischild-2012.
55. Tulane University—Frequently Asked Questions [Internet]. Tulane.edu. 2016 [cited 6 May 2016]. https://tulane.edu/tnprc/outreach/public-faq/#q20. Accessed.
56. Ape versus machine [Internet]. BBC Nature. 2012 [cited 6 May 2016]. http://www.bbc.co.uk/nature/16832378. Accessed.
57. Christakis DA, Zimmerman FJ, DiGiuseppe DL, McCarty CA. Early television exposure and subsequent attentional problems in children. Pediatrics. 2004;113(4):708–13.

58. Gentile DA, Choo H, Liau A, Sim T, Li D, Fung D, Khoo A. Pathological video game use among youths: a two-year longitudinal study. Pediatrics. 2011 Jan 12; peds-2010.
59. Hastings EC, Karas TL, Winsler A, Way E, Madigan A, Tyler S. Young children's video/computer game use: relations with school performance and behavior. Issues Ment Health Nurs. 2009;30(10):638–49.
60. Green CS, Bavelier D. Action video game modifies visual selective attention. Nature. 2003;423(6939):534–7.
61. Green CS, Bavelier D. Effect of action video games on the spatial distribution of visuospatial attention. J Exp Psychol Hum Percept Perform. 2006;32(6):1465.
62. Green CS, Bavelier D. Action-video-game experience alters the spatial resolution of vision. Psychol Sci. 2007;18(1):88–94.
63. Blumberg FC, Altschuler EA, Almonte DE, Mileaf MI. The impact of recreational video game play on children's and adolescents' cognition. New Dir Child Adolesc Dev. 2013;2013(139):41–50.
64. Gentile DA, Lynch PJ, Linder JR, Walsh DA. The effects of violent video game habits on adolescent hostility, aggressive behaviors, and school performance. J Adolesc. 2004;27(1):5–22.
65. Cummings HM, Vandewater EA. Relation of adolescent video game play to time spent in other activities. Arch Pediatr Adolesc Med. 2007;161(7):684–9.
66. Cordes C, Miller E. Fool's gold: a critical look at computers in childhood.
67. Corbett AT, Koedinger KR, Hadley WH. Cognitive tutors: from the research classroom to all classrooms. Technol Enhanced Learn Opportunities Change. 2001;1:235–63.
68. Gentile DA, Gentile JR. Violent video games as exemplary teachers: a conceptual analysis. J Youth Adolesc. 2008;37(2):127–41.
69. Tandon PS, Zhou C, Lozano P, Christakis DA. Preschoolers' total daily screen time at home and by type of child care. J Pediatr. 2011;158(2):297–300.
70. Beyens I, Eggermont S. Putting young children in front of the television: antecedents and outcomes of parents' use of television as a babysitter. Commun Q. 2014;62(1):57–74.
71. Zimmerman FJ, Christakis DA, Meltzoff AN. Television and dvd/video viewing in children younger than 2 years. Arch Pediatr Adolesc Med. 2007;161(5):473–9.
72. Evans CA, Jordan AB, Horner J. Only two hours? A qualitative study of the challenges parents perceive in restricting child television time. J Fam Issues. 2011;32(9):1223–44.
73. Pagani LS, Fitzpatrick C, Barnett TA, Dubow E. Prospective associations between early childhood television exposure and academic, psychosocial, and physical well-being by middle childhood. Arch Pediatr Adolesc Med. 2010;164(5):425–31.
74. Brown A, Shifrin D, Hill D. Beyond 'turn it off': How to advise families on media use. AAP News [Internet]. 2015 [cited 13 May 2016];36(10):54–54. http://www.aappublications.org/content/36/10/54.full. Accessed.
75. Funk JB, Brouwer J, Curtiss K, McBroom E. Parents of preschoolers: expert media recommendations and ratings knowledge, media-effects beliefs, and monitoring practices. Pediatrics. 2009;123(3):981–8.
76. Gentile DA. The multiple dimensions of video game effects. Child Dev Perspect. 2011;5(2):75–81.
77. Pies R. Should DSM-V designate "internet addiction" a mental disorder? Psychiatry. 2009;6(2):1550–5952.
78. Jago R, Fox KR, Page AS, Brockman R, Thompson JL. Parent and child physical activity and sedentary time: do active parents foster active children? BMC Public Health. 2010;10(1):1.
79. Barradas DT, Fulton JE, Blanck HM, Huhman M. Parental influences on youth television viewing. J Pediatr. 2007;151(4):369–73.
80. Salmon J, Timperio A, Telford A, Carver A, Crawford D. Association of family environment with children's television viewing and with low level of physical activity. Obes Res. 2005;13(11):1939–51.

81. Carlson SA, Fulton JE, Lee SM, Foley JT, Heitzler C, Huhman M. Influence of limit-setting and participation in physical activity on youth screen time. Pediatrics. 2010;126(1):e89–96.
82. Hattersley LA, Shrewsbury VA, King LA, Howlett SA, Hardy LL, Baur LA. Adolescent-parent interactions and attitudes around screen time and sugary drink consumption. In: Palmer SD, editor. Social work and community practice. Apple Academic Press; 2011. pp. 158–172.

Chapter 13
School Refusal

Overview

Children in the United States are required, by law, to attend school. This has been the case since 1944 [1]. The term **absenteeism** refers to all child absences from school, whether excused or unexcused, and applies primarily refers to children and adolescents in elementary through high school [2]. Because attendance in this age group is compulsory, absenteeism is often considered within the societal-legal realm [3]. Absenteeism directly impedes children from accessing education, so it has clear academic implications as well. Beyond academic services, modern schools also provide children with social, emotional, and health services they may not receive otherwise [1]. Attending school therefore conveys many more benefits than educational attainment alone. Accordingly, absenteeism nearly always indicates the presence of an underlying issue of health or safety. Prolonged absence from school has proven adverse consequences [3].

Legitimate absences include genuine illness, religious occasions, family obligations (such as funerals), and dangerous weather [4]. Most other reasons for missing school are generally considered illegitimate [4]. This chapter focuses on illegitimate absenteeism driven by children. First, however, it is necessary to briefly describe **school withdrawal**, a parent-driven form of missing school about which physicians should be aware.

School withdrawal occurs when a parent encourages a child to stay home from school or directly prevents a child from attending [4]. These parents may be maltreating their children, or they may have other reasons for wanting their child out of school [4]. For example, some parents may want their adolescents to financially contribute to the household [4]. They may want to prevent an estranged spouse from taking the child from school [4]. Some parents suffer from separation anxiety, panic attacks, or other psychiatric illness for which they prefer their child's company [4]. Regardless of the reason, school withdrawal is handled differently

© Springer International Publishing AG 2017
C.A. Di Bartolo and M.K. Braun, *Pediatrician's Guide to Discussing Research with Patients*, DOI 10.1007/978-3-319-49547-7_13

than child-directed absence. Clinicians should attempt to identify its occurrence whenever possible for the purposes of providing appropriate intervention.

School Refusal Behaviors

School refusal behaviors are defined as child-driven refusal to attend school, difficulties remaining in classes for an entire day, or both [5]. This expression encompasses the multiple terms pertaining to children's nonattendance at school that have sprung up throughout the past one hundred years: truancy, school refusal, and "school phobia" [2]. As we will review in depth, children exhibiting school refusal behaviors vary widely in their clinical presentations and in their reasons for avoiding school [4]. Accordingly, school refusal manifests in widely varying behaviors. Some children may beg and plead not to attend but ultimately do so [2]. Others actively engage in problematic behaviors in the morning to avoid school, such as tantrums, hiding, and noncompliance. Attendance, but with morning tardiness, is another presentation. Children may sporadically skip some classes or miss days altogether. They can also repeatedly miss classes or days. At the most severe end, children may be completely absent. Absences last for either a certain period within the school year or for an extended period of time [2]. In the face of this heterogeneity, all children and adolescents who display school refusal behaviors share the goal of removing regular school attendance from a daily routine [4]. Because school is the primary occupation of children in developed nations, school refusal indicates a clinically significant impairment in functioning and coping with a developmentally appropriate task.

Despite all the challenges school refusal presents, it is not a distinct diagnosis within the Diagnostic and Statistical Manual of Mental Disorders. This is not because the field of mental health finds school refusal unimportant. On the contrary, school refusal is included as a symptom of other disorders. As such, children who exhibit school refusal behaviors are often diagnosed with preexisting psychiatric conditions [2]. The diagnoses most commonly observed among children who refuse school are anxiety, depression, and disruptive behavior disorders [6, 7]. Both depression and anxiety are characterized by the presence of internalizing symptoms—symptoms that distress the child [8]. Disruptive behavior disorders (such as Oppositional Defiant Disorder and Conduct Disorder) are characterized by their externalizing symptoms—impulsivity, defiance, and noncompliance [8, 9]. Clinicians and researchers often attempt to categorize children based on the differentiation between internalizing and externalizing symptoms as either anxious school refusers or truant school refusers [3]. Truancy is conceptualized as nonattendance driven by a disinterest in school itself and/or defiance of adult authority [3]. This chapter explores the differences between these two types of school refusers and the validity of this distinction between classifications.

Many school-refusing children present with psychiatric symptoms without meeting the eligibility criteria needed to receive a diagnosis [1]. Among a sample of children who were referred to a specialized outpatient unit for missing school, almost one-third did not meet criteria for any psychiatric disorder [10]. Among those who met criteria, the most common diagnosis was separation anxiety disorder (22.4%); this was followed by generalized anxiety disorder (10.5%) [10]. Almost 5% met criteria for depression [10]. Oppositional defiant disorder criteria were met for 8.4% of the sample [10]. Other researchers studied a group of children and adolescents in a general population who refused school. In this group, approximately three-quarters of participants were not diagnosed with a psychiatric disorder [11].

While most children attend school regularly, a portion of students is consistently absent year to year [1]. Absenteeism rates have remained relatively consistent since 1994, with 7% of fourth graders and eighth graders missing at least 5 school days in the past month [12]. Among children chronically absent in kindergarten, over half will go on to be chronically absent in first grade [12]. Among absentee children, researchers estimate that the prevalence of school refusal is approximately 5% among school-aged children, with higher rates observed in urban settings [13–15]. In the general population, prevalence rates of anxious school refusal were found to be between 1 and 2% [11]. Prevalence rates in clinical populations have been observed anywhere between 5 and 15% [16].

Epidemiologists have studied school refusal with regard to basic demographic characteristics. Gender differences have not been found in absenteeism rates or prevalence of school refusal [12, 17]. Certain ages or life stages are associated with higher rates of school refusal behavior [3]. By age, the highest rates of school refusal are seen among 5 to 6 and 10 to 11-year-old children [18]. Nationally, 11% of kindergarteners miss at least 18 days of school per year [12]. Peak incidence rates for school refusal have been found at transition points for children and adolescents as they move from life stage to another: starting a new academic course, moving to a new school, or moving up to a new school by moving through grades [19]. These contextually influenced peaks in school refusal highlight the multidetermined nature of the behavior [20].

Historically, school refusal is notable only within a context of mandated school attendance. In the late nineteenth century, industrialization led to child labor laws that sought to direct the time children were to spend working or studying [4]. Additionally, the evolving sociopolitical atmosphere was thought to require increased social order and a trained workforce, goals supposedly achievable through widespread education [4]. By 1918, nearly every state in the United States had enacted compulsory school attendance legislation [4]. Children who did not attend school were described as "truants," a term that remains popular today [4]. Truancy was seen as an aspect of delinquency [4]. Not until the 1930s was an alternative explanation for children's absences considered [4]. Specifically, three articles were published that proposed that some underlying anxious temperament was implicated in school refusal [4, 21–23], one of which first put forth the idea of "school phobia" [23]. This term persisted for decades despite very little evidence that children who refuse school are directly afraid of school itself [4]. This article also described an enmeshment between the parent and school-refusing child, which served to bring separation anxiety into the discussion [23]. In the decades following, researchers and clinicians continued to attribute a child's refusal to attend school to an overly attached relationship between an anxious mother and child [4].

Over the ensuing decades, researchers attempted to categorize school refusal behaviors, using concepts such as chronic versus acute and anxious versus truant [4]. Very few of the proposed typologies were subsequently empirically supported [4]. Largely, the misconceptions regarding school refusal that parents currently hold reflect the theories researchers posited prior to finding evidence to the contrary [4]. In this chapter, we review what current research tells us about school refusal behavior, rather than what theories suggest.

Common Parental Concerns

Absenteeism Creates Short-Term and Long-Term Problems

In the short term, children's absence from school causes parents and school personnel stress [3, 24]. Considerable challenges arise when attempting to resolve the issue [24]. The stress of these difficulties has been found to cause family conflict [25]. In managing the crisis, the family sometimes displaces their stress onto the school staff [24]. School refusal is also associated with negative peer interactions and poor academic performance [26, 27]. A follow-up study was conducted 7 years after children were treated for school refusal. For some, the treatment was successful, and they returned to school, while others did not improve [28]. Those who did not return to school displayed more antisocial behavior after 7 years than those who returned [28]. With regard to academics, researchers estimate that about half of children who are regularly absent will not reach their academic potential [29].

When a child is not consistently present at school, his or her social and educational development nearly always suffers [30]. Later in life, school-refusing children have reduced access to higher education, more employment challenges, more social problems, and an increased risk for development of psychiatric illnesses [31–33]. Absenteeism in general is a risk factor for other adverse life events such as suicide, teenage pregnancy, and substance use [2]. Chronic absenteeism is a risk factor in later dropping out completely from school, which is associated with financial, marital, social, and psychiatric problems later in life [2, 34]. Swedish researchers used the national registry data to find that school refusers were more likely to live with their parents as adults and were seen for psychiatric consultations at higher rates than the general population [32]. In sum, parents of children who are consistently refusing school are correct to be concerned about the implications for both short-term and long-term functioning.

Absenteeism Is Worse Among Adolescents

Parents are justifiably concerned when their adolescent children refuse to attend school. The symptoms of school-refusing adolescents are more severe than those exhibited by younger children [35]. Adolescents also present with complex diagnostic profiles, with depression or depressive symptoms in greater evidence than in younger children [36, 37]. Adolescents with anxiety may have more to legitimately fear about school than younger children because the high school environment is more demanding academically and socially than elementary school [35]. Adolescents are more likely to resist their parents' attempts to return them to school [38].

Treatment for school refusal in adolescents generally yields less successful outcomes than treatment for younger children [35]. The age difference holds for cognitive behavioral therapy (CBT) as well as non-CBT interventions studied [35]. Researchers and clinicians have been working on adapting CBT for use with adolescent school refusers, but no definitive protocol has yet been established [35].

Common Misconceptions

School refusal is a commonly occurring childhood phenomenon; as such, it doesn't require treatment

It is true that almost all children are absent from time to time [39]. Anywhere from 5 to 28% of children are likely to demonstrate some kind of school refusal at some point in their lives [40]. Some school refusal is short in duration and remits without treatment [4]. Any absenteeism that resolves within 2 weeks is called **self-corrective school refusal** [4]. For example, school refusal behavior is a common response to starting a new school or wanting to test parents' limits [4]. When parents consistently enforce attendance during these times, the behavior typically resolves rapidly [4]. Self-corrective school refusal has been observed in as much as 80% of the population [41].

However, some children display school refusal behaviors that do not resolve as quickly. Children absent due to illegitimate reasons for anywhere between 2 weeks to 12 months are said to have acute school refusal, while incidents lasting more than 1 year are chronic [4]. Students whose absenteeism affects at least 2 academic years suffer worse prognostic outcomes than children with shorter durations of absenteeism [4]. Ultimately, while some school refusal behavior is common, resistance that lasts for longer than 2 weeks indicates that treatment should be sought.

Children with school refusal behaviors have separation anxiety or a "school phobia"

As an initial point of clarification, the main cause for school absence—extended or otherwise—is chronic illness [2]. A leading contributor to school absence is asthma [42]. Children with asthma miss between 1.5 and 3.0 times as many school days than their non-asthmatic peers [43–46]. Missing school for a medical illness is considered a legitimate reason for absence. As we will see, some children who initially experience medical symptoms learn over time that their symptoms may elicit responses from their parents that allow them to stay home even when they could attend. The line between legitimate reasons for absenteeism and illegitimate reasons that become school refusal is often ambiguous. The same child can at some times legitimately be unable to attend school and at other times use a medical diagnosis to avoid school.

As discussed in the overview, past understandings of absenteeism first focused on truancy as the sole reason children avoided school [4]. With time, others began to write about an anxious profile among children who did not attend school [23]. The conception of an anxious child, overly attached to his mother, who refuses to go to school, has persisted for decades. However, an analysis found that internalizing symptoms such as those found in anxiety did not predict absenteeism among adolescents [39]. Meanwhile, externalizing symptoms, family, and school factors did predict absenteeism [39]. Another study of over 800 absentee children found that three-quarters did not meet criteria for any psychiatric disorder [11]. While some children may refuse school due to anxiety, this is clearly not the only reason.

Among children who avoid school due to anxiety, the anxiety rarely centers on parental separation [11]. In part, this misconception that school refusal is a direct result of separation anxiety may be due to the behaviors displayed by young children when first attending daycare or preschool. Learning to separate from one's primary caregiver is a developmental task that children must learn, and it commonly occurs with some distress. We reviewed self-corrective school refusal, which affects a great number of children for short periods of time. While this form of school refusal may be tied closely to separation difficulties, longer term school refusal is influenced by a number of factors and psychiatric diagnoses, of which separation anxiety may or may not be one.

Some children refuse to attend school in order to avoid school itself, as found in 35% of anxious school refusers in one study [11]. Researchers still could not conclude those children had a "school phobia" [11]. This is because school sometimes does pose a situation to be feared, as in cases where school provides opportunities for bullying, gang violence, or other negative external situations [47]. As for "school phobia" itself, a true phobia of school is exceptionally rare; as such, most children who refuse school are not actually "school phobic" [48, 49].

Children with school refusal behaviors are either anxious or truants

Clearly some, but not all, school-refusing children experience anxiety. Combined with the fact that many children refuse to attend school for reasons associated with truancy (lack of interest in school, a defiance of authority, etc.) there is a strong tendency to divide children into one of these 2 types [11]. However, this categorization is not supported by research. A large epidemiological study found that children who did not attend school primarily due to anxiety also showed a high prevalence of the externalizing disorders erroneously attributed only to truant children [11]. On the other hand, symptoms commonly associated with anxious school refusers (such as nervousness) were also observed in truant children upon the prospect of returning to school [11]. That neither diagnostic criteria nor symptomatology sufficiently distinguishes these groups indicates that school refusers cannot be differentiated according to these constructs. Even more tellingly, this categorization has not been found effective in assessment or treatment planning among the population [50]. If a categorization cannot accurately differentiate between groups or assist assessment and treatment planning, then it should be discarded as a classification system.

A valid categorization would account for the heterogeneity of school refusers' behaviors and symptoms [2]. Researchers designed and tested a model that accounts for the differences among school refusers according to the function nonattendance serves [2]. The function served by avoiding school essentially answers the question: "What does this child stand to gain by not attending school?" In some cases, the gain is the attainment of a positive experience (e.g., parental attention, time on more pleasurable activities than schoolwork) [10]. This function represents the positive reinforcement of the school refusal behavior. In other cases, the gain is avoiding an undesired experience (e.g., escape from a dangerous school setting, avoidance of feared social interactions) [10]. School refusal behavior is here maintained through negative reinforcement. This model has been established as better able to predict absenteeism rates than the traditional anxious versus truant distinction [51].

Current Research

Risk Factors

School refusal behavior has risk factors at the individual, family, school, and community levels [52, 53]. Illnesses and chronic diseases are the main individual factors that influence absenteeism [2]. Among adolescent anxious school refusers, individual differences were found to influence which children attend school and which stay home [54]. Type of anxiety disorder, presence of behavioral problems, substance abuse, psychiatric severity, perception of health, and number of friends all differentiate between those who attend despite their anxiety and those who stay home [54]. Attendees were not as socially anxious as absentee students [54]. They were less afraid of their own anxious symptoms [54]. Attenders also had more friends [54].

Among the family, it is suspected that parents contribute to school refusal behavior, or reduce its impact, depending upon how they respond [3]. Among families in which a child has already begun to refuse school, difficulties in family functioning have been found [55]. However, few studies examine family functioning using validated measures [3]. Even among these studies, a glaring limitation exists in that once a child has begun to refuse school, disturbances in family functioning are nearly guaranteed to occur. The oft-repeated refrain that "correlation does not equal causation" applies here because it is unclear whether dysfunctional families contribute to school refusal or families become dysfunctional as a result of school refusal. It is also possible that both can be true: dysfunctional families may be more likely to have children who refuse school, who in turn, create more stress on their families with their refusal. Regardless of which occurred first, it is presumed that parents and children (particularly adolescents) could benefit from treatments that include an emphasis on improved communication and problem solving [35].

Even in cases of medical illness, parents play a role in how much school their children attend [56]. After accounting for the child's level of pain and depressive symptomatology, one study found that parents' protectiveness and catastrophizing reactions to their children's pain influenced how much school their child attended [56]. Higher intensity of parental protective behaviors and catastrophizing thoughts were more likely to lead to less school attendance [56]. Researchers proposed that child illness elicits responses from parents that convey some social reward to the child, such as increased attention, time with parents, and expressions of support [56]. Over time, children learn to associate their illness with positive interactions with their parents [56]. Just as the toddler looks at his mother after falling to gauge her reaction before crying, older children look to their parents' reactions to decide how ill they are. As such, this family factor has the capacity to influence school refusal.

School environments also influence absenteeism rates [39]. Bullying and violence in school increase the risk of absenteeism [39]. Schools that inconsistently enforce attendance policies also experience higher rates of absenteeism [57]. While the interactions between school refusal and psychiatric diagnoses have been widely studied, not enough attention has been paid to the relationship between learning or language disorders and school refusal [3]. Children with learning or language disorders experience significant frustration when engaging in academic tasks [3]. In an inpatient setting, adolescents with depression and school refusal behavior were found to have significantly more challenges with learning and language than other psychiatry patients [27]. These diagnoses are hypothesized to add another risk factor for school refusal, because these disorders make school that much more challenging [3]. In the community, children who live in chaotic, dangerous, or unsupportive neighborhoods with low parental monitoring of school attendance are at considerably higher risk of absenteeism [58–61].

Treatment

Possibly as a result of these systemic factors, treatments involving more than just the child have been found to have greater effect than treatments working with the child or adolescent alone [62]. Treating school refusal behavior in children should therefore include the family extensively in therapeutic work [3]. One review of the literature found that more than two-thirds of patients recovered with the help of behavioral family therapy, which was significantly better than the improvement rate of children who received individual treatment [63]. Recommended interventions include CBT strategies, family therapy, social skills training (for refusers with social anxiety), and ongoing collaboration with treatment providers and school providers [40, 64–67]. Behavioral family therapy includes gradually exposing the child to the feared stimulus, relaxation training, social skills training, and contingency management procedures with the family (e.g., rewards for attendance, loss of privileges for nonattendance) [68].

In general, the first component of treatment should involve a careful assessment of the situations that the child finds most distressing and the barriers that have gotten in the way of school attendance in the past [62]. Because children refuse school for different reasons, treatment should be selected to ensure that it addresses what motivates the child's refusal [69]. Physicians can administer the School Refusal Assessment Scale-Revised to assess which functions a child's refusal serves [2]. This scale has been found to successfully guide treatment planning that is appropriately tailored to the child's specific school refusal behavior characteristics [2]. The measure adequately distinguishes between the different motivators for refusing school described above (avoiding negative experiences that occur at school, obtaining positive experiences caused by staying home, or both). Children may then receive coaching in relaxation techniques, coping skills, and social skills to address anxiety symptoms they may experience upon returning to school [62]. Parents and school staff learn how to prompt children to use these skills and provide additional positive feedback when children use them [62]. All involved parties develop a plan for returning to school [62].

As far as individual treatment, clinicians began treating anxious school refusers with CBT as far back as the 1980s [68]. CBT was originally conceptualized as a treatment for individuals with depression and anxiety, so it was presumed that anxious school-refusing children could benefit from it. Most of the 5 CBT manuals for school-refusing youth include some aspects of psychoeducation, problem solving, and family communication strategies [68]. Despite a number of research trials, CBT does not appear to be the obvious treatment of choice for school refusal. One study compared CBT to educational support therapy and found no benefit to CBT relative to educational support therapy [70]. Even when only anxious school refusers are treated with CBT, approximately one-third to one-half of treated children show little or no response to treatment [70–73]. Because of this suboptimal response to CBT, researchers have begun studying which aspects of the treatment may help children return to school. One set of researchers hypothesized that self-efficacy, a person's beliefs about their ability to perform as they intend to in situations, may influence whether or not children return to school [74, 75]. That is, they proposed that the more self-efficacy adolescents gained from CBT, the more likely they were to return to school [75]. In a study of 19 adolescents treated with CBT, self-efficacy did mediate outcome [75]. One possible conclusion of this finding is that the more quickly an intervention succeeds in returning a child to school, the sooner the child receives the information that they can indeed tolerate being in school.

Some pharmacotherapy has been studied for school refusal behavior [3]. While medications may be considered as part of a multicomponent approach such as the one described above, they are not to be prescribed independent of other concurrent therapy [76].

Homeschooling is not a recommended response to school refusal [3]. Children who refuse school due to anxiety will not learn how to manage their anxiety if they remain home. On the contrary, symptoms associated with a feared stimulus increase more when the stimulus is avoided [77]. This has wide-ranging implications as children age and encounter numerous challenging situations requiring adequate anxiety management. Children who refuse school to avoid peer interactions will similarly not gain the skills needed to develop positive peer relationships if they stay home. Those who refuse school to obtain additional parental attention will be reinforced for this desire if homeschooled. Children who refuse school to obtain other experiences are not likely to submit to tutoring from their parents as they age. Because homeschooling does not address any of the underlying functions for school refusal, it is therefore not a productive school refusal response.

Conclusion

Researchers have long struggled to define, classify, study, assess, and treat children with school refusal behavior [4]. Meta reviews are scarce, in part because researchers in different fields use varying terms to describe what appear to be the same phenomena [54]. At other times, different definitions are used for the same term [78]. Comparisons between studies cannot be performed with validity if the terms are not clearly and consistently defined [54]. Despite the known heterogeneity of school refusers, a common misconception still persists that children are either anxious or truant. Focusing on symptoms has not led to clarity, but assessing children's reasons (or functions for refusing school) provides a more accurate depiction [4]. If physicians do not have access to the School Refusal Assessment Scale-Revised, they should be aware that researchers have found a triad of challenges that, when combined, indicate high likelihood of the presence of a psychiatric disorder: school refusal, sleep difficulties, and somatic complaints [11]. In light of this finding, any kind of school refusal should be addressed when it occurs in conjunction with these other conditions.

Pediatricians tend to encounter children who display somatic complaints associated with school refusal (e.g., chronic stomachaches that present in the morning before school) [79]. The general practitioner's role is to explore possible medical causes and remain cognizant of possible psychological, family, school, and community factors that may influence these symptoms [79]. In particular, anxiety symptoms often manifest as somatic complaints in children. As such, pediatricians should consider whether abdominal pain, vomiting, or headaches are medical or psychological symptoms [79]. If chronic school refusal is suspected, physicians should initiate referral to a mental healthcare provider [79]. As a trusted part of their child's health team, pediatricians can support families in returning their children to school [79].

References

1. Gresham FM, Vance MJ, Chenier J, Hunter K. Assessment and treatment of deficits in social skills functioning and social anxiety in children engaging in school refusal behaviors. In: Handbook of assessing variants and complications in anxiety disorders. New York: Springer; 2013. p. 15–28.
2. Kearney CA. School absenteeism and school refusal behavior in youth: a contemporary review. Clin Psychol Rev. 2008;28(3):451–71.
3. King NJ, Bernstein GA. School refusal in children and adolescents: a review of the past 10 years. J Am Acad Child Adolesc Psychiatry. 2001;40(2):197–205.
4. Kearney CA. What is school refusal behavior? American Psychological Association; 2001.
5. Kearney CA, Silverman WK. A preliminary analysis of a functional model of assessment and treatment for school refusal behavior. Behav Modif. 1990;14(3):340–66.
6. Silove D, Manicavasagar V, Drobny J. Associations between juvenile and adult forms of separation anxiety disorder: a study of adult volunteers with histories of school refusal. J Nerv Ment Dis. 2002;190(6):413–5.
7. Tramontina S, Martins S, Michalowski MB, Ketzer CR, Eizirik M, Biederman J, Rohde LA. School dropout and conduct disorder in Brazilian elementary school students. Can J Psychiatry. 2001;46(10):941–7.
8. Young JG, Brasic JR, Kisnadwala H. Strategies for research on school refusal and related nonattendance at school. 1990.
9. Wood JJ, Lynne-Landsman SD, Langer DA, Wood PA, Clark SL. Mark Eddy J, Ialongo N. School attendance problems and youth psychopathology: structural cross-lagged regression models in three longitudinal data sets. Child Dev. 2012;83(1):351–66.
10. Kearney CA, Albano AM. The functional profiles of school refusal behavior diagnostic aspects. Behav Modif. 2004;28(1):147–61.
11. Egger HL, Costello JE, Angold A. School refusal and psychiatric disorders: a community study. J Am Acad Child Adolesc Psychiatry. 2003;42(7):797–807.
12. Rooney P, Hussar W, Planty, M, Choy, S, Hampden-Thompson, G, Provasnik, S, Fox, MA. The condition of education 2006.In: National center for education statistics.US: Institute of Education Sciences, DC, Washington: Department of Education; NCES 2006–071.
13. Burke AE, Silverman WK. The prescriptive treatment of school refusal. Clin Psychol Rev. 1987;7(4):353–62.

14. Kearney CA, Robleck, TL. Parent training in the treatment of school refusal behavior. In: Briesmeister JM, Schaefer CD, editors. Handbook of parent training: parents as co-therapists for children's behavior problems. 2nd ed. New York: Wiley; 1997.
15. King NJ, Ollendick TH, Tonge BJ. School refusal: assessment and treatment. Allyn & Bacon; 1995.
16. Heyne D, King NJ. Treatment of school refusal. Handb Interventions Work Child Adolesc: Prev Treat. 2004;9:243–72.
17. Granell de Aldaz E, Vivas E, Gelfand DM, Feldman L. Estimating the prevalence of school refusal and school-related fears: a Venezuelan sample. J Nerv Ment Dis. 1984.
18. Ollendick TH, Mayer JA. School phobia. In: Turner SM, editor. Behavioral theories and treatment of anxiety. New York: Plenum; 1984.
19. Pina AA, Zerr AA, Gonzales NA, Ortiz CD. Psychosocial interventions for school refusal behavior in children and adolescents. Child Dev Perspect. 2009;3(1):11–20.
20. Thambirajah MS, Grandison KJ, De-Hayes L. Understanding school refusal: a handbook for professionals in education, health and social care. Jessica Kingsley Publishers; 2008.
21. Broadwin IT. A contribution to the study of truancy. Am J Orthopsychiatry. 1932;2(3):253.
22. Partridge JM. Truancy. Br J Psychiatry. 1939;85(354):45–81.
23. Johnson AM, Falstein EI, Szurek SA, Svendsen M. School phobia. Am J Orthopsychiatry. 1941;11(4):702.
24. McAnanly E. School phobia: the importance of prompt intervention. J Sch Health. 1986;56(10):433–6.
25. McShane G, Walter G, Rey JM. Characteristics of adolescents with school refusal. Aust N Z J Psychiatry. 2001;35(6):822–6.
26. Last CG, Strauss CC. School refusal in anxiety-disordered children and adolescents. J Am Acad Child Adolesc Psychiatry. 1990;29(1):31–5.
27. Naylor MW, Staskowski M, Kenney MC, King CA. Language disorders and learning disabilities in school-refusing adolescents. J Am Acad Child Adolesc Psychiatry. 1994;33(9):1331–7.
28. Valles E, Oddy M. The influence of a return to school on the long-term adjustment of school refusers. J Adolesc. 1984;7(1):35–44.
29. Chazan M. School phobia. Br J Educ Psychol. 1962;32(P3):209–17.
30. Berg I, Nursten JP. Unwillingly to school. Springer Science & Business; 1996.
31. Buitelaar JK, van Andel H, Duyx JH, van Strien DC. Depressive and anxiety disorders in adolescence: a follow-up of adolescents with school refusal. Acta Paedopsychiatrica: Int J Child Adolesc Psychiatry. 1994.
32. Flakierska-Praquin N, Lindström M, Gillberg C. School phobia with separation anxiety disorder: a comparative 20-to 29-year follow-up study of 35 school refusers. Compr Psychiatry. 1997;38(1):17–22.
33. Kearney CA, Albano AM. When children refuse school: a cognitive-behavioral Therapy approach therapist guide. Oxford University Press; 2007.
34. Christle CA, Jolivette K, Nelson CM. School characteristics related to high school dropout rates. Rem Spec Educ. 2007;28(6):325–39.
35. Heyne D, Sauter FM, Ollendick TH, Van Widenfelt BM, Westenberg PM. Developmentally sensitive cognitive behavioral therapy for adolescent school refusal: rationale and case illustration. Clin Child Fam Psychol Rev. 2014;17(2):191–215.
36. Baker H, Wills U. School phobia: classification and treatment. Br J Psychiatry. 1978;132(5):492–9.
37. Kearney CA. Depression and school refusal behavior: a review with comments on classification and treatment. J Sch Psychol. 1993;31(2):267–79.
38. Hansen C, Sanders SL, Massaro S, Last CG. Predictors of severity of absenteeism in children with anxiety-based school refusal. J Clinical Child Psychol. 1998;27(3):246–54.
39. Ingul JM, Klöckner CA, Silverman WK, Nordahl HM. Adolescent school absenteeism: modelling social and individual risk factors. Child Adolesc Mental Health. 2012;17(2):93–100.

40. Kearney CA, Bates M. Addressing school refusal behavior: suggestions for frontline professionals. Child Sch. 2005;27(4):207–16.

41. Watters J. School refusal. BMJ. Br Med J. 1989;298(6666):66.

42. Borrego LM, César M, Leiria-Pinto P, Rosado-Pinto JE. Prevalence of asthma in a Portuguese countryside town: repercussions on absenteeism and self-concept. Allergol Immunopathol. 2005;33(2):93–9.

43. Fowler MG, Davenport MG, Garg R. School functioning of US children with asthma. Pediatr. 1992;90(6):939–44.

44. Bonilla S, Kehl S, Kwong KY, Morphew T, Kachru R, Jones CA. School absenteeism in children with asthma in a Los Angeles inner city school. J Pediatr. 2005;147(6):802–6.

45. Moonie SA, Sterling DA, Figgs L, Castro M. Asthma status and severity affects missed school days. J Sch Health. 2006;76(1):18–24.

46. Silverstein MD, Mair JE, Katusic SK, Wollan PC, O'Connell EJ, Yunginger JW. School attendance and school performance: a population-based study of children with asthma. J Pediatr. 2001;139(2):278–83.

47. Maughan B. Conduct disorder in context. Conduct Disord Childhood Adolesc. 2001:169–201.

48. Hanna GL, Fischer DJ, Fluent TE. Separation anxiety disorder and school refusal in children and adolescents. Pediatr Rev. 2006;27(2):56.

49. Suveg C, Aschenbrand SG, Kendall PC. Separation anxiety disorder, panic disorder, and school refusal. Child Adolesc Psychiatr clin N Am. 2005;14(4):773–95.

50. Kearney CA. Bridging the gap among professionals who address youths with school absenteeism: overview and suggestions for consensus. Prof Psychol: Res Pract. 2003;34(1):57.

51. Kearney CA. Forms and functions of school refusal behavior in youth: an empirical analysis of absenteeism severity. J Child Psychol Psychiatry. 2007;48(1):53–61.

52. Heyne D, King NJ, Ollendick T. School refusal. In: Graham P, editor. Cognitive behaviour therapy for children and families. 2nd ed. Cambridge: Cambridge University Press; 2004. p. 320–41.

53. Heyne D. School refusal. In: Fisher JE, O'Donohue WT, editors. Practitioner's guide to evidence-based psychotherapy. New York: Springer; 2006. p. 599–618.

54. Ingul JM, Nordahl HM. Anxiety as a risk factor for school absenteeism: what differentiates anxious school attenders from non-attenders? Ann Gen Psychiatry. 2013;25(12):25.

55. Hersov L. School refusal. In: Rutter M, Hersov L, editors. Child and adolescent psychiatry: modern approaches. 2nd ed. Oxford, England: Blackwell Scientific Publications; 1985. p. 382–99.

56. Logan DE, Simons LE, Carpino EA. Too sick for school? Parent influences on school functioning among children with chronic pain. Pain. 2012;153(2):437–43.

57. Stickney MI, Miltenberger RG. School refusal behavior: prevalence, characteristics, and the schools' response. Educ Treat Child. 1998;1:160–70.

58. Chapman MV. Poverty level and school performance: using contextual and self-report measures to inform intervention. Child Sch. 2003;25(1):5–17.

59. Crowder K, South SJ. Neighborhood distress and school dropout: the variable significance of community context. Soc Sci Res. 2003;32(4):659–98.

60. Henry KL. Who's skipping school: characteristics of truants in 8th and 10th grade. J Sch Health. 2007;77(1):29–35.

61. Reid K. The Causes, Views and Traits of School Absenteeism and Truancy An Analytical Review. Res Educ. 2005;74(1):59–82.

62. Carr A. The evidence base for family therapy and systemic interventions for child-focused problems. J Fam Ther. 2014;36(2):107–57.

63. Heyne DA, Sauter FM. The Wiley-Blackwell handbook of the treatment of childhood and adolescent anxiety. School Refusal: Wiley, Chichester; 2013.

64. Gosschalk PO. Behavioral treatment of acute onset school refusal in a 5-year old girl with separation anxiety disorder. Educ Treat Child. 2004;1:150–60.

65. Lauchlan F. Responding to chronic non-attendance: a review of intervention approaches. Educ Psychol Pract. 2003;19(2):133–46.
66. Moffitt CE, Chorpita BF, Fernandez SN. Intensive cognitive-behavioral treatment of school refusal behavior. Cogn Behav Pract. 2004;10(1):51–60.
67. Place M, Hulsmeier J, Davis S, Taylor E. School refusal: a changing problem which requires a change of approach? Clin Child Psychol Psychiatry. 2000;5(3):345–55.
68. Maynard BR, Heyne D, Brendel KE, Bulanda JJ, Thompson AM, Pigott TD. Treatment for School Refusal Among Children and Adolescents A Systematic Review and Meta-Analysis. Res Soc Work Pract. 2015;10:1049731515598619.
69. Inglés CJ, Gonzálvez-Maciá C, García-Fernández JM, Vicent M, Martínez-Monteagudo MC. Current status of research on school refusal. Eur J Educ Psychol. 2015;8(1):37–52.
70. Last CG, Hansen C, Franco N. Cognitive-behavioral treatment of school phobia. J Am Acad Child Adolesc Psychiatry. 1998;37(4):404–11.
71. Heyne D, Sauter FM, Van Widenfelt BM, Vermeiren R, Westenberg PM. School refusal and anxiety in adolescence: non-randomized trial of a developmentally sensitive cognitive behavioral therapy. J Anxiety Disord. 2011;25(7):870–8.
72. Heyne D. KIng NJ, Tonge BJ, Rollings S, Young D, Pritchard M, Ollendick TH. Evaluation of child therapy and caregiver training in the treatment of school refusal. J Am Acad Child Adolesc Psychiatry. 2002;41(6):687–95.
73. King NJ, Tonge BJ, Heyne D, Pritchard M, Rollings S, Young D, Myerson N, Ollendick TH. Cognitive-behavioral treatment of school-refusing children: a controlled evaluation. J Am Acad Child Adolesc Psychiatry. 1998;37(4):395–403.
74. Bandura A. Self-efficacy. In: Ramachaudran VS, editor. Encyclopedia of human behavior. vol. 4, p. 71–81).
75. Maric M, Heyne DA, MacKinnon DP, Van Widenfelt BM, Westenberg PM. Cognitive mediation of cognitive-behavioural therapy outcomes for anxiety-based school refusal. Behav Cogn Psychother. 2013;41(05):549–64.
76. Bernstein GA, Shaw K. Practice parameters for the assessment and treatment of children and adolescents with anxiety disorders. J Am Acad Child Adolesc Psychiatry. 1997;36(10):69S–84S.
77. Deacon B, Maack DJ. The effects of safety behaviors on the fear of contamination: an experimental investigation. Behav Res Ther. 2008;46(4):537–47.
78. McCune N, Hynes J. Ten year follow-up of children with school refusal. Ir J Psychol Med. 2005;22(02):56–8.
79. Katz F, Leith E, Paliokosta E. Fifteen-minute consultation for a child not attending school: a structured approach to school refusal. Arch Dis Child-Educ Pract Ed. 2016;101(1):21–5.

Chapter 14
Infectious Diseases

Overview

The human body contains millions of organisms that generally live in symbiosis with their host. The host provides an environment for the organisms to colonize and grow, and the organisms contribute to necessary human functions such as digestion and immunity. When these organisms instead cause harm to the host, they are said to produce infectious diseases. Parents may refer to these as communicable or contagious diseases because they spread when organisms are transferred from the infected individual to a new host. A century ago, epidemics of diseases such as tuberculosis, smallpox, polio, and tetanus raged simultaneously, killing young and old in alarming numbers [1]. Since then, medical care in developed countries has continued to improve, and individuals on average will experience fewer illnesses and live longer than prior generations [2]. When otherwise healthy individuals now encounter infectious diseases, they rarely die from them. Only two communicable diseases—influenza and pneumonia—made the list of top 10 causes of death in the United States in 2013 (the most recent year for which data are available) [3]. The deaths due to those diseases largely affected the elderly rather than children or healthy adults [4].

Despite the positive prognosis for the general population, people feel more vulnerable to infectious diseases than ever before [2]. Diseases with terrifying side effects capture the public's attention and incite fear [5]. Evidence suggests that people overestimate the likelihood of experiencing rare events (such as Ebola) and underestimate the likelihood of far more mundane yet deadly ailments (such as heart disease) [5]. Given that contracting a life-threatening communicable disease is a rare event from an individual standpoint, it follows that many overestimate the likelihood of this outcome [6].

Rare infectious diseases still require attention during pediatric office visits from time to time. If a child or adolescent is more likely to contract the disease (e.g.,

© Springer International Publishing AG 2017
C.A. Di Bartolo and M.K. Braun, *Pediatrician's Guide to Discussing Research with Patients*, DOI 10.1007/978-3-319-49547-7_14

an adolescent leaving for college contracting meningitis) physicians should vaccinate, emphasize effective preventative measures, and provide education regarding warning signs. However, many other diseases are unlikely to affect an individual patient (e.g., a resident of Kentucky with no ties to international health care workers contracting Ebola). In these cases, the physician's role is to educate patients about their risk profile, explain any preventative measures that can be taken, and dissuade patients from taking unproven cautionary measures.

Other infectious diseases are far less dangerous and exceedingly more prevalent, such as the common cold. Despite the relative safety of these diseases, parents still naturally become worried when their children are ill [7]. Medical professionals must know where parents' concerns lie in order to appropriately address their anxieties [7]. Without adequate knowledge, people are known to engage in untested or ineffectual procedures to reduce symptoms, attempt a cure, and prevent reoccurrence. A number of these ineffectual responses can serve to worsen the child's condition. For common diseases, physicians can provide rationale for focusing on effective responses by clarifying the mechanisms that cause these diseases and allow them to propagate.

This chapter reviews parents' concerns regarding frightening diseases and their children's susceptibility to contracting common diseases. We present the evidence regarding the effectiveness and limitations of hand washing as a method for preventing the spread of infectious disease. Physicians are likely to encounter erroneous beliefs regarding the causes and treatment for the common cold and fevers, and we discuss frequently encountered misconceptions and provide accurate clarifications. We conclude with current research regarding the media's influence on the perception of medical risks, as well as the physician's role in assuaging the resulting fears.

Common Parental Concerns

Infectious Disease Public Panic

Rare yet dramatic diseases inspire great fear among patients [5]. These diseases usually involve terrifying symptoms, high rates of death, or both [1]. People become concerned that these frightening diseases will spread far and wide [1]. The paradox of infectious diseases is that the likelihood of spreading decreases as symptom severity increases, because victims of diseases that cause rapid and severe symptoms, such as Ebola, are quickly relegated to care and quarantine [1]. Diseases that lie dormant or do not present symptoms serious enough to warrant immediate medical attention are more likely to spread, as is the case with the common cold [1]. This inverse association between symptom severity and ability to propagate holds even within one disease type. The most dangerous strains of a disease such as influenza eventually winnow out and leave only the more mild versions affecting humans [1]. At this stage, those who are immunologically vulnerable (e.g., the elderly) are most susceptible to the remaining strains [1].

Medical practitioners are tasked with the balance of dispersing sufficient information for people to take precautionary measures without unnecessarily frightening them. Patients often view infectious disease agents as having all powerful capabilities, but the organisms that cause infectious diseases have biological constraints, just as humans do [1]. To counter the fear of vulnerability, physicians can explain the organisms' weaknesses and the preventative measures that can be taken to exploit them [1]. Without knowledge of effective measures and the rationale for them, people will often engage in ineffectual preventative measures out of a need to feel in control in the midst of a frightening situation.

One infectious disease that presents a risk to older adolescents, particularly college students, is meningitis. Meningitis causes a swelling of the brain and spinal cord [8]. Meningitis is relatively rare; approximately between 600 and 1,000 people contract meningococcal disease in the United States each year, 21% of whom are preteenagers, teenagers, and young adults [9]. Different types of organisms cause meningitis, but the 2 most common agents are viruses and bacteria [8]. The viral form is typically less severe and can remit without medical intervention [8]. The bacterial form is highly contagious among people who come in close personal contact [10]. Invasive meningococcal disease progresses rapidly from initial symptom onset to extremely severe outcomes, including brain damage or death [11–13]. The initial symptoms are nonspecific and often described as "flu-like" [11]. This lack of clarity can cause individuals suffering from a common cold or flu to believe their symptoms indicate the onset of meningitis. Because the symptoms can progress in a matter of hours, there is little opportunity for testing when an individual develops the more general symptoms [10]. The initial symptoms progress to specific indicators: vomiting or nausea, stiff neck, confusion, and a purple/reddish pink rash that appears on the lower extremities or lower arms or hands [10].

Meningitis incidence peaks in adolescents and young adults [14, 15]. College students in particular engage in activities that promote meningococcal transmission, such as close personal contact, drinking from the same beverage glasses, and sharing cigarettes [10]. Many colleges require that their students receive the meningitis vaccine prior to enrolling in classes. In these cases, the pediatrician's role in explaining the benefits of the vaccine is relatively straightforward. Adolescents who are not planning on attending college may still engage in behaviors that increase transmission. Without an educational institution requiring their vaccination, these patients may need to be told more explicitly that the vaccine is crucial in preventing many types of meningitis.

While vaccines are available for most serogroups of the bacterial form, not all serogroups have vaccines approved for use in the United States [10]. Therefore, even vaccinated students should understand what preventative measures are worthwhile to take if their campus experiences an outbreak [10]. Most cases of meningitis on campuses are isolated and do not transmit to other students [16]. The disease cannot spread through casual contact, such as handshakes [10]. Nor can someone contract meningitis by breathing the air where an infected individual has been [10]. Still, the activities that promote transmission are common among college students, and an outbreak of meningitis itself is likely to be the inducement students need to reduce these behaviors [10]. Before patients leave for college, pediatricians should inform them to immediately reduce forms of close personal contact if the school announces an outbreak. More anxious adolescents can be shown images of the meningitis rash so that common rashes that occur in the absence of a meningitis outbreak do not unduly alarm them.

Many infectious diseases that inspire public panic require no such preventative measures, as they are extremely rare. Panic arises when individuals believe there is some risk that they will become infected, whether that risk assessment is accurate or not. For example, the Ebola Virus Disease (referred to colloquially as "Ebola") had claimed hundreds of lives in Africa without garnering an international response [17]. Only after health officials determined it was possible for Ebola to infect individuals outside of Africa did international bodies declare Ebola a public health emergency [17]. Once the chance of contraction entered the consciousness of the Western public, details of the virus emerged to fan the flames of panic. Panic produces "irrational" fears and "overreactions" in preventative measures [17]. One such overreaction occurred when school administrators in New Jersey banned students from Rwanda, even though this country is 1,700 miles from the outbreak region, a distance roughly equivalent to that from New York City to New Orleans [17]. Ebola panic spread more quickly and widely than the disease itself [17].

During an outbreak of a relatively new infectious disease, the lack of available research compounds public panic. Without studies to clarify the causes, treatment, and effective prevention of the disease, physicians have less information to relay to worried parents. Searching for answers and reassurance, the public relies on the media to deliver breaking news as groups such as the Centers for Disease Control and Prevention publish information as soon as it becomes available. Yet as is always the case with scientific research, new findings can contradict older information. The iterative nature of research always unfolds in this manner, but it usually does so largely outside of the public's awareness. When placed within the context of panic, the public is even less tolerant of the imperfections that characterize research investigations. Without understanding the nature of the scientific process, parents may erroneously believe that the organizations producing these new, more accurate findings were "wrong" before, reducing their overall confidence in the organizations.

Children's Susceptibility to Infectious Disease

Generally, children are more susceptible than adults to contracting infectious diseases. First, young children have poor personal hygiene [18]. They tend to put their hands and other objects into their mouths [18]. Second, children's emerging immune systems are not yet as effective as those of adults [18]. As a result of these factors, parents views that their children are more vulnerable to contracting illnesses than adults is, on average, accurate.

While parents may be concerned about the striking diseases highlighted in the media, children are significantly more likely to contract gastrointestinal diseases (such as diarrhea), upper respiratory tract infections (when caused by a strain of the rhinovirus, called the "common cold"), and acute otitis media (referred to as "ear infections"). These common ailments result in high usage of medical services. Upper respiratory infections confer heavy health care usage and economic burdens [19]. Because they are so prevalent, focusing efforts on preventing the spread of these diseases can reduce suffering and costs to families.

Parents want to know which environments may increase their children's chances of contracting an illness. Day care centers have been of particular interest, especially as an increasing number of children are cared for in these settings. There is evidence that children who attend day care centers are at higher risk of contracting infectious diseases, although the risk has not been proven across all common ailments [18]. The most common syndrome that affects children who attend day care is the upper respiratory infection [18]. The incidence of this common cold is 1.6 times higher in children who are in day care than in children who do not attend day care [20–25]. In real numbers, this translates to an average of 7 or 8 colds per year for children under the age of 2 years who attend day care centers [20, 21]. Children who attend day care centers are also at higher risk of contracting acute otitis media [26]. On average, as the number of children present at the center increases, so does the risk of contraction [26].

The centers themselves are not considered to blame for disease transmission. Day care centers are specifically designed for children, who are already, as highlighted above, more susceptible to contracting illnesses. Two additional factors that generally contribute to the spread of illness are also present in this type of environment [18]. The day care environment provides ample opportunities for direct physical contact between children, easily aiding host-to-host transmission [18]. Also, children can be contagious while asymptomatic, permitting a disease to transmit before the day care center staff has time to implement any response to reduce the spread [18]. These same factors impact other environments where young children congregate, such as parks, camps, and preschools. In large part, the more time children spend with other children in close settings, the higher their risk for contracting an infectious disease [18].

The most important factor in the reduction of common infectious diseases is proper hand washing, including the method, frequency, and timing [18, 27]. A meta-analysis of various hand hygiene methods found that education about proper hand washing technique and the use of regular soap was efficacious in the prevention of gastrointestinal and respiratory illness [27]. Day care centers that initiated hand washing training programs saw a 50% reduction in diarrheal illness [28]. The Centers for Disease Control and Prevention recommend individuals wash their hands with soap and water for 20 seconds [29]. They should lather the soap by rubbing their hands together, rinse the soap off completely with water, and dry their hands completely [29].

This meta-analysis found no evidence supporting the use of antibacterial soap over regular, nonantibacterial soap [27]. Antibacterial soap, by definition, would not be expected to have any impact on viral illnesses, but bacterial illnesses affect a great number of children worldwide [27]. The study authors, however, found no evidence in their data supporting the hypothesis that antibacterial soaps were more effective in preventing transmission of these illnesses [27]. Not only do antibacterial soaps fail to convey extra protection against infectious diseases when used in the community, laboratory studies have found evidence that these products contribute to the development of bacteria that are resistant to antibacterial soaps and medications [30–32]. Due to the lack of evidence in favor of anti-bacterial hand soaps and the increasing evidence that the chemicals used in many of them pose public health risks, the U.S. Food and Drug Administration (FDA) banned the sale of products containing some of the most common antibacterial agents. While consumers may, for a time, still be able to purchase products containing other permitted antibacterial agents, a clear trend away from these products is emerging. As such, pediatricians should be prepared to address parents' questions about the removal of these products, and assure parents that use of regular hand soap is effective.

In general, hand washing has been found to be slightly more effective in the prevention of gastrointestinal diseases than respiratory diseases, suggesting that other preventative measures are needed to supplement proper hand washing [27]. For example, hand washing is not particularly effective in reducing the transmission of influenza. While influenza can spread via direct physical contact and touching objects the infected individual has handled, it also spreads through droplets in the air [33]. Hand washing would influence the first modes of transmission, but not the aerosol mode of transmission. Recommendations to supplement hand washing include promoting higher uptakes of the influenza vaccine for young children [33]. Other preventative measures include increasing ventilation and separating infected individuals from other children while they remain contagious [34, 35].

Despite the popularity of alcohol-based hand sanitizers for personal use (i.e., not in hospitals), the meta-analysis did not return strong associations between such products and reductions in gastrointestinal or respiratory illness [27]. Within health care settings, alcohol sanitizers have been shown to prevent infections [29]. The difference between these findings is hypothesized to be a result of the differences between the practices and habits of people in the general population and those trained in health care fields [27]. As such, suggesting that people in the community use hand sanitizers is not a particularly helpful recommendation. The FDA is examining hand sanitizers and is expected to then rule as to whether they will permit the continued sale of these products.

In addition to antibacterial soaps, parents buy other antibacterial products aimed at disinfecting the common household [36]. These products are typically applied to surfaces within the household with the aim of inhibiting bacterial growth [36]. While these products are not directly designed to reduce illness, people who buy them may believe they are promoting healthy living among their family members [36]. While antibacterial products can protect vulnerable patients from bacteria that cause infectious disease, these products are limited in their influence on lives of typical, healthy individuals [36]. As with antibiotic medications, antibacterial products can only inhibit the growth of bacteria; they play no role in viral illness transmission [36]. These products also are static—developers select a few bacteria to target [36]. Meanwhile, bacteria are constantly growing and adapting, rendering these products effective among some bacteria for only a limited time [36]. Finally, not all bacteria cause illness in a human host [36], and humans should not attempt to kill all bacteria they come into contact with. This would be impossible in any case, but it is important for people to remember that bacteria are a crucial part of the human biosphere. Bacteria support the development of the human immune system and aid other crucial functions, such as digestion [37]. While the relationship between bacteria and health is still being studied extensively, some researchers have found a connection between higher rates of allergies in individuals who practice excessive hygienic practices [37–40]. The physician's role is to promote effective and reasonable prevention methods for common diseases while discouraging parents from engaging in any unnecessary or overly cautious practices.

Common Misconceptions

Don't go outside with wet hair. It's cold out; you'll catch a cold if you don't wear a coat

The "common cold" is indeed common, with children suffering an average of 6 to 10 colds per year [41]. A group of viruses called rhinoviruses infiltrates the upper respiratory system and causes this contagious infectious disease [42]. Most parents identify a common cold by a mixture of symptoms that may include runny nose, sore throat, congestion, coughing, fever, and fatigue. Colds present varying symptoms and severity. These differences in presentation are a result of the approximately 200 different strains of virus that can cause the illness [41]. Differences in the child's immunity also contribute to the diversity of experiences with the common cold [41]. Parents may be surprised to learn that their child may be infected with a rhinovirus and show no symptoms at all [41].

Understanding the scientific causes of the common cold is thought to be an important step in increasing the use of preventative measures [42]. If parents hold inaccurate views about causes, they may avoid certain situations or engage in other behaviors that are ineffective in helping them achieve their goal of preventing colds. So-called **folk beliefs**—commonly accepted wisdom with no scientific basis—about the causes of the common cold have persisted for generations. Some of these are erroneous beliefs about what causes colds, such as changes in the weather, cold weather itself, not wearing enough clothing in cold weather, going outside in cold weather with wet hair, sleeping with wet hair, teething, and walking outside barefoot [42, 43]. Some may also believe that sharing food or utensils with a sick individual can transmit the rhinovirus. However, the virus does not thrive in saliva or normal human body temperatures [44]. Folk beliefs regarding the causes of the common cold remain common in the twenty-first century [43]. Among a sample of nearly 200 parents of children younger than 5 years, 25% believed in five or more of these erroneous notions about colds [43]. Parents who follow these folk beliefs sometimes engage in practices that are ineffective at reducing transmission of the common cold.

Once a child is already sick, misconceptions also prompt parents to make ineffective and sometimes dangerous treatment choices. On the less dangerous end, parents may be under the impression that dietary supplements such as Vitamin C, Emergen-C, and Airborne reduce the severity of cold symptoms [42]. However, there is no evidence to support these claims [44]. Many of these products are taken with water or dissolved in water. As adequate hydration is crucial for immune support during an illness, parents can save their money on these products and instead ensure that their children drink enough water when ill. More dangerously, many parents purchase and administer over-the-counter (OTC) products containing antihistamines and decongestants to their young children [45]. Many parents are familiar with OTC antihistamine and decongestant products because they take them themselves. The U.S. Food and Drug Administration (FDA) approves these OTC medications for use in adults [45]. Parents may assume that the products are safe for children [45]. The labels of the products often seem to confirm this misconception. One study found that the labels of many OTC cough and cold products include wording and images that imply safe use among children [45]. The 3 label attributes that most commonly influenced parents in this study to believe the product was safe for children were the word "infant" on the label, infant-related images (such as teddy bears or infants themselves), or other wording implying that the product is appropriate for children (such as "pediatrician recommended") [45]. In addition to the labels, studies have found that up to half of pediatricians have endorsed these products to parents for use among children [46, 47].

Parents and teachers, who are in positions to prevent and manage symptoms of children afflicted with common colds, should ideally understand the causes and symptom management of these illnesses [42]. Physicians should correct folk beliefs when parents express them. For example, while colds appear more common in cold weather, the temperature is not directly to blame [42]. Instead, the cold weather influences people to spend more time indoors, in close quarters, assisting the rhinovirus in transmitting from host to host [42]. Additionally, many people inaccurately self-diagnose themselves with allergies in the summer, further contributing to the impression that colds are a cold weather phenomenon [48].

There is novel yet preliminary research conducted on human cells that indicates colder temperatures lessen the immune system's ability to kill human cells as a method for preventing the spread of the rhinovirus [49]. While an intriguing finding, this research is still limited in its clinical or practical applications. The results pertain only to the spread of an already present rhinovirus, so it is not pertinent to prevention. Also, while cold temperatures may affect one mechanism to prevent and inhibit the spread of infection throughout the body, it may not affect other aspects of immune functioning. Finally, as preliminary research, this study was performed on human cells rather than humans. Until the field understands more, physicians can encourage parents to reduce the spread of the rhinovirus with proper hand washing rather than focusing on bundling children up in cold temperatures [42].

As for treatment, both parents and pediatricians should be clear that the FDA recommends against the use of antihistamines or decongestants in response to a common cold in any child younger than 6 years of age [50]. Not only have studies failed to find clinical efficacy for the use of these products in children, they are also implicated in adverse events resulting in emergency room visits and death [45]. These products' labels and inserts typically include language that advises parents to seek consultation from a pediatrician prior to administration in children younger than 24 months [45]. These injunctions confuse matters further, because they imply that there are cases when a pediatrician would approve the use of these products in very young children [45]. Yet to do so would ignore the research that has found no evidence that these products are safe and effective for that age group [45]. Consequently, pediatricians should carefully advise against the use of these products in children younger than 6 years of age [45].

Fevers are dangerous and should be reduced at any cost

Among acute illness in children less than 5 years old, fever is a leading cause for concern among parents [7]. Parents may, in part, be concerned with temperature because it is regularly assessed by medical professionals: pediatricians often inquire about temperature and take temperatures during routine office visits; discharge instructions often include directing parents to return if a fever emerges [51]. An emphasis on temperature without an accompanying explanation creates high vigilance about fever [51]. Parents often attempt to manage their child's fever in an effort to exert personal control over a frightening situation [7]. Regrettably, a number of common false beliefs prompt many parents to excessively monitor or manage their children's fevers even when these actions, at best, do not improve medical outcomes or, at worst, put their children at greater risk than they were before these interventions were attempted [7]. A common misconception is that fever is a disease rather than the body's immunologic response to a threat [51]. Due to this one false belief, parents subsequently may hold other misconceptions about the causes of a fever, fever's role in the healing process, the long-term effects of a high fever, and the difference between heating due to fever and overheating due to external circumstances (e.g., a hot day) [7, 51]. As such, it is crucial that physicians correctly communicate the causes and recommended symptom management of fevers to parents.

An important component of the immunologic response, fever inhibits the growth and spread of viral and bacterial organisms [51]. A fever is a controlled process with multiple physiological safeguards that prevent the child's temperature from rising to a degree that could cause harm [52]. Pediatric fevers usually arise in response to viral infections [53]. Among infants younger than 6 weeks old, a fever is considered a medical emergency, nearly always requiring further testing of blood, urine, and spinal fluid. Fevers may be one of the first warning signs of serious illnesses including meningitis, and physicians may request testing to ensure the fever is not linked to meningitis [51]. As such, testing itself may increase parents' fears about fevers [51]. Parents also worry about febrile convulsions (FC) [54], which are seizures accompanying fevers that have no defined cause (e.g., they are not indicators of epilepsy, meningitis, etc.) [55, 56]. These convulsions typically occur in children ages 6 months through 5 years and are associated with a slightly elevated risk of developing epilepsy [54].

Research indicates that parental fears about acute illness stem from beliefs that these conditions could cause their children to suffer long-term bodily harm or possibly die. In one study of parents of young children, parents reported initial fear when they perceive their children are in discomfort. Once parents believe that discomfort has advanced to suffering, their anxiety may increase to fear. Many parents in this study viewed suffering as an indication that the illness is severe enough to cause irreparable harm. When children suffer from high fevers, parents may worry about insidious causes or lasting damage. Parents and physicians alike are concerned when fevers are not accompanied by other symptoms of a cold [7]. In the absence of viral symptoms, physicians are tasked with identifying less common sources of infection, such as urinary tract infections, otitis media, or other potentially dangerous conditions.

A common belief among parents is that fevers initiated in response to an infection can spiral "out of control" without intervention [51]. This fear may stem from parents' awareness that children exposed to overly hot external environments (such as being left in a car in the sun) can overheat [51]. The difference between the body's internal febrile mechanisms and a body overheating as a result of the environment should be made clear. As such, in otherwise healthy children, there are no negative effects of fever and fever need not be "treated" [57]. Unnecessary monitoring or "prevention" of fever may impede the naturally occurring healing process. In a sample of over 300 parents, 52% said they would check their child's temperature at least once an hour to monitor their child's fever [51]. Waking a child every hour will disrupt the body's ability to fight the infection that initiated the febrile response.

In responding to fevers, physicians sometimes recommend cooling via sponging or antipyretics [7]. Cooling is suggested for the purpose of keeping a febrile child comfortable [7]. Neither sponging nor antipyretics are needed to prevent an impending fever or a current fever from rising because fever is already a controlled process [7]. Even if external cooling was effective in reducing core body temperature, fevers arise to meet the demands of the immune system [7]. This crucial element of the child's recovery should not be removed. Maintaining children's comfort throughout fevers is the paramount goal. Uncomfortable children, especially infants, tend to drink less water, eat less, and sleep less than those who are kept as comfortable as possible. As hydration, nourishment, and sleep are key to immunologic functioning, physicians should recommend supporting these processes by keeping children comfortable.

Without understanding the rationale behind such recommendations, parents may interpret cooling recommendations as advice administered to "control" the fever [7]. Nearly a quarter of parents in one study reportedly sponged their children in response to normal temperatures (i.e., 100 degrees or cooler) [51]. Parents also reported using cool water for sponging, which initiates an unpleasant shivering response in febrile children [51]. As cooling is only helpful for reducing discomfort, initiating more through shivering is counterproductive. Dangerously, 18% of parents in this study reported using alcohol to sponge their children [51]. Alcohol should not be used for sponging because it can cause dehydration and hypoglycemia in young children [51].

Parents may also administer antipyretics, thinking the medication will "control" the fever [7]. Antipyretic medications are frequently misused and overused, possibly as a result of parents' anxiety to reduce a fever at any cost [58]. Pediatricians should clarify with parents that antipyretics are an option to make their child more comfortable, but the data are still unclear as to whether they can be used as fever reducers per se [52]. For example, the still unclear etiology of FCs means antipyretics are not indicated for this condition, and research shows such medications are largely ineffective in reducing the frequency of FC occurrence [59, 60]. Misconceptions affect clinicians as well as parents. One study found that 50% of pediatricians advised their patients to follow the unproven practice of alternating the administration of acetaminophen and ibuprofen to treat fever [61]. Instead, parents should be informed that there is no research indicating a benefit from alternating doses of acetaminophen with ibuprofen [51]. Troublingly, 85% of parents in one study said they would wake their child during the night to administer antipyretics [51]. Similar to the drawbacks of waking a child to monitor temperature, disturbing the sleep of a sick child impedes the immune system's ability to function maximally. An already sleeping child is unlikely to benefit from any reduction in discomfort an antipyretic can bring.

Many parents are afraid that FC can cause long-term harm to their children [54]. A large proportion of parents with children who experienced FC believed their children might likely die [54]. Parents of children with FC overestimated the risk that their child would later develop epilepsy [54]. Parents also overestimated the correlation between repeated FCs and brain damage [54]. Many physicians are unaware their patients have such extreme fears [54]. In fact, research has found very few negative outcomes associated with either one or multiple febrile convulsions—there is no established increased risk of death, serious injury, brain damage, or learning disorders [62–64].

Current Research

A great deal is known about prevention, treatment, and symptom management of the infectious diseases most likely to affect an individual child. Physicians may find they need to correct misconceptions about overzealous and generally useless prevention strategies among healthy children, such as supplements, antibacterial soap, and other antibacterial cleaning products. Parents may not be aware of the limitations of hand washing in decreasing susceptibility to airborne illnesses, and thus lack understanding of the recommendation for vaccination against such diseases (e.g., influenza). Pediatricians may also need to clarify the difference between symptom management (i.e., reducing discomfort) and treatment or cure. In particular, many parents cool their children because they believe they are controlling the fever, often at the expense of their child's comfort. While it is emotionally upsetting to watch one's child suffer, symptom reducers such as decongestants and antihistamines should not be used among very young children, due to the risk of overuse and adverse events associated with these medications.

Despite advances in medicine, people view themselves as more at risk than ever before [65]. Journalists and scholars have suggested that the media contributes to this paradox by overemphasizing events that are dramatic, new, and rare rather than those most likely to pose an actual risk to the audience [66, 67]. The practice of devoting proportionally more airtime and column inches to relatively uncommon phenomena, simply because these stories easily capture the attention of the audience, has been called **selective amplification** [68]. Many parents have a general understanding that the media is prone to this bias. Despite this conscious knowledge, repeatedly hearing about a frightening prospect has a way of heightening concern even among those who logically understand it is unlikely to affect them directly. Consequently, there is an established relationship between level of public concern regarding a particular situation and media coverage of that event [69]. Conversely, there is little to no relationship between media coverage of a phenomenon and its lethality [69]. The hypothesized interpretation of these 2 facts is that people become worried by events or conditions they encounter the most, which are not necessarily those that are the most dangerous to the average individual.

Worrying about unlikely phenomena presents 2 challenges. The first is that pediatricians spend limited time reassuring parents that the newest, most feared infectious disease is unlikely to affect their child and that, in fact, their prevention strategies may be causing more harm than good. The second is that people's attention is diverted from the conditions that do require their focus [5]. Physicians can take their patients' fears seriously by responding with the information the media often omits, thus directing parents' efforts to more productive activities. For example, fears about meningitis are likely exacerbated by media coverage of the disease [7]. Journalists may report that one of the first symptoms of meningitis is a rash, without providing images of a meningitis-specific rash [7]. As rashes are extremely common in children, this partial reporting causes fear and false positives [7]. In addition to assuring parents that meningitis is quite rare, pediatricians can take the parents' fears seriously by showing images of rashes due to meningitis [7]. In this fashion, clinicians can assuage parents' fears while giving them a greater sense of control through the dispersal of accurate and complete information.

Conclusion

Physicians are generally not in a position to influence the information their patients hear about infectious disease through the media. Clearly there is a delicate balance between informing the public about interesting, low-probability events and reporting high-probability events that are more likely to affect greater numbers [70]. The media have a responsibility to communicate risk accurately to their audience as to avoid inciting panic [70]. Given the statistics on media reporting and public fear, clinicians can assume that if a story went viral on the Internet, parents will ask them about it. When fearful parents inquire about the "disease du jour," pediatricians can first situate the information from the media within the broader context of likelihood. They can then direct parents to focus on evidence-based preventions and treatments. If none are yet established for a new disease, pediatricians should share best practices.

References

1. Gladwell M. This is the original book that explained the ebola virus [Internet]. New Republic. 2014 [cited 22 June 2016]. https://newrepublic.com/article/118972/ebola-virus-obsession.
2. Young ME, King N, Harper S, Humphreys KR. The influence of popular media on perceptions of personal and population risk in possible disease outbreaks. Health Risk Soc. 2013;15(1):103–14.
3. Xu J, Murphy SL, Kochanek KD, Bastian BA. Deaths: final data for 2013. National vital statistics reports. 2016. http://www.cdc.gov/nchs/data/nvsr/nvsr64/nvsr64_02.pdf.
4. Mokdad AH, Marks JS, Stroup DF, Gerberding JL. Actual causes of death in the United States, 2000. JAMA. 2004;291(10):1238–45.
5. Gwyn R. 'Killer bugs', 'silly buggers' and 'politically correct pals': competing discourses in health scare reporting. Health. 1999;3(3):335–46.
6. Frost K, Frank E, Maibach E. Relative risk in the news media: a quantification of misrepresentation. Am J Public Health. 1997;87(5):842–5.
7. Kai J. What worries parents when their preschool children are acutely ill, and why: a qualitative study. BMJ. 1996;313(7063):983–6.
8. Meningitis. Centers for disease control and prevention. 2016 [cited 22 June 2016]. https://www.cdc.gov/meningitis/.
9. Statistics and disease facts [Internet]. National meningitis association. 2016 [cited 22 June 2016]. http://www.nmaus.org/disease-prevention-information/statistics-and-disease-facts/.

10. Schaffner W, Baker CJ, Bozof L, Engel J, Offit PA, Turner JC. Addressing the challenges of serogroup B meningococcal disease outbreaks on campuses. Infect Dis Clin Pract. 2014;22(5):245–52.
11. Pace D, Pollard AJ. Meningococcal disease: clinical presentation and sequelae. Vaccine. 2012;30(30):B3–9.
12. Edwards MS, Baker CJ. Complications and sequelae of meningococcal infections in children. J Pediatr. 1981;99(4):540–5.
13. Kirsch EA, Barton RP, Kitchen L, Giroir BP. Pathophysiology, treatment and outcome of meningococcemia: a review and recent experience. Pediatr Infect Dis J. 1996;15(11):967–79.
14. Froeschle JE. Meningococcal disease in college students. Clin Infect Dis. 1999;29(1):215–6.
15. Harrison LH, Dwyer DM, Maples CT, Billmann L. Risk of meningococcal infection in college students. JAMA. 1999;281(20):1906–10.
16. Brooks R, Woods CW, Benjamin DK, Rosenstein NE. Increased case-fatality rate associated with outbreaks of Neisseria meningitidis infection, compared with sporadic meningococcal disease, in the United States, 1994–2002. Clin Infect Dis. 2006;43(1):49–54.
17. Karamouzian M, Hategekimana C. Ebola treatment and prevention are not the only battles: understanding Ebola-related fear and stigma. Int J Health Policy Manag. 2015;4(1):55.
18. Thacker SB, Addiss DG, Goodman RA, Holloway BR, Spencer HC. Infectious diseases and injuries in child day care: opportunities for healthier children. JAMA. 1992;268(13):1720–6.
19. Freid VM, Makuc DM, Rooks RN. Ambulatory health care visits by children: principal diagnosis and place of visit. Vital Health Stat Ser 13, Data from the national health survey. 1998;137:1–23.
20. Wald ER, Guerra N, Byers C. Frequency and severity of infections in day care: three-year follow-up. J Pediatr. 1991;118(4):509–14.
21. Loda FA, Glezen WP, Clyde WA. Respiratory disease in group day care. Pediatrics. 1972;49(3):428–37.
22. Fleming DW, Cochi SL, Hightower AW, Broome CV. Childhood upper respiratory tract infections: to what degree is incidence affected by day-care attendance? Pediatrics. 1987;79(1):55–60.
23. Hurwitz ES, Gunn WJ, Pinsky PF, Schonberger LB. Risk of respiratory illness associated with day-care attendance: a nationwide study. Pediatrics. 1991;87(1):62–9.
24. Bell DM, Gleiber DW, Mercer AA, Phifer R, Guinter RH, Cohen AJ, Epstein EU, Narayanan M. Illness associated with child day care: a study of incidence and cost. Am J Public Health. 1989;79(4):479–84.
25. Denny FW, Collier AM, Henderson FW. Acute respiratory infections in day care. Rev Infect Dis. 1986;8(4):527–32.
26. Uhari M, Mäntysaari K, Niemelä M. Meta-analytic review of the risk factors for acute otitis media. Clin Infect Dis. 1996;22(6):1079–83.
27. Aiello AE, Coulborn RM, Perez V, Larson EL. Effect of hand hygiene on infectious disease risk in the community setting: a meta-analysis. Am J Public Health. 2008;98(8):1372–81.
28. Black RE, Dykes AC, Anderson KE, Wells JG, Sinclair SP, Gary GW, Hatch MH, Gangarosa EJ. Handwashing to prevent diarrhea in day-care centers. Am J Epidemiol. 1981;113(4):445–51.
29. Boyce JM, Pittet D. Guideline for hand hygiene in health-care settings: recommendations of the healthcare infection control practices advisory committee and the HICPAC/SHEA/APIC/IDSA hand hygiene task force. Am J Infect Control. 2002;30(8):S1–46.
30. Aiello AE, Larson E. Antibacterial cleaning and hygiene products as an emerging risk factor for antibiotic resistance in the community. Lancet Infect Dis. 2003;3(8):501–6.
31. Aiello AE, Larson EL, Levy SB. Consumer antibacterial soaps: effective or just risky? Clin Infect Dis. 2007;45(Supplement 2):S137–47.
32. Levy SB. Antimicrobial consumer products: where's the benefit? what's the risk? Arch Dermatol. 2002;138(8):1087–8.

33. Wong VW, Cowling BJ, Aiello AE. Hand hygiene and risk of influenza virus infections in the community: a systematic review and meta-analysis. Epidemiol Infect. 2014;142(05):922–32.

34. Lowen A, Palese P. Transmission of influenza virus in temperate zones is predominantly by aerosol, in the tropics by contact. PLoS currents influenza. 2009.

35. Yang W, Marr LC. Dynamics of airborne influenza a viruses indoors and dependence on humidity. PLoS ONE. 2011;6(6):e21481.

36. Levy SB. Antibacterial household products: cause for concern. Emerg Infect Dis. 2001;7(3 Suppl):512.

37. Rook GA, Stanford JL. Give us this day our daily germs. Immunol Today. 1998;19(3):113–6.

38. Strachan DP. Hay fever, hygiene, and household size. BMJ. Brit Med J. 1989;299(6710):1259.

39. Braun-Fahrländer CH, Gassner M, Grize L, Neu U, Sennhauser FH, Varonier HS, Vuille JC, Wüthrich B. Prevalence of hay fever and allergic sensitization in farmer's children and their peers living in the same rural community. Clin Exp Allergy. 1999;29(1):28–34.

40. Matricardi PM, Rosmini F, Riondino S, Fortini M, Ferrigno L, Rapicetta M, Bonini S. Exposure to foodborne and orofecal microbes versus airborne viruses in relation to atopy and allergic asthma: epidemiological study. BMJ. 2000;320(7232):412–7.

41. Larson EL, Ferng YH, McLoughlin JW, Wang S, Morse SS. Effect of intensive education on knowledge, attitudes, and practices regarding upper respiratory infections among urban Latinos. Nurs Res. 2009;58(3):150–7.

42. Johnson ML, Bungum T. Identifying and reconstructing common cold misconceptions among developing K–12 educators. Am J Health Educ. 2013;44(3):169–75.

43. Lee GM, Friedman JF, Ross-Degnan D, Hibberd PL, Goldmann DA. Misconceptions about colds and predictors of health service utilization. Pediatrics. 2003;111(2):231–6.

44. Muha L. Hot on the trial of the common cold. Biography. 2000;4:60–7.

45. Lokker N, Sanders L, Perrin EM, Kumar D, Finkle J, Franco V, Choi L, Johnston PE, Rothman RL. Parental misinterpretations of over-the-counter pediatric cough and cold medication labels. Pediatrics. 2009;123(6):1464–71.

46. Cohen-Kerem R, Ratnapalan S, Djulus J, Duan X, Chandra RV, Ito S. The attitude of physicians toward cold remedies for upper respiratory infection in infants and children: a questionnaire survey. Clin Pediatr. 2006;45(9):828–34.

47. Gadomski AM, Rubin JD. Cough and cold medicine use in young children: a survey of Maryland pediatricians. Maryland medical journal (Baltimore, Md.: 1985). 1993;42(7):647–50.

48. Rodriguez D. Summer cold or simply summer allergies? [Internet]. EverydayHealth.com. 2016 [cited 22 June 2016]. Available from:http://www.everydayhealth.com/cold-flu/summer-cold-or-simply-summer-allergies.aspx.

49. Foxman EF, Storer JA, Vanaja K, Levchenko A, Iwasaki A. Two interferon-independent double-stranded RNA-induced host defense strategies suppress the common cold virus at warm temperature. In: Proceedings of the national academy of sciences of the United States of America; 2016.

50. Garbutt JM, Sterkel R, Banister C, Walbert C, Strunk RC. Physician and parent response to the FDA advisory about use of over-the-counter cough and cold medications. Acad Pediatr. 2010;10(1):64–9.

51. Crocetti M, Moghbeli N, Serwint J. Fever phobia revisited: have parental misconceptions about fever changed in 20 years? Pediatrics. 2001;107(6):1241–6.

52. Purssell E, Collin J. Fever phobia: the impact of time and mortality–a systematic review and meta-analysis. Int J Nurs Stud 2015.

53. Adam HM. Fever and host responses. Pediatr Rev/Am Acad Pediatr. 1996;17(9):330.

54. Huang MC, Liu CC, Huang CC, Thomas K. Parental responses to first and recurrent febrile convulsions. Acta Neurol Scand. 2002;105(4):293–9.

55. Hirtz DG. Febrile seizures. Pediatr Rev. 1997;1(18):5–9.

56. Provisional committee on quality improvement. Practice parameter the neurodiagnostic eval-
    uation of the child with. Pediatrics. 1996;97(5):769.
57. National Collaborating Centre for Women's and Children's Health (UK. Feverish illness in
    children: assessment and initial management in children younger than 5 years.
58. Teagle AR, Powell CV. Is fever phobia driving inappropriate use of antipyretics? Arch Dis
    Child 2014:archdischild-2013.
59. Hopkins A. For Ddebate-Guidelines for the management of convulsions with fever. Br Med
    J. 1991;303(6803):634–6.
60. Purssell E. The use of antipyretic medications in the prevention of febrile convulsions in chil-
    dren. J Clin Nurs. 2000;9(4):473–80.
61. Mayoral CE, Marino RV, Rosenfeld W, Greensher J. Alternating antipyretics: is this an alter-
    native? Pediatrics. 2000;105(5):1009–12.
62. Leung AK, Robson WL. Febrile convulsions. How dangerous are they? Postgrad Med.
    1991;89(5):217–8.
63. Verity CM, Greenwood R, Golding J. Long-term intellectual and behavioral outcomes of
    children with febrile convulsions. N Engl J Med. 1998;338(24):1723–8.
64. Knudsen FU. Febrile seizures—treatment and outcome. Brain and development.
    1996;18(6):438–49.
65. Kasperson RE, Renn O, Slovic P, Brown HS, Emel J, Goble R, Kasperson JX, Ratick S. The
    social amplification of risk: a conceptual framework. Risk Anal. 1988;8(2):177–87.
66. Adams WC. The role of media relations in risk communication. Public Rel Q. 1992;37(4):28.
67. Singer E, Endreny PM. Reporting on risk: how the mass media portray accidents, diseases,
    disasters and other hazards. Risk. 1994;5:261.
68. Murdock G, Petts J, Horlick-Jones T. After amplification: rethinking the role of the media in
    risk communication. Soc Amplification Risk. 2003;10:156–78.
69. Slovic P, Weber EU. Perception of risk posed by extreme events. In: Applegate, Gabba,
    Laitos, and Sachs, editors. Regulation of toxic substances and hazardous waste. 2nd ed.
    Foundation Press, Forthcoming; 2002.
70. Cooper CP, Roter DL. "If it bleeds it leads"? Attributes of TV health news stories that drive
    viewer attention. Public Health Rep. 2000;115(4):331.

Index

© Springer International Publishing AG 2017
C.A. Di Bartolo and M.K. Braun, *Pediatrician's Guide to Discussing
Research with Patients*, DOI 10.1007/978-3-319-49547-7

Printed in the United States
by Bookmasters

Printed in the United States
By Bookmasters